CLINICAL CASES
Anesthesiology

CLINICAL CASES
Anesthesiology

Lydia Conlay, MD, PhD, MBA
Formerly Professor of Anesthesiology
Baylor College of Medicine
Houston, Texas
Currently Russell and Mary Shelden Professor of Anesthesiology
University of Missouri College of Medicine
Columbia, Missouri

Julia Pollock, MD
Program Director, Anesthesia Residency
Staff Anesthesiologist
Virginia Mason Medical Center
Seattle, Washington

Mary Ann Vann, MD
Instructor in Anesthesia
Harvard Medical School
Beth Israel Deaconess Medical Center
Boston, Massachusetts

Sheela Pai, MD
Associate Director, Residency Program
Assistant Professor
Temple University School of Medicine
Philadelphia, Pennsylvania

Eugene C. Toy, MD
The John S. Dunn, Senior Academic Chair and Program Director
The Methodist Hospital Ob/Gyn Residency Program
Houston, Texas
Vice Chair of Academic Affairs
Department of Obstetrics and Gynecology
The Methodist Hospital
Houston, Texas
Associate Clinical Professor and Clerkship Director
Department of Obstetrics and Gynecology
University of Texas–Houston Medical School
Houston, Texas
Associate Clinical Professor
Weill Cornell College of Medicine
New York, New York

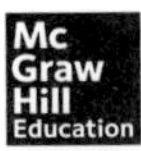

McGraw Hill Education (India) Private Limited
NEW DELHI

McGraw Hill Education Offices
New Delhi New York St Louis San Francisco Auckland Bogotá Caracas
Kuala Lumpur Lisbon London Madrid Mexico City Milan Montreal
San Juan Santiago Singapore Sydney Tokyo Toronto

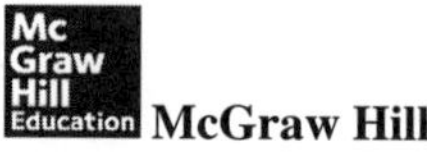

McGraw Hill Education (India) Private Limited

Clinical Cases: Anesthesiology

Notice

Medicine is an ever-changing science. As new research and clinical experience broaden our knowledge, changes in treatment and drug therapy are required. The authors and the publisher of this work have checked with sources believed to be reliable in their efforts to provide information that is complete and generally in accord with the standards accepted at the time of publication. However, in view of the possibility of human error or changes in medical sciences, neither the authors nor the publisher nor any other party who has been involved in the preparation or publication of this work warrants that the information contained herein is in every respect accurate or complete, and they disclaim all responsibility for any errors or omissions or for the results obtained from use of the information contained in this work. Readers are encouraged to confirm the information contained herein with other sources. For example and in particular, readers are advised to check the product information sheet included in the package of each drug they plan to administer to be certain that the information contained in this work is accurate and that changes have not been made in the recommended dose or in the contraindications for administration. This recommendation is of particular importance in connection with new or infrequently used drugs.

McGraw Hill Education (India) Edition 2013

RZZYCDRODRRRR

Reprinted in India by arrangement with The McGraw Hill Companies, Inc., New York

Sales territories: India, Pakistan, Nepal, Bangladesh, Sri Lanka and Bhutan

Library of Congress Cataloging-in-Publication Data

Clinical Case: Anesthesiology / Lydia Conlay … [et al.].
p. ; cm
Other title: Anesthesiology
Includes bibliographical references and index.
ISBN 978-0-07-160639-4 (pbk.: alk paper)
ISBN 0-07-160639-4 (pbk.: alk paper)
I Anesthesia—Case studies. I. Conlay, Lydia Ann. II. Title: Anesthesiology.
[DNLM: 1. Anesthesia—Case Reports. 2. Anesthesia—Problems and Exercises. 3. Anesthetics—Case Reports. 4. Anesthetics—Problems and Exercises.
WO 18.2 C3365 2011]
RD82.45.C375 2011
617.9'6—dc22 2010018793

ISBN-13: 978-93-5134-338-7
ISBN-10: 93-5134-338-3

Published by McGraw Hill Education (India) Private Limited, P-24, Green Park Extension, New Delhi 110 016, and printed at Rajkamal Electric Press, Kundli-131028, Haryana

DEDICATION

This book is dedicated to the Educational Scholars' Fellowship Program (ESFP), a combined effort of Baylor College of Medicine and the University of Texas at Houston, to recognize and train individuals in educational pursuits. It was at the ESFP that Drs. Conlay and Toy met, and where this book was conceived. We also dedicate this book to educators everywhere, who work so tirelessly to see that the craft of anesthesiology is perpetuated for generations to come.

CONTENTS

CONTENTS

CONTRIBUTORS

Kamardeen Alao, MD
Assistant Professor of Anesthesiology
Temple University School of Medicine
Philadelphia, Pennsylvania

Amit Asopa, MD
Resident in Anesthesia
Beth Israel Deaconess Medical Center
Boston, Massachusetts

Prasad Atluri, MD
Associate Professor of Anesthesiology
Baylor College of Medicine
Chief, Anesthesiology Service Line
Michael E. DeBakey Veterans Affairs Medical Center
Houston, Texas

Heather Ballard, MD
Resident in Anesthesia
Beth Israel Deaconess Medical Center
Boston, Massachusetts

Holly Barko, MD
Resident in Anesthesia
Beth Israel Deaconess Medical Center
Boston, Massachusetts

Sheila Ryan Barnett, MD
Associate Professor of Anesthesiology
Harvard Medical School
Beth Israel Deaconess Medical Center
Boston, Massachusetts

Ruma Bose, MD
Instructor in Anesthesia
Harvard Medical School
Beth Israel Deaconess Medical Center
Boston, Massachusetts

Asher Cantor, MD
Resident in Anesthesiology
Virginia-Mason Medical Center
Seattle, Washington

Corey E. Collins, DO
Instructor in Anesthesia
Harvard Medical School
Assistant Anesthesiologist
Massachusetts Eye and Ear Infirmary
Boston, Massachusetts

Lydia A. Conlay, MD, PhD, MBA
Formerly Professor of Anesthesiology
Baylor College of Medicine
Houston, Texas
Currently Russell and Mary Shelden Professor of Anesthesiology
University of Missouri College of Medicine
Columbia, Missouri

Melanie Darke, MD
Anesthesiologist
St John Hospital and Medical Center
Detroit, Michigan

Thomas Dean, MD
Resident in Anesthesiology
Virginia-Mason Medical Center
Seattle, Washington

Christina Fidkowski, MD
Attending Anesthesiologist
Henry Ford Hospital
Detroit, Michigan

Paul G. Firth, MBChB
Instructor in Anesthesia
Harvard Medical School
Attending in Anesthesia, Massachusetts General Hospital
Massachusetts Eye and Ear Infirmary
Boston, Massachusetts

Adam Fleckser, MD
Assistant Professor, Department of Anesthesiology
Temple University School of Medicine
Philadelphia, Pennsylvania

Matthew Fritsch, MD
Clinical Fellow in Anesthesia
Department of Anesthesia, Critical Care, and Pain Medicine
Beth Israel Deaconess Medical Center
Boston, Massachusetts

Matthew Hansen, MD
Resident in Anesthesia
Department of Anesthesia, Critical Care, and Pain Medicine
Beth Israel Deaconess Medical Center
Boston, Massachusetts

Ellen Hauck, MD, PhD
Assistant Professor, Department of Anesthesiology
Temple University School of Medicine
Philadelphia, Pennsylvania

James D. Helman, MD
Staff Anesthesiologist
Section Head, Cardiac Anesthesiology
Virginia-Mason Medical Center
Seattle, Washington

Raegan Hicks, MD
Resident in Anesthesiology
Virginia-Mason Medical Center
Seattle, Washington

Stephanie B. Jones, MD
Associate Professor of Anesthesia
Harvard Medical School
Residency Program Director and Vice Chair for Education
Department of Anesthesia, Critical Care, and Pain Medicine
Beth Israel Deaconess Medical Center
Boston, Massachusetts

Ihab Kamel, MD
Assistant Professor, Department of Anesthesiology
Temple University School of Medicine
Philadelphia, Pennsylvania

Swaminathan Karthik, MD
Instructor in Anesthesia
Harvard Medical School
Beth Israel Deaconess Medical Center
Boston, Massachusetts

David Kim, MD
Assistant Professor, Department of Anesthesiology
Temple University School of Medicine
Philadelphia, Pennsylvania

Lisa Kunze, MD
Instructor in Anesthesia
Harvard Medical School
Beth Israel Deaconess Medical Center
Boston, Massachusetts

Julia Labovsky, MD
Department of Anesthesia and Surgical Services
National Institutes of Health Clinical Center
Bethesda, Maryland

Laura Leduc, MD
Clinical Fellow in Anesthesia
Children's Hospital of Boston
Boston, Massachusetts

Susan Lin, MD
Anesthesiologist
Good Samaritan Medical Center
Brockton, Massachusetts

Devi Mahendren, MBChB
Resident in Anesthesia
Beth Israel Deaconess Medical Center
Boston, Massachusetts

John D. Mitchell, MD
Instructor in Anesthesia
Harvard Medical School
Associate Residency Program Director
Beth Israel Deaconess Medical Center
Boston, Massachusetts

Vivek Moitra, MD
Assistant Professor of Anesthesiology, Division of Critical Care
Columbia University College of Physicians and Surgeons
New York, New York

Jennifer D. Nguyen, MD, MEd
Associate Professor of Anesthesiology
Baylor College of Medicine
Director of Pre-Operative Evaluation Clinic
Michael E. DeBakey Veterans Affairs Medical Center
Houston, Texas

Sheela Pai, MD
Associate Director, Residency Program
Assistant Professor, Department of Anesthesiology
Temple University School of Medicine
Philadelphia, Pennsylvania

Julia Pollock, MD
Staff Anesthesiologist
Program Director Anesthesia Residency
Virginia-Mason Medical Center
Seattle, Washington

Norma J. Sandrock, BSChE, MD
Instructor in Anesthesia
Harvard Medical School
Director, Acute Pain Service
Beth Israel Deaconess Medical Center
Boston, Massachusetts

Wyndam Strodtbeck, MD
Staff Anesthesiologist
Virginia-Mason Medical Center
Seattle, Washington

Lila Sueda, MD
Staff Anesthesiologist
Virginia-Mason Medical Center
Seattle, Washington

Eswar Sundar, MD
Instructor in Anesthesia
Harvard Medical School
Director of Post-Anesthesia Care Units
Beth Israel Deaconess Medical Center
Boston, Massachusetts

Eugene C. Toy, MD
The John S. Dunn, Senior Academic Chair and Program Director
The Methodist Hospital Ob/Gyn Residency Program, Houston, Texas
Vice Chair of Academic Affairs
Department of Obstetrics and Gynecology
The Methodist Hospital-Houston
Associate Clinical Professor and Clerkship Director
Department of Obstetrics and Gynecology,
University of Texas–Houston Medical School
Houston, Texas
Associate Clinical Professor
Weill Cornell College of Medicine
New York, New York

Mary Ann Vann, MD
Department of Anesthesia, Critical Care, and Pain Medicine
Beth Israel Deaconess Medical Center
Instructor in Anesthesia
Harvard Medical School
Boston, Massachusetts

Anu Vasudevan, MD, FRCA
Instructor in Anesthesia
Harvard Medical School
Beth Israel Deaconess Medical Center
Boston, Massachusetts

Sherien Verchere, MD
Clinical Assistant Professor of Anesthesiology
Baylor College of Medicine
Staff Anesthesiologist
Michael E. DeBakey Veterans Affairs Medical Center
Houston, Texas

Wade Weigel, MD
Staff Anesthesiologist
Virginia-Mason Medical Center
Seattle, Washington

Zdravka Zafirova, MD
Associate Director, Anesthesia Perioperative Medicine Clinic
Assistant Professor, Department of Anesthesia and Critical Care
University of Chicago
Chicago, Illinois

PREFACE

We appreciate all the kind remarks and suggestions from the many medical students over the past 7 years regarding the Clinical Cases series. Your positive reception has been an incredible encouragement, especially in light of the short life of the Clinical Cases series. In this first edition of *Clinical Cases: Anesthesiology*, the basic format of the other books in the series has been retained, with some unique twists to be best suited to the field of anesthesiology. Cases 1-9 are deemed "Anesthesiology 101," which reviews the basics such as machine setup, preoperative evaluation, and how to troubleshoot an intraoperative emergency. This first section grew from an initial draft of a few key concepts to 9 independent clinical cases because we wanted to ensure that students fully grasped the significance of each teaching point. The remaining cases are organized by surgical or organ system to aid the student in the general approach to physiology and pathophysiology. The case listing in the back of the book and the index will allow a student quickly to reference similar situations for the sake of comparison. The multiple choice questions have been carefully reviewed and rewritten to ensure that they comply with the National Board and USMLE Step 2 format. As with any first edition, this undertaking has required more effort, yet with the toil comes much satisfaction with the end product. We hope that the reader will enjoy learning anesthesiology through the simulated clinical cases and that this text will help in organizing the information and clinical approach in such a challenging specialty. It is certainly a privilege to be a teacher for so many students, and it is with humility that we present this book.

The Authors

PREFACE

ACKNOWLEDGMENTS

The curriculum that evolved into the ideas for this series was inspired by two talented and forthright students, Philbert Yao and Chuck Rosipal, who have since graduated from medical school. It has been a tremendous joy to work with my friend and colleague Lydia Conlay, a brilliant anesthesiologist and medical educator, and the many excellent contributors. I am greatly indebted to my editor, Catherine Johnson, whose exuberance, experience, and vision helped to shape this series. I appreciate McGraw-Hill's believing in the concept of teaching through clinical cases. I am also grateful to Catherine Saggese for her excellent production expertise. At Methodist Hospital, I appreciate the great support from Drs. Marc Boom, Dirk Sostman, Alan Kaplan, and Karin Larsen-Pollock. Likewise, without Ayse McCracken, David Campbell, and Linda Swagger for their advice and support, this book may never have been completed. Without my dear colleagues, Drs. Konrad Harms, Jeané Holmes, and Priti Schachel, this book could not have been written. Most of all, I appreciate my loving wife, Terri, and my four wonderful children, Andy, Michael, Allison, and Christina, for their patience and understanding.

Eugene C. Toy

INTRODUCTION

Mastering the cognitive knowledge within a field such as anesthesia is a formidable task, especially for the new learner. It is even more difficult to draw on that knowledge, procure and filter through the clinical and laboratory data, develop a differential diagnosis, and finally form a rational treatment plan. To gain these skills, the student often learns best at the bedside (or for anesthesia, most often the operating table), guided and instructed by experienced teachers and inspired toward self-directed, diligent reading. Clearly, there is no replacement for education in the operating room or bedside. Unfortunately, clinical situations usually do not encompass the breadth of the specialty. Perhaps the best alternative is a carefully crafted patient case designed to stimulate the clinical approach and decision making. In an attempt to achieve this goal, we have constructed a collection of clinical vignettes to teach diagnostic or therapeutic approaches relevant to the field of anesthesia. Most importantly, the explanations for the cases emphasize the mechanisms and underlying principles rather than merely rote questions and answers.

This book is organized for versatility: to allow the student "in a rush" to go quickly through the scenarios and check the corresponding answers, and to provide more detailed information for the student who wants thought-provoking explanations. The answers are arranged from simple to complex: a summary of the pertinent points, the bare answers, an analysis of the case, an approach to the topic, a comprehension test at the end for reinforcement and emphasis, and a list of resources for further reading. The clinical vignettes are purposely arranged in a systematic manner to more easily allow the student to learn and integrate the mechanisms. A listing of cases is included in Section IV to aid the student who desires to test his or her knowledge of a certain area or to review a topic, including basic definitions. Finally, we intentionally did not primarily use a multiple-choice question format because clues (or distractions) are not available in the real world. Nevertheless, several multiple-choice questions are included at the end of each scenario to reinforce concepts or introduce related topics.

HOW TO GET THE MOST OUT OF THIS BOOK

Each case is designed to simulate a patient encounter and includes open-ended questions. At times, the patient's complaint differs from the issue of most concern, and sometimes extraneous information is given. The answers are organized into four different parts:

PART I

1. **Summary:** The salient aspects of the case are identified, filtering out the extraneous information. The student should formulate his or her summary from the case before looking at the answers. A comparison with the summation in the answer helps to improve one's ability to focus on the important data while appropriately discarding irrelevant information, a fundamental skill required in clinical problem solving.
2. A **straightforward answer** is given to each open-ended question.
3. An **analysis of the case,** which consists of two parts:
   a. **Objectives:** A listing of the two or three main principles that are crucial for a practitioner in treating a patient. Again, the student is challenged to make educated "guesses" about the objectives of the case after an initial review of the case scenario, which helps to sharpen his or her clinical and analytical skills.
   b. **Considerations:** A discussion of the relevant points and a brief approach to a **specific** patient.

PART II

An **approach to the disease process,** consisting of two distinct parts:

1. **Definitions:** Terminology pertinent to the disease process.
2. **Clinical approach:** A discussion of the approach to the clinical problem in general, including tables, figures, and algorithms.

PART III

Comprehension questions: Each case includes several multiple-choice questions that reinforce the material or introduce new and related concepts. Questions about material not found in the text are explained in the answers.

PART IV

Clinical pearls: A listing of several clinically important points, which are reiterated as a summation of the text and to allow for easy review, such as before an examination.

SECTION I

How to Approach Clinical Problems

- Part 1. Approach to the Patient
- Part 2. Approach to Clinical Problem Solving
- Part 3. Approach to Reading

Part 1. Approach to the Patient

The transition from textbook or journal article learning to an application of the information in a specific clinical situation is one of the most challenging tasks in medicine. It requires retention of information, organization of the facts, and recall of a myriad of data with precise application to the patient. In anesthesiology, this application of information acquires an additional dimension: time. **Time** is an ever present consideration for anesthesiologists because in the most dire situations such as the inability to secure an airway or to preserve cardiac output, life is sustained for only minutes, not hours.

The purpose of this text is to facilitate this process. The first step is gathering information, also known as establishing the **database**. This includes recording the patient's history; performing the physical examination; and obtaining selective laboratory examinations and/or imaging tests. Of these, the historical examination is the most important and most useful in aiding the anesthesiologist's assessment of risks to the patient, and the formulation of plans to mitigate those risks. However, unlike many specialties, when an acute problem becomes apparent, the patient is usually anesthetized and unable to provide verbal information. In this setting, an assessment of vital signs, gas analysis, lab tests, and imaging guide the diagnosis.

Clinical Pearl

- When an acute problem becomes apparent and the patient is anesthetized, an assessment of vital signs, gas analysis, lab tests, and imaging often guide the diagnosis.

Anesthesiologists also face an additional challenge in their approach to a patient: a short period of time to develop the physician-patient relationship. While patients will most likely have had multiple interactions with most of their physicians including their surgeon, anesthesiologists are all too often strangers who appear seemingly out of nowhere, and of whose activities patients are largely unaware. Taking the time for an unhurried introduction and actively working to develop a rapport go a long way toward inspiring a patient's confidence. "Little things" such as providing a warm blanket, or inquiring about a patient's fears are especially welcome. In contrast to the prevailing opinion that anesthesiologists are impersonal and only monitor physiological processes, the skilled anesthesiologist must be able to "read" many different types of patients during stressful times and develop a trusting relationship in a short time frame. In the preoperative period, patients are often anxious, and acutely aware of their interactions with the anesthesiologist, everyone, and everything.

Clinical Pearl

> ➤ Since anesthesiologists often have a short period of time to develop the physician-patient relationship, this activity requires special attention.

Part 2. Approach to Clinical Problem Solving

There are generally seven distinct steps that an anesthesiologist takes to systematically solve most clinical problems:

1. Vigilance: discovering an abnormal, unusual, or changing condition.
2. Assessing the situation.
3. Considering the treatment of the clinical sign(s) even before reaching the diagnosis.
4. Formulating a differential diagnosis.
5. Initiating treatment based on the probability of occurrence.
6. Formulating a backup plan.
7. Observing the patient's response.

Then the cycle may begin all over again.

1. DETECTING AN ABNORMAL, UNUSUAL, OR CHANGING CONDITION

Anesthesia is a discipline of vigilance. During an operative case, the anesthesiologist frequently—if not almost constantly—scans the anesthesia machine and evaluates the displaying of the patient's vital signs, oxygen saturation, and the concentration of gases at the end of expiration (end-tidal CO_2, or end-tidal desflurane, etc.), and the patient's physical signs such as papillary dilatation, sweating, tearing, the position of his or her extremities, the extent of his or her neuromuscular blockade, the progress of the surgery, etc.

Clinical Pearl

> ➤ The most important part of clinical problem solving during anesthesiology is **vigilance.** Vigilance allows the detection of information that is abnormal, and which requires prompt assessment by the anesthesiologist.

2. ASSESSING THE SITUATION

When anything is unusual, the anesthetist promptly assesses the situation. This involves integrating the patient's current clinical information with pre-existing information obtained during the preoperative evaluation. It is important to quickly determine "how bad" the situation is, and whether it is likely to be a "big" problem (implying a situation that is life threatening or can degenerate into a situation that is life threatening), or a "little" problem which can be fixed with "fine-tuning." For example, the appearance of new premature ventricular arrhythmias (PVAs) could be a "big problem" representing a myocardial event, or a "little problem" resulting from an endotracheal tube tickling the carina, or hypoventilation-induced hypercarbia which is easily corrected by changing the ventilator settings. Similarly, the new onset of unifocal premature ventricular complexes (PVCs) in a frequency of 3 to 5 per minute is a very different situation from the onset of frequent runs of ventricular tachycardia.

Clinical Pearl

- The second step in clinical problem solving during anesthesiology is **assessing the situation and the severity of the problem.**

3. CONSIDER TREATING THE ABNORMAL CLINICAL SIGN

Because of the urgent nature of complications, anesthesiology is one of the few specialties where treatment is often initiated prior to obtaining a diagnosis, or indeed, even establishing a differential. This practice reflects the fact that abnormalities in some of the physical signs such as blood pressure, heart rate, and oxygen saturation, for example, can be harmful and even life threatening in and of themselves. For example, if a patient with coronary artery disease becomes hypotensive, the hypotension can reduce coronary blood flow to vulnerable areas of the myocardium and result in ischemia. Thus a vasopressor would often be administered, even before the cause of the hypotension was determined. In addition to preventing the ischemia, treating the hypotension would also "buy time" to allow the formulation of a differential diagnosis.

Clinical Pearl

- The third step in clinical problem-solving is to consider treating the abnormal clinical sign in order to mitigate any potential complications from the abnormality and "buy time" to establish a differential diagnosis.

4. FORMULATING A DIFFERENTIAL DIAGNOSIS

A diagnosis is made by a prompt evaluation and analysis of the available information, assessing the risk factors, and developing the list of possibilities (the differential diagnosis). Experience, knowledge, and years of training help the anesthetist to "key in" on the most important possibilities. A long list of possible diagnoses is usually pared down to two or three that are the most likely for the given situation. For example, a patient who experiences tachycardia under anesthesia may be too "light" and require more anesthesia, or hypovolemic, perhaps secondary to a bowel prep prior to surgery and require fluids, or be manifesting signs of malignant hyperthermia, more likely if the patient also presents with muscular dystrophy.

Clinical Pearl

- The fourth step in clinical problem solving in anesthesiology is **formulating a differential diagnosis.**

5. TREATING BASED ON PROBABILITY

Many illnesses are stratified according to severity because the prognosis and treatment often vary based on the severity. In anesthesiology, because of the importance of time in life-threatening situations, the treatment is based on the most likely diagnosis. But since the most likely diagnosis is not necessarily the only possible diagnosis, the patient's response to treatment must be carefully observed. For example, if a patient is hypotensive early in the course of a colectomy, and the most likely diagnosis is considered to be a high concentration of an inhalation agent such as isoflurane, it is important to observe whether the hypotension abates as the concentration of isoflurane is reduced.

Clinical Pearl

- The fifth step in most cases is tailoring the treatment to most likely diagnosis.

6. FORMULATING A BACKUP PLAN

The steps of **treating based on probability and formulating a backup plan** are naturally interconnected. As the most likely diagnosis and its treatment are determined, it is natural to concurrently formulate a backup plan. The anesthetist must be prepared to know what to do if the patient does not respond according to what is expected. Is the next step to treat again and if so, how and when? Or is the next step to reassess the diagnosis, or to follow up with another more specific test? For example, if the patient undergoing colectomy does not respond to reducing the concentration of isoflurane, then perhaps he is hypovolemic secondary to dehydration from his bowel prep.

Because the abnormalities in physical signs can be harmful, it is common to undertake the treatment plan and the backup plan almost simultaneously. But at this time, a "backup" to the "backup" is always in mind. As in the game of chess, the anesthesiologist is trained to think of alternatives and the appropriate response several steps ahead. For example, in the colectomy patient, the isoflurane would be reduced and fluids would be administered at almost the same time.

Clinical Pearl

- Clinical problem solving in anesthesiology involves thinking several steps ahead.

7. FOLLOWING THE RESPONSE TO TREATMENT

The final step in the approach to disease is to follow the patient's response to the therapy. The "measure" of response is recorded and monitored. Some responses are clinical, such as improvement (or lack of improvement) in a patient's blood pressure, or oxygen saturation. Other responses can be followed by invasive monitors, such as pulmonary artery wedge pressure, continuous cardiac output, or transesophageal echocardiography.

Clinical Pearl

- **The seventh step** in clinical problem-solving **is to monitor treatment response or efficacy,** which can be measured in different ways.

Part 3. Approach to Reading

The clinical problem-oriented approach to reading is different from the classic "systematic" research of a disease. A patient's presentation rarely provides a clear diagnosis; hence, the student must become skilled in applying textbook information to the clinical setting. Furthermore, one retains more information when one reads with a purpose. In other words, the student should read with the goal of answering specific questions. There are seven fundamental questions that facilitate **clinical thinking:**

1. What is the most likely diagnosis?
2. How can you confirm the diagnosis?

3. What should be your next step?
4. What is the most likely mechanism for this disease process?
5. What are the risk factors for this disease process?
6. What are the complications associated with this disease process?
7. What is the best therapy?

Clinical Pearl

- Reading with the purpose of answering the seven fundamental clinical questions improves retention of information and facilitates the application of book knowledge to clinical knowledge.

WHAT IS THE MOST LIKELY DIAGNOSIS?

The method of establishing the diagnosis has been covered in the previous section. One way of attacking this problem is to develop standard approaches to common clinical problems. It is helpful to understand the most common causes of various presentations, such as the fact that "the most common locations of a leak in the breathing circuit begin at the patient, and become less frequent the farther away from the patient and closer to the anesthesia machine."

The clinical scenario might be "A 38-year-old woman undergoing breast biopsy under general anesthesia has a leak in the breathing circuit, noted by a failure of the ventilator bellows to rise. The patient is not receiving an adequate tidal volume, and the oxygen saturation is beginning to decline. Where should the student check first? What is the most likely location for the leak?"

With no other information to go on, the student uses the "most common cause" information, makes an educated guess that the patient has a leak in the endotracheal tube cuff, and adds more air to the cuff's balloon.

Then student uses the clinical pearl: "When detecting a leak in the breathing circuit, start at the patient and work back toward the machine."

Clinical Pearl

- When detecting a leak in the breathing circuit, start at the patient and work back toward the machine. Thus, the first step in detecting the location of the leak is to add air to the endotracheal tube's cuff. If the leak continues, move one step toward the machine, and check the connection of the endotracheal tube, followed by the connection of the end-tidal CO_2 tubing, etc.

HOW CAN YOU CONFIRM THE DIAGNOSIS?

In the scenario in the preceding discussion, it is suspected that the leak is located in the endotracheal tube cuff. As the additional air is added, all eyes are on the capnograph, which shows that end-tidal CO_2 is present. The diagnosis is confirmed by looking at the chest which does not rise, and listening to breathe sounds by auscultation, though none are heard. This patient has an esophageal intubation, and instead of coming from the lungs, the CO_2 measured by the capnograph originated from a gastric bubble. The student should strive to know the limitations of various diagnostic tests and equipment, especially when used in the context of a potentially life-threatening situation.

WHAT SHOULD BE YOUR NEXT STEP?

This question is difficult because the next step has many possibilities; the answer may be to obtain more diagnostic information, introduce therapy, or even query a consultant in another field. It is often a more challenging question than, "What is the most likely diagnosis?" because there may be insufficient information to make a diagnosis and the next step may be to obtain more data. Or, the most appropriate answer may be to begin treatment. Hence, based on the clinical data, a judgment needs to be rendered regarding how far along one is in the following sequence.

(1) Make a diagnosis →(2) Determine the urgency and severity of the situation →(3) Decide to treat or support →(4) Follow the response.

Frequently, students are taught to "regurgitate" information that they have read about a particular disease but are not skilled at identifying the next step. This talent is learned optimally at the bedside in a supportive environment with the freedom to take educated guesses and receive constructive feedback. In anesthesiology, it is learned in the operating room, an environment that carries with it the constraint of potential harm to the patient. Nevertheless, a sample scenario might describe a student's thought process as follows:

1. **Make a diagnosis:** "Based on the information I have, I believe that Mr. Smith is hypertensive *because* of light anesthesia." His heart rate is also elevated, and he is producing tears from the corner of his eyes.
2. **Determine the severity and urgency of the situation:** "I do not believe that this hypertension is severe, because it is only 160/80, although it has risen from his starting pressure of 120/65." Similarly, there is no urgency to treat his blood pressure (this answer might be different as the patient is under observation for an expanding thoracic aneurysm).
3. **Decide to treat or support:** "Therefore, my next step is to deepen the anesthetic by increasing the concentration of isoflurane."
4. **Follow the response:** "I want to follow the treatment by assessing his blood pressure, heart rate, and other signs of sympathetic stimulation such as tearing, sweating, and pupillary dilatation."

In a similar patient, when the clinical presentation is unclear, perhaps the best next step is a diagnostic one such as checking his bispectral EEG to determine the depth of anesthesia.

Clinical Pearl

> ➤ The vague question, "What is your next step?" is often the most difficult one because the answer may be diagnostic, supportive, or therapeutic.

WHAT IS THE LIKELY MECHANISM FOR THIS DISEASE PROCESS?

This question goes further than making the diagnosis and requires the student to understand the underlying mechanism of the process. For example, a clinical scenario may describe a 22-year-old man with non-Hodgkin lymphoma who is short of breath at rest, and who cannot lie flat. When first seen by the anesthetist, he is sitting forward in his bed. The patient's inability to lie flat is suggestive of a mediastinal mass, and the mechanism of his shortness of breath is tracheal or bronchial compression by a large mediastinal tumor. If the compression is distal to the endotracheal tube, then inducing anesthesia and laying the patient flat could quickly result in death. A more prudent approach would be to cannulate the patient's groin under local anesthesia and be prepared to institute cardiopulmonary bypass if the patient cannot be ventilated. Thus, the student is advised to learn the mechanisms of each disease process and not merely to memorize a constellation of symptoms. Furthermore, in anesthesiology, it is crucial for students to understand the anatomy, function, and how the problem can be corrected.

WHAT ARE THE RISK FACTORS FOR THIS DISEASE PROCESS?

Understanding the risk factors helps the practitioner to establish a diagnosis and to determine how to interpret test results. For example, understanding the risk factor analysis may help in the treatment of a 55-year-old man who suddenly becomes hypotensive during a general anesthesia for an esophagectomy. If the patient has risk factors for a pneumothorax (such as emphysematous blebs or in this case, the surgical procedure itself), it may be appropriate to insert a chest tube. Otherwise, hypovolemia would be a common etiology. If he has just received a dose of fentanyl, that may be the cause.

Clinical Pearl

> ➤ A knowledge of the risk factors can be a useful guide in testing and in developing the differential diagnosis.

WHAT ARE THE COMPLICATIONS OF THIS DISEASE PROCESS?

Clinicians must be cognizant of the complications of a disease so that they can understand how to follow and monitor the patient, and so they can choose the optimal anesthetic agent for a given procedure. Sometimes, the student has to make a diagnosis from clinical clues and then apply his or her knowledge of the consequences of the pathologic process. For example, a 68-year-old woman, who presents for a nephrectomy, complains of a 7-month history of dizziness with occasional blackouts. On ECG, she is determined to have a bifascicular block. The long-term complications of this process include complete heart block, and inhalation agents can impair myocardial conduction. Understanding the types of consequences also helps the clinician to become aware of the dangers to the patient. The ready availability of external pacing or a transvenous pacemaker may be indicated, and require preparation as well as some setup time.

WHAT IS THE BEST THERAPY?

To answer this question, the clinician not only needs to reach the correct diagnosis and assess the severity of the condition but also must weigh the situation to determine the appropriate intervention. For the student, knowing exact dosages is not as important as understanding the best medication, route of delivery, mechanism of action, and possible complications. It is important for the student to be able to verbalize the diagnosis and the rationale for the therapy.

Clinical Pearl

- Therapy should be logical based on the severity of the disease and the specific diagnosis. An exception to this rule is in an urgent situation such as severe hypotension, when the clinical sign such as blood pressure must be treated even as the etiology is being investigated.

SUMMARY

1. The anesthesiologist must be astute in discerning a patient's concerns and fears, and engendering trust.
2. There is no replacement for a meticulous history and physical examination. However, anesthesiologists must often rely on other means of achieving a differential diagnosis in an urgent situation.
3. There are seven steps in the clinical approach to the patient: discovering an abnormal, unusual, or changing condition, assessing the situation, considering the treatment of the clinical sign(s), formulating a differential

diagnosis, treating based on the probability of occurrence while formulating a backup plan, and observing the patient's response.

4. There are seven questions that help to bridge the gap between the textbook and the clinical arena.

REFERENCES

Doherty GM. Preoperative care. In: Doherty GM, Way LE, eds. *Current Surgical Diagnosis and Treatment*. 12th ed. New York, NY: McGraw-Hill Publishers; 2005: 6-13.

Englebert JE, Way LW. Approach to the surgical patient. In: Doherty GM, Way LE, eds. *Current Surgical Diagnosis and Treatment*. 12th ed. New York, NY: McGraw-Hill Publishers; 2005: 1-5.

SECTION II

Fundamental Information

Part 1. Anesthetics

Case 1

A 6-year-old child is scheduled for an MRI to rule out a possible brain tumor. The child is terrified by the scanner's noise and the closed space, and refuses to hold still. The patient is scheduled for general anesthesia. However, an anesthesia machine cannot be brought into the same room with the magnet.

➤ How can this patient safely receive general anesthesia?

ANSWER TO CASE 1: Intravenous Anesthesia

Summary: A 6-year-old child needs an MRI scan and cannot hold still. The general anesthesia machine cannot be brought into the room due to the magnet.

➤ **Method of Anesthesia:** Intravenous anesthetics are used for a pleasant, rapid induction of general anesthesia. Intravenous agents are also useful in lower doses for sedation. They may also be used for maintenance of anesthesia in conjunction with inhalational anesthetics, or instead of inhalational anesthetics when the later are contraindicated (such as in malignant hyperthermia, case on strabismus) or where it is impractical for an anesthesia machine to be present.

ANALYSIS

Objective

Introduce the student to the more common intravenous anesthetics including their properties, uses, and potential side effects.

Considerations

This patient can have an anesthetic cream placed on the arm, and then an i.v. placed with minimal pain. During the procedure, he will be anesthetized with a continuous infusion of propofol, an intravenous agent, and intubated with an endotracheal tube prior to entering the MRI machine. A continuous infusion such as this does not require metal equipment such as an anesthesia machine, and is thus an option in this circumstance.

"Intravenous anesthetics" do not necessarily include intravenous opioids. Opioids are analgesics, and do not cause general anesthesia per se, unless used in very large doses. However, an opioid (eg, fentanyl) is often combined with an intravenous hypnotic drug for prevention of a response to a noxious stimulus (such as movement), and can thus aid in providing a rapid awakening and spontaneous ventilation at the end of a surgical procedure.

APPROACH TO Intravenous Anesthesia

DEFINITIONS

Pharmacodynamics: The effects of a drug on the body, or relationship between the plasma concentration of a drug and the pharmacologic response to it.

Pharmacokinetics: The effects of the body on a drug, and are determined by the volume of distribution for the drug (V_d) and clearance of that drug from the body. Intravenous anesthetics exhibit multi-compartmental pharmacokinetics: that is, the drugs are distributed into peripheral tissues, and at the same time cleared from the body. The administration of an intravenous anesthetic obviously increases the plasma concentration. The concentration of the agent next peaks in the "vessel rich" group of tissues, such as liver and spleen, followed by the "muscle group," and then, finally, into fat. (Please see Figure 1–1.) Plasma concentrations of intravenous agents are also affected by tissue uptake, renal excretion, and hepatic metabolism.

Volume of distribution (V_d): The volume that relates the plasma concentration of a drug to the total amount of drug in the body. It can be thought of as the "size of the tank." By rearranging the terms defining concentration, V_d becomes the dose of drug given intravenously divided by its plasma concentration.

Clearance: The amount of a drug removed by the kidneys and/or metabolized in the liver during a specified period of time (eg, mL/min).

Context-sensitive half-time: The time for the plasma concentration of a drug to decrease by 50% from an infusion that maintains a constant concentration. The context is the duration of the infusion.

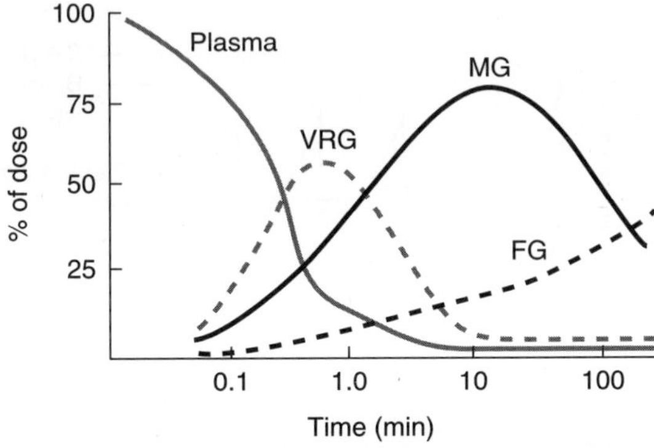

Figure 1–1. Concentrations of anesthetics peak first in plasma, then in the "vessel rich group" (VRG), next the muscle group (MG), then in the fat group (FG). *(Reprinted by permission from Macmillan Publishers Ltd.: Price HL, et al. The uptake of thiopental by body tissues and its relation to the duration of narcosis.* Clin Pharmacol Ther. *1960;1:16.)*

CLINICAL APPROACH

Propofol

Propofol is the most commonly used intravenous drug for induction of anesthesia. It has gained its popularity because it is associated with a pleasant, rapid loss of consciousness, rapid awakening, and seemingly fewer residual effects on patient's brain. Its chemical structure is an alkyl phenol, and some of its behavioral effects seem to resemble those observed with alcohol.

Propofol is used as a bolus for the induction of anesthesia, in doses ranging from 1.5 to 2.5 mg/kg. The administration of propofol can cause significant pain upon injection, which can be attenuated by using an intravenous placed in a large vein, and/or administering lidocaine 0.5 to 1.0 mg/kg i.v. just prior to injecting the propofol. It is also advisable to warn the patient that some burning might occur during injection.

Propofol can also be used for the maintenance of anesthesia. While it is possible to administer propofol for maintenance in multiple boluses, it is best used as continuous infusion since it has a short context-sensitive half-time. Perhaps surprisingly, administering propofol by multiple boluses actually consumes more of the drug than a continuous infusion (please see Figure 1–2). For the maintenance of anesthesia, a loading dose of 1 to 2 mg/kg can be followed by an infusion of 100 μg/kg/min to be titrated to effect.

Propofol is also useful in lower doses for sedation during regional and monitored anesthesia care, and for patients in the intensive care unit. Propofol has never been associated with a case of malignant hyperthermia; so it is the agent of choice for general anesthesia in this setting.

Etomidate

Etomidate is distinguished from the other intravenous agents by its paucity of effects on the cardiovascular system. It causes little or no change in systemic

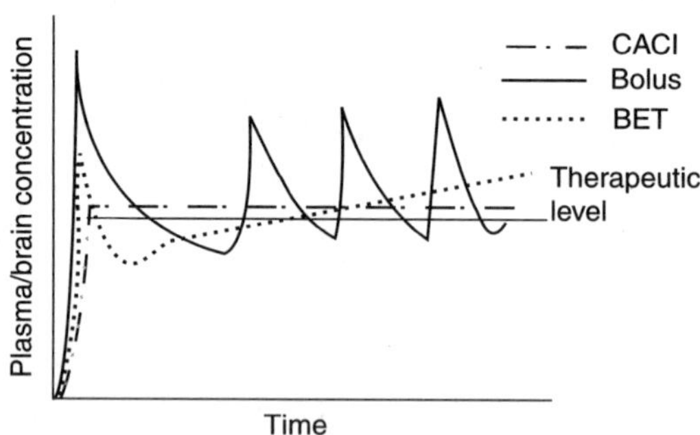

Figure 1–2. Administering an intravenous anesthetic using multiple boluses actually consumes more of the drug than a continuous infusion. *(Reprinted from Reeves JG. Profiles in anesthetic practice: Rational administration of intravenous anesthesia. In: Morgan GE Jr, Mikhail MS, Murray MJ, eds. Clinical Anesthesiology, 4th ed. New York, NY: McGraw-Hill, 2006:190-191.)*

or pulmonary artery pressure, little or no change in heart rate, and only a mild effect on cardiac output. Thus, etomidate is the agent of choice whenever cardiovascular stability is potentially an issue. The possible side effects of etomidate are adrenocortical suppression, myoclonus, and the activation of seizure foci.

Thiopental

Originally known as "sodium pentothal," thiopental is mainly used for induction of anesthesia in patients undergoing neurosurgery. Thiopental reduces the brain's oxygen consumption, and may reduce ischemia-induced brain damage. It is also used intraoperatively for burst suppression, and for the treatment of increased intracranial pressure. There is absolutely no merit in the concept that thiopental was a "truth serum."

Ketamine

Ketamine is an intravenous hypnotic drug that is chemically related to LSD. It produces a dissociative state accompanied by analgesia, unawareness, and nystagmus. When used for induction, it can be associated with "bad dreams" or emergence delirium, although this side effect can be prevented by pretreatment with a benzodiazepine.

Ketamine increases systemic blood pressure, heart rate, and cardiac output. It has no effect on ventilation, although pretreatment with an antisialagogue (eg, glycopyrrolate) may be warranted as ketamine causes an increase in respiratory secretions. Ketamine is contraindicated in patients with intracranial pathology, as it increases intracranial pressure and cerebral blood flow.

Comprehension Questions

1.1. A 60-year-old man undergoing an inguinal hernia repair is induced with propofol. Which of the following is most likely to be observed?

A. Hyperthermia
B. Hypetension
C. Apnea
D. Prolonged sedation

1.2. Match the anesthetic (A-D) to its effect (1-4).

A. Propofol	1. "Bad dreams"
B. Sodium pentothal	2. Pleasant emergence and slight euphoria
C. Ketamine	3. Long-term sedation
D. Etomidate	4. Few hemodynamic effects

ANSWERS

1.1. **C.** Hypotension and apnea are the most common side effects of propofol. Answers A and D are incorrect. Propofol does not cause hyperthermia, indeed, it is the anesthetic of choice in patients at risk for malignant hyperthermia. Propofol is associated with a fast emergence, which is also an advantage of the drug.

1.2. **A, 2.** Propofol is known for its pleasant anesthetic properties and occasional euphoria.
B, 3. Sodium pentothal is a barbiturate known for its long-term sedation.
C, 1. Ketamine is chemically related to LSD and is sometimes associated with "bad dreams."
D, 4. Etomidate is associated with the fewest cardiovascular side effects.

Clinical Pearl

➤ Intravenous anesthetics have life-threatening complications, so they should always be used in an environment with appropriately trained personnel and monitoring.

REFERENCES

Glass PSA, Shafer SL, Reeves JG. Intravenous drug delivery systems. In: Miller, R. ed. *Anesthesia.* 5th ed. Philadelphia, PA: Churchill Livingstone; 2000: 390-398.

Shafer SL, Varel JR. *Anesthesiology*. 1991;74:53-63.

Case 2

A 6-year-old child is to undergo bilateral placement of ear tubes under general anesthesia, a 5-minute procedure. Not unlike many children of this age, he has a significant fear of needles. His mother states that he will under no circumstance hold still for the placement of an i.v.

➤ How can this child be anesthetized safely without an intravenous?

ANSWER TO CASE 2: Inhalation Anesthetics

Summary: A 6-year-old child is to undergo bilateral placement of ear tubes under general anesthesia. He has a significant fear of needles and will not hold still for the placement of an i.v.

➤ **Best anesthetic technique:** Inhalation anesthesia

ANALYSIS

Objectives

1. Be familiar with the nomenclature regarding inhalation anesthetics.
2. Introduce the types of equipment used to administer inhalation anesthetics.
3. Become familiar with some of the advantages and disadvantages unique to individual inhalation anesthetics.

Considerations

This patient can be easily anesthetized using an inhalation induction, where the child inspires an anesthetic vapor. First, in order to reduce the child's anxiety when asked to breathe through a mask, flavors are placed in the mask such as grape, bubble gum, peppermint, etc. If possible, monitors are placed prior to induction. If this is not possible, monitors are placed as soon as the child allows. Since this patient is healthy and the duration of the procedure is only about 5 minutes, an intravenous line will probably not be required.

APPROACH TO Inhalation Anesthesia

The first anesthetics, ether and chloroform, were inhaled anesthetics. Indeed, inhaled aesthetics are commonly used today. Their applications range from use as induction agents (as in the vignette described earlier), to more commonly, for the maintenance of anesthesia. The most commonly used inhalational anesthetics are nitrous oxide, isoflurane, sevoflurane, desflurane, and in children, halothane.

A simple approach to understanding clinical pharmacology is to consider the qualities of an ideal anesthetic, and how the currently-used inhaled anesthetics use either meet these requirements or fall short. These qualities of an ideal anesthetic agent involve the anesthesia machine and the breathing circuit, the lungs and breathing, the cardiovascular system, other organ systems, and finally the central nervous system.

DEFINITIONS

Minimum alveolar concentration (MAC): Minimum alveolar concentration (MAC) is the alveolar concentration of an inhaled anesthetic that prevents movement in 50% of patients in response to a stimulus (such as surgical stimulation). It can also be considered an anesthetic's ED_{50}. The goal of an anesthetic is obviously not MAC, since 50% of patients move in response to a stimulus at this concentration.

Partial pressure: The pressure of an ideal gas if it occupied a fixed volume alone. Gases dissolve, diffuse, and react according to their partial pressures, and not necessarily according to their concentrations in a gaseous mixture, although the two terms are often used interchangeably. Gases always flow or equilibrate from a region of higher partial pressure to one of lower pressure.

Blood/gas partition coefficient or solubility is the ratio of the partial pressures of the anesthetic in the blood and alveolar gas at equilibrium.

Blood/fat partition coefficient or solubility is the ratio of the partial pressures of the anesthetic in the blood and fat at equilibrium.

CLINICAL APPROACH

Desirable Properties of an Inhaled Anesthetic

1. **Involving the anesthesia machine and breathing circuit**
   - 1.1. Lack of flammability: Three of the volatile anesthetics (isoflurane, sevoflurane, and desflurane) are not flammable in clinically relevant concentrations. Nitrous oxide (N_2O) does support combustion, which is of concern in procedures using lasers or cautery in air spaces which could contain the drug.
   - 1.2. Ease of vaporization at room temperature: Three of the anesthetics are volatile, and can be supplied as bottled liquids, which can be easily transformed into a much larger volume of gas. Vaporizers, specific for each anesthetic, accomplish this task. Each vaporizer converts its liquid into the anesthetic vapor, which is then delivered in a specified quantity to the patient along with oxygen through the breathing circuit. Desflurane is especially volatile and requires a special heated

and pressurized vaporizer. Nitrous oxide, the one nonvolatile anesthetic, is supplied as a compressed gas (in a blue tank) and can be delivered along with oxygen in the breathing circuit.

1.3. Chemical stability: The anesthesia machine includes a canister of a carbon dioxide absorbent (such as soda lime) to prevent the accumulation of CO_2 in the breathing circuit. All of the volatile inhaled anesthetics are somewhat unstable when exposed to soda lime and form small amounts of toxic substances. A nephrotoxic vinyl compound is formed from sevoflurane, and carbon monoxide is formed from desflurane, and to a lesser extent isoflurane. Nevertheless, the stability of these newer anesthetics when exposed to soda lime is much improved when compared to some of the older anesthetics. When trichloroethylene was exposed to soda lime, the result was significant quantities of phosgene gas.

2. Desirable properties involving the lungs and breathing

2.1. Rapid induction and emergence influence both patient satisfaction, and their ease of use. The speed of an inhaled anesthetic's induction is directly related to the rate of rise of its concentrations in the alveolus. Indeed, the anesthetic's partial pressure in the alveolus governs its partial pressure in all tissues in the body, since all ultimately equilibrate with the partial pressure of the gas in the alveolus.

However, these compounds also dissolve in blood, thus "partitioning" the anesthetic between the soluble and insoluble portions. The more a compound dissolves in blood, the slower its concentration can rise in the alveolus, which determines the amount of the gaseous form of the anesthetic transmitted to organs like the brain. Conversely, the more insoluble the gas that's inhaled, the quicker its alveolar and gaseous plasma concentrations rise, and the more rapid its action. Nitrous oxide and desflurane are very insoluble, and thus have the fastest rate of rise in alveolus. Sevoflurane is next, and isoflurane has the slowest rate of rise. (please see Table 2–1 for the blood:gas solubilities of the inhaled anesthetics.)

Lipid solubility also affects the speed of an anesthetic's onset (or conversely, off set), since lipid solubility enables the anesthetic to cross membranes and equilibrate between the blood and the brain. Isoflurane and sevoflurane are quite lipid soluble, followed by desflurane and nitrous oxide, which are not (Please see Table 2–1). However, lipid solubility is a double-edged sword. If an anesthetic is soluble in fat, then body fat can act as a depot in which the anesthetic can accumulate, thus slowing emergence. Since the fat cells have little blood flow, accumulation in fat occurs over a long period of time.

2.2. Lack of airway irritation: A lack of airway irritation is a plus for sevoflurane and nitrous oxide; these two agents could be used along with oxygen for a pleasant mask induction in children. Isoflurane and desflurane have a pungent odor, are quite irritating, and may

Table 2–1 COMPARATIVE SOLUBILITIES AND MINIMAL ALVEOLAR CONCENTRATIONS OF THE INHALED ANESTHETICS

INHALED ANESTHETIC	BLOOD:GAS SOLUBILITY	FAT:BLOOD SOLUBILITY	MINIMAL ALVEOLAR CONCENTRATION (MAC)
Desflurane	0.45	27	6%
Nitrous oxide	0.47	2.3	1.04%
Sevoflurane	0.65	48	2.05%
Isoflurane	1.4	45	1.15%

cause coughing and even laryngeal spasm. For this reason, desflurane is used only for the maintenance of anesthesia.

2.3 Bronchodilation: Bronchodilation is helpful in patients with reactive airway disease, and is a plus for sevoflurane and isoflurane. Desflurane has no effect on airway resistance in nonsmokers, but produces bronchoconstriction in smokers. Nitrous oxide has no effect on airway resistance.

2.4. Lack of respiratory depression: Unfortunately, all of the inhaled anesthetics are respiratory depressants. Their effects may be summarized according to "3 Rs": rapid respiration, reduced tidal volume, and of regular duration with loss of the awake respiratory variability. All of the inhaled anesthetics also increase arterial carbon dioxide (except nitrous oxide), depress the ventilatory response to hypercarbia in anesthetic concentrations, and most importantly, depress the ventilatory response to hypoxia even in sub-anesthetic concentrations.

3. Desirable properties involving the cardiovascular system

3.1. Maintenance of mean arterial pressure: Unfortunately, all of the volatile inhaled anesthetics reduce arterial pressure in a dose-dependent fashion. Nitrous oxide is the only inhaled anesthetic that does not drop the blood pressure.

3.2. Suppression of sympathetic nervous system activity: Three inhaled anesthetics, nitrous oxide, isoflurane, and desflurane, actually increase sympathetic activity, usually in a dose-dependent fashion.

3.3. Maintenance of heart rate: All of the inhaled anesthetics tend to increase the heart rate, at least at some concentrations. These effects are complicated, and may represent sympathetic stimulation, a reflex tachycardia from the reduction in arterial pressure, or actions on the baroreceptors.

4. Desirable properties involving other organ systems

4.1. Low solubility in skeletal muscle and fat: When inhaled anesthetics get into the blood stream, they are distributed or absorbed into skeletal muscle and fat. This volume of distribution can be large, providing a significant depot which must be cleared so the patient can emerge from the anesthetic. Because nitrous oxide and desflurane are insoluble in blood, smaller quantities are stored in the body during a given anesthetic, thus shortening the time for emergence.

4.2. Direct skeletal muscle relaxation: Desflurane and sevoflurane cause the most relaxation of skeletal muscles, followed closely by isoflurane. Nitrous oxide has little effect on skeletal muscles.

4.3. Not being a trigger for malignant hyperthermia (MH): Malignant hyperthermia is a rare, genetically-based disorder of calcium metabolism, which usually presents as a complication of anesthesia. Unfortunately, all of the volatile inhaled anesthetics—isoflurane, sevoflurane, and desflurane—can trigger a malignant hyperthermia crisis, and must be scrupulously avoided if a patient has a history or family history of malignant hyperthermia.

4.4. Low hepatic metabolism: A simple mnemonic to remember the hepatic metabolism of inhaled anesthetics is the so-called "Rule of 2's." Halothane is roughly 20% metabolized, enflurane 2%, isoflurane 0.2%, desflurane 0.02%, and sevoflurane roughly 4% (2%   2). The hepatic metabolism of nitrous oxide is negligible. Of the inhaled anesthetics that are now available clinically, sevoflurane undergoes the most hepatic metabolism.

4.5. Lack of organ toxicity: Unfortunately, all of the inhaled anesthetics have the potential to cause different types of organ toxicity. Hepatic toxicity is a concern with isoflurane and desflurane, renal toxicity is a concern with sevoflurane, and bone marrow toxicity is a concern with nitrous oxide. If a patient has a history of inhaled anesthetic-induced hepatitis, it is recommended to avoid all of the volatile inhaled anesthetics—isoflurane, desflurane, and sevoflurane.

5. Desirable properties involving the central nervous system

5.1. Analgesia: Of all the inhaled anesthetics, only nitrous oxide is analgesic. This property is blocked with naloxone.

5.2. Potency: The potency of an inhaled anesthetic is indicated by its MAC, or the partial pressure of an inhaled anesthetic that prevents movement in 50% of patients in response to a painful stimulus. Of the volatile inhaled anesthetics, isoflurane is the most potent (MAC = 1.15%), followed by sevoflurane (MAC = 2.05%) and desflurane (MAC = 6%). Nitrous oxide has the highest MAC (104%); it is not potent enough to be used alone and must be used in combination with other anesthetics. Some of the advantages and disadvantages of nitrous oxide, isoflurane, sevoflurane, and desflurane are summarized in Tables 2–2 to 2–5.

Table 2–2 SOME ADVANTAGES AND DISADVANTAGES OF NITROUS OXIDE

ADVANTAGES	DISADVANTAGES
Analgesia	Nauses and vomiting
Fastest induction and emergence	Low potency (high MAC)
Negligible hepatic metabolism	Sympathetic stimulation
Not pungent	Bone marrow toxicity
Less hypotension	Expands closed air spaces
Less cardiac depression	Supports combustion
Less respiratory depression	

Table 2–3 SOME ADVANTAGES AND DISADVANTAGES OF ISOFLURANE

ADVANTAGES	DISADVANTAGES
Potency (low MAC)	Slower induction and emergence
Low hepatic metabolism	Highly soluble in fat and muscle
Bronchodilator	Pungent odor
Inexpensive	Hypotension (strong vasodilator)
	Trigger for malignant hyperthermia

Table 2–4 SOME ADVANTAGES AND DISADVANTAGES OF DESFLURANE

ADVANTAGES	DISADVANTAGES
Fastest induction and emergence	Very pungent odor
Lowest blood:gas solubility	Bronchoconstriction (in smokers)
Very low hepatic metabolism	CO formed in CO_2 absorbent
	Needs special heated vaporizer
	Sympathetic stimulation
	Hypotension (strong vasodilator)
	Trigger for malignant hyperthermia

Table 2–5 SOME ADVANTAGES AND DISADVANTAGES OF SEVOFLURANE

ADVANTAGES	DISADVANTAGES
Faster induction and emergence	High hepatic metabolism (about 4%)
Pleasant odor (not pungent)	High inorganic fluoride ion levels
Suitable for mask induction (in children)	Compound A formed in CO_2 absorbent
Bronchodilator	Potential renal toxicity
	Most soluble in fat and muscle
	Hypotension (vasodilator)
	Trigger for malignant hyperthermia

Comprehension Questions

2.1. A 30-year-old man presents for open reduction and internal fixation of a left radius fracture as an outpatient. He has smoked 1 pack of cigarettes per day for 12 years. The plan is general anesthesia with endotracheal intubation. Which one of the following agents is most appropriate for him?

A. Isoflurane
B. Sevoflurane
C. Desflurane
D. Nitrous oxide

2.2 A 42-year-old woman presents for laparoscopic gastric bypass. She weighs 191 kg (420 lb) and is 165 cm (5 ft and 5 in) tall. She has a history of hypertension, diabetes mellitus, obstructive sleep apnea, and acid reflux. Because of the sleep apnea, there is concern about mild pulmonary hypertension. Which of the following agents is most likely to produce the most rapid emergence in this patient?

A. Isoflurane
B. Sevoflurane
C. Desflurane
D. Nitrous oxide

2.3. A 38-year-old man presents for ventral hernia repair. He had a malignant hyperthermia crisis during a prior surgery. Which of the following inhaled anesthetics would be appropriate for this patient?

A. Isoflurane
B. Sevoflurane
C. Desflurane
D. Nitrous oxide

ANSWERS

2.1 **B.** Although all agents could be used, sevoflurane would be the preferred choice. Sevoflurane could be used in combination with nitrous oxide. Desflurane has a lower blood:gas solubility that would provide rapid awakening, but desflurane is irritating to inhale and can cause bronchoconstriction in smokers. Isoflurane could also be used, but because of its high blood:gas solubility it may delay emergence.

2.2. **C.** Desflurane has the lowest blood:gas partition coefficient of all agents listed. In addition, desflurane has a lower fat:blood solubility, which may help in this case because of the patient's morbid obesity. Under usual circumstances, nitrous oxide could be used in combination with desflurane; however, in this situation, nitrous oxide is contraindicated since the patient likely has pulmonary hypertension.

2.3. **D.** Malignant hyperthermia (MH) is a life-threatening hypermetabolic state of skeletal muscle that is triggered by the volatile inhaled anesthetics—isoflurane, desflurane, and sevoflurane—and by the depolarizing muscle relaxant succinylcholine. Malignant hyperthermia presents as an increase in carbon dioxide production, acidosis, cardiac arrhythmias, muscle rigidity, and hyperthermia. Death can occur if the MH crisis is not managed appropriately and early in the course of the episode. The mainstay of treatment is i.v. dantrolene. Of the inhaled anesthetics, only nitrous oxide is not contraindicated in malignant hyperthermia. An alternative anesthetic plan would be to employ nitrous oxide in combination with propofol (an intravenous anesthetic), fentanyl (an opioid analgesic), and vecuronium or rocuronium (competitive, nondepolarizing muscle relaxants).

Clinical Pearl

- Like most general classes of anesthetics, inhalation anesthetics vary in their properties. Some are desirable; some are not. Thus, their use is tailored to a specific patient, or a specific situation.

REFERENCES

Eger II EI. Uptake and redistribution. In: Miller RD, ed. *Miller's Anesthesia*. 6th ed. Philadelphia, PA: Churchill Livingstone; 2005:131-153.

Farber NE, Pagel PS, Warltier DC. Pulmonary pharmacology. In: Miller RD, ed. *Miller's Anesthesia*. 6th ed. Philadelphia, PA: Churchill Livingstone; 2005:155-189.

Forman SA, Mashour GA. Pharmacology of inhalational anesthetics. In: Longnecker DE, ed. *Anesthesiology*. New York, NY: McGraw-Hill Companies; 2008: 739-766.

Case 3

A 25-year-old, 75-kg man presents for open appendectomy. The surgery is performed under general anesthesia, without complications. After the specimen is removed, the attending surgeon leaves the operating room to dictate the operative report, leaving the intern and medical student to close the skin. Upon leaving, the surgeon asks them to "inject some local anesthetic into the wounds." The intern turns to you and asks which local anesthetic you suggest and how much to inject.

- ➤ What are the benefits of local anesthetic infiltration?
- ➤ What attributes are you looking for in a local anesthetic in this case?
- ➤ Which agent would you choose and what is the maximum dose?

ANSWERS TO CASE 3: Local Anesthetic Infiltration

Summary: A 25-year-old healthy male undergoes uneventful laparoscopic appendectomy. Local anesthetic infiltration of surgical sites is requested.

- **Benefits of local anesthetic infiltration:** Decreased pain and narcotic usage
- **Local anesthetic attributes:** Long-acting, inexpensive, with addition of vasoconstrictor to decrease toxicity and in some cases increase duration
- **Agent of choice:** Bupivacaine with epinephrine, with a maximum dose of 225 mg bupivacaine

ANALYSIS

Objectives

1. Review pharmacology of local anesthetics.
2. Describe the various ways that local anesthetics can be used for surgical anesthesia.

Considerations

For this application, a long-acting local anesthetic is injected, in an amount that is determined by the toxicity of the drug. As mentioned earlier, bupivacaine is chosen. Epinephrine is added in an attempt to prolong its action.

APPROACH TO Local Anesthesia

Local anesthetic agents have been used for surgical anesthesia for over 100 years. The prototypical local anesthetic is cocaine, first incorporated into surgical practice in 1884 by Carl Koller for use in ophthalmic surgery. Cocaine has fallen out of favor as a primary local anesthetic because of its undesirable systemic effects and its abuse potential, but is still used today for otolaryngology cases where its topical anesthetic action and vasoconstriction capabilities are desirable.

Modern local anesthetics are used in a wide array of situations for surgery. Local anesthetics can be used as the sole anesthetic agent for abdominal and lower extremity procedures in the form of a neuraxial block technique (spinal anesthesia or epidural anesthesia). These techniques are overwhelmingly more common for obstetric anesthesia, and are also the technique of choice for joint replacement of the lower extremity in many anesthesia practices.

Local anesthetics have long been used as a part of a multimodal approach for postoperative pain control. Instillation of local anesthetic at the surgical site has commonly been used, but more recently, continuous infusions of local anesthetics in the forms of patient-controlled epidural anesthesia (PCEA) for thoracic and abdominal procedures as well as continuous peripheral nerve catheters are increasingly being used for postprocedural pain control and have been shown to decrease postoperative pain, as well as narcotic-associated morbidity. A thorough understanding of local anesthetics allows the anesthesiologist to tailor the correct drug, formulation, and technique to each clinical situation.

Historically, the maximal acceptable dose of local anesthetics, as well as adjuvants (such as opiates), have been based on a patient's weight. This practice is somewhat controversial since these different compounds are absorbed from different sites in the body at different rates. For example, the systemic absorption of local anesthetics is very high in vascular regions of the body such as the intercostal space for intercostals nerve blocks, but very low in the regions in which a sciatic nerve bloc is performed. To date, no studies have determined the actual "safe" doses of local anesthetics. However, if body weight is used to estimate the maximal safe dose, it seems more appropriate to base dosing on lean body weight rather than actual weight.

Local anesthetics are similar in their chemical structure and mechanism of action. These agents are amphipathic molecules consisting of three moieties: a lipophilic aromatic region (benzene ring), connected to a hydrophilic tertiary amide group, via an intermediate chain. Local anesthetics block neural transmission by blocking voltage-gated sodium (Na^+) channels. By binding to the Na^+ channel, the local anesthetic blocks Na^+ influx, thus abolishing membrane depolarization, action potential generation, and neural transmission.

Local anesthetics are weak bases, with pKa's ranging from 7.6 to 9.0. Therefore, both the ionic (protonated) and anionic forms are present at physiologic pH. However, only the nonanionic form can cross a cell's lipid bilayer and gain access to its site of action on the intracellular domain of the sodium channel protein. Because a low pH favors the ionized or ineffective form of the local anesthetic, its injection into an acidotic environment such as an abscess, will prove ineffective since the ion cannot enter the neuronal cells.

The anesthetic molecule preferentially binds to the open sodium channel; therefore, local anesthetics preferentially act upon rapidly-firing nerves, so-called "state-dependent blockade." This property is important when local anesthetics are used as antiarrhythmics to abolish ventricular tachycardia as they preferentially act on the rapidly depolarizing foci. As anesthetic agents, local anesthetics also show "state-dependent blockade," but other factors such as nerve diameter and degree of myelination predominate as determinants of nerve fiber blockade. Smaller, unmyelinated fibers are typically blocked before larger, myelinated ones. These properties explain the predictable sequence of nerve function blockade beginning with sympathetic fibers, progressing to pain and temperature fibers, followed by proprioception, then touch and pressure, before finally, motor transmission impairment. The sequence of block resolution is the same, but regression is in reverse order.

There are two classes of local anesthetics: the esters, and the amides, based on its intermediate chain. The **esters,** such as procaine, benzocaine, and tetracaine, are more likely to cause an allergic reaction because of their cross reactivity to para-aminobenzoic acid (PABA). Metabolized by plasma esterase, ester anesthetics tend to have a shorter duration of action. The **amide local anesthetics**, such as lidocaine and bupivacaine, have an intermediate chain linkage that is an amide group. Amides undergo hepatic metabolism in the form of N-dealkylation followed by hydrolysis. Allergic reactions to amide anesthetics are rare.

Local anesthetic formulations are reported as percent solutions, or grams of material per 100 mL solution. Thus a 1% solution contains 1 g of material per 100 mL of solution, or 10 mg material per mL solution. Therefore, 0.5% bupivacaine contains 5 mg/mL, and a total of 45 mL would have to be infiltrated to reach the maximum dose of 225 mg.

PHYSIOCHEMICAL PROPERTIES AND CLINICAL EFFECT

Physiochemical properties of local anesthetics predict their pharmacokinetic and pharmacologic properties.

pKa

An agent's pKa determines the onset of action. The pKa is the pH at which a local anesthetic is present in both charged and uncharged forms in equal amounts. As mentioned earlier, only the anionic form of a local anesthetic can gain access to the binding site on the sodium channel, which is located on the intracellular portion of the protein. Local anesthetics with a pKa closer to 7.4 will have a greater percentage of molecules in the anionic form compared to those with higher pKa's, and therefore will have a quicker onset of action. The notable exceptions to this rule are procaine and chloroprocaine both of which have a high pKa but very rapid onset of action.

Lipid Solubility

Lipid solubility is directly correlated with potency. More lipophilic agents more easily cross the lipid bilayer and become pharmacodynamically active.

Protein Binding

The degree of protein binding is a primary determinant of duration of action for local anesthetics. The higher the degree of protein binding, the longer it engages the sodium channel, and longer is its duration of action. Protein binding in the serum is most commonly to α_1-acid glycoprotein and albumin, which leads to sequestration of the local anesthetic and prevents it from being metabolized, extending its plasma half-life.

In addition to the physiochemical properties, other factors affect the properties of neural blockade.

Dose

The higher the dose, the faster the onset of action and the longer the duration of neural blockade.

Site of Injection

Common sites of local anesthetic injection vary in degrees of vascularity leading to differing pharmacokinetics of these injections. **The more vascular the area of injection, the higher the peak plasma level of local anesthetic, the higher the potential for toxicity, and the shorter the duration of blockade.** The peak plasma levels of local anesthetic depending on site of injection are in descending order: intravenous, intercostal, caudal, epidural, upper extremity (brachial plexus), lower extremity (sciatic/femoral).

Anesthetic Adjuvants

Addition of adjuvant drugs can favorably affect the pharmacokinetics and pharmacodynamics of local anesthetics.

Sodium Bicarbonate

Most local anesthetic formulations are prepared with a pH of 4 to 6; as a result, most of the molecules are present in the poorly lipid-soluble ionic form. **The addition of sodium bicarbonate to local anesthetic preparations raises the pH of the solution and increases the percentage of anionic local anesthetic molecules, and thus speeds the onset of action.** There is also data to suggest that by increasing the pH, the addition of sodium bicarbonate decreases the pain of injection.

Epinephrine

The addition of epinephrine to local anesthetic solutions has a myriad of benefits. **One of the most useful applications of epinephrine-containing preparations compared to plain solutions is the ability to rapidly detect an intravascular—specifically an intra-arterial—injection.** Even relatively small amounts of local anesthetic, if injected directly into the vasculature can lead to toxicity (see Case 15). If a local anesthetic containing epinephrine is injected into a blood vessel, a 10% to 20% increase in heart rate and/or blood pressure will result. Thus it is a common practice to include epinephrine in the small or "test" dose which precedes the injection of any large amount of

Table 3–1 PROPERTIES OF COMMONLY USED LOCAL ANESTHETICS

DRUG	CLASS	pKa	POTENCY	ONSET OF ACTION	DURATION OF ACTION	MAXIMUM DOSE (PLAIN)	MAXIMUM DOSE (EPINEPHRINE ADDED)
2-Chloroprocaine	Ester	8.7	Low	Very Rapid	Short	800 mg	1,000 mg
Procaine	Ester	8.9	Very low	Rapid	Short	400 mg	600 mg
Tetracaine	Ester	8.5	High	Slow	Very long	100 mg	200 mg
Lidocaine	Amide	7.72	Moderate	Rapid	Moderate	300 mg	500 mg
Mepivacaine	Amide	7.7	Moderate	Moderate	Moderate	400 mg	550 mg
Ropivacaine	Amide	8.1	High	Slow	Long	225 mg	225 mg
Bupivacaine	Amide	8.1	High	Slow	Very Long	175 mg	225 mg

local anesthetic. If a rise in heart rate and/or blood pressure is observed, the injection should be halted and the needle/catheter repositioned before continuing. The addition of epinephrine to the test dose lends an increased sensitivity to intravascular injection when compared to aspiration before injection.

The addition of epinephrine to local anesthetics also leads to local vasoconstriction, less systemic uptake of the local anesthetic, and a decreased risk of toxicity. The duration of action of long-acting agents such as bupivacaine are not affected by the addition of epinephrine. However, the decreased systemic absorption can extend the clinical effect of shorter acting agents such as lidocaine and chloroprocaine.

Epinephrine can also potentiate the analgesic action of local anesthetics through alpha-2 receptor-mediated action.

Comprehension Questions

3.1. A 48-year-old woman presents for laparoscopic cholecystectomy. Her past medical history is significant only for prior tonsillectomy and adenoidectomy as a child. She states that she has an allergy to local anesthetics. Upon further questioning, she states that she received Novocain (procaine) at the dentist and her "heart began to race and she became light-headed." Which of the following conditions most likey explains this patient's reaction?

A. A true allergic reaction to the amide local anesthetic procaine
B. An allergic reaction to a breakdown product of procaine
C. A side effect of epinephrine, which was added to the Novocain preparation
D. A somatization of the patient's apprehension toward dental procedures
E. A side effect of phenylephrine, which was added to the Novocain preparation

3.2. A 60-kg 17-year-old man presents for open reduction and internal fixation of an ankle fracture. You discuss a general anesthetic for intraoperative management with a sciatic block via the popliteal approach. You decide to use 20 mL of 0.5% bupivacaine with 1:200,000 of epinephrine. How many mL of 1:1000 epinephrine should you add to your bupivacaine to reach the appropriate concentration?

A. 0.05 mL
B. 0.1 mL
C. 0.02 mL
D. 0.2 mL
E. 0.04 mL

ANSWERS

3.1. **C.** The patient's reaction is most likely a representation of the side effects of epinephrine that is often added to local anesthetic preparations in order to increase duration of action and reduce systemic absorption of the local anesthetic. The patient's symptoms of tachycardia are more consistent with the sympathetic sequelae from epinephrine injection rather than a true allergic reaction (bronchospasm and urticaria). Procaine is an ester local anesthetic, which is more likely to cause an allergic reaction than amide local anesthetics, although the incidence of ester-mediated allergic reaction is very rare. Ester local anesthetics are broken down to para-aminobenzoic acid (PABA), a known allergen. Further, certain preservatives in local anesthetics such as methylparaben and sulfites can cause an allergic response.

3.2. **B.** A 1:1000 solution of epinephrine contains 1 mg/mL epinephrine. Twenty mL of 1:200,000 solution would contain 100 g of epinephrine (1 g epinephrine/200,000 mL 20 mL = 0.0001 g or 100 g, or 0.1 mg). To add 100 g epinephrine, one would need to add 0.1 mL of 1:1000 epinephrine (100 g 1 mg/1000 g 1 mL/ 1 mg = 0.1 mL).

Clinical Pearls

- Local anesthetics will not work in acidotic tissues.
- Factors determining the onset, duration, and potential complications of a regional block with local anesthetics include the site of injection, the dose of local anesthetics, the volume of the local anesthetic, and its physiochemical properties.
- The addition of epinephrine to local anesthetics is useful to detect intravascular injection, to increase duration of the blockade, and to prevent systemic absorption and toxicity.

REFERENCES

Haddad T, Min J. Local anesthetics. In: Hurford, WE, Bail MT, Daviso JK, Haspel KL, Rosow C, Vassallo SA, eds. *Clinical Anesthesia Procedures of the Massachusetts General Hospital*. 6th ed. Philadelphia, PA: Lippincott Williams & Wilkins; 2002: 220-230.

Miller RD, Katzung BG. Local anesthetics. In: Katzung, BG, ed. *Basic and Clinical Pharmacology*. 8th ed. New York, NY: Lange medical books/McGraw-Hill; 2001: 436-445.

Viscomi CM. Pharmacology of local anesthetics. In: Rathmell JP, Neal JM, Viscomi CM, ed. *Regional Anesthesia: The Requisites in Anesthesiology*. Philadelphia, PA: Elsevier Mosby; 2004: 13-24.

Case 4

A 47-year-old patient is undergoing the clipping of an intracranial aneurysm of the anterior communicating artery. The surgery is being performed under a microscope, so even the smallest movement by the patient could have devastating consequences.

➤ How can the patient be protected and the surgery allowed to proceed?

ANSWER TO CASE 4:
Muscle Relaxants (Neuromuscular Junction Blockers)

Summary: A 47-year-old patient is undergoing intracranial surgery, performed under a microscope, requiring the patient to be completely still.

➤ **Best method to protect the patient:** Neuromuscular blockade leading to muscle paralysis

ANALYSIS

Objectives

1. Introduce the student to the uses for neuromuscular blockers (relaxants) during general anesthesia.
2. Acquaint the student with the various classes of muscle relaxants.
3. Review some of the most common side effects associated with the use of a neuromuscular blocker.

Considerations

During intracranial aneurysm surgery, the patient is positioned with the head stabilized by pins. Moreover, the surgery is exquisitely delicate and typically performed under a microscope. Because of the necessity of keeping the patient still, she will receive vecuronium, a nondepolarizing neuromuscular blocker. This surgery usually takes many hours. However, at the end of the procedure, the patient's paralysis will be reversed, she will be allowed to awaken, and will be extubated to allow her participation in a neurological examination.

APPROACH TO
Muscle Relaxants

CLINICAL APPROACH

Clinical Pharmacology of the Neuromuscular Blockers

Neuromuscular blockers (NMB) or muscle relaxants are intravenous drugs that are used for muscle relaxation and paralysis by interrupting the transmission of action potentials at the neuromuscular junction. They act predominantly by binding post-junctional nicotinic receptors on skeletal muscle, thereby blocking the nerve depolarization caused by acetylcholine.

There are three main indications for neuromuscular blockade:

- To facilitate tracheal intubation
- To optimize surgical conditions, for example, during intra-abdominal, intrathoracic, and intracranial procedures
- To optimize ventilation in a patient who requires controlled mechanical ventilation

Muscle relaxants (or NMBs) block the transmission of action potentials at the neuromuscular junction. NMBs only produce paralysis; they have no intrinsic anesthetic or sedative effects. Paralysis with insufficient anesthesia or sedation is an unpleasant and frightening event. In rare cases, surgery has continued in paralyzed patients who are insufficiently anesthetized, leading to "awareness under anesthesia."

Two Classes of Muscle Relaxants

NMBs are divided into two classes: depolarizing, and nondepolarizing. The only depolarizing NMB is succinylcholine. Succinylcholine acts at the nicotinic receptor to produce an initial depolarization manifested by transient skeletal muscle fasciculations, later followed by repolarization and paralysis (Figure 4–1).

Since succinylcholine is a depolarizing muscle relaxant, it causes the release of potassium in a manner similar to that observed when a neuron actually fires.

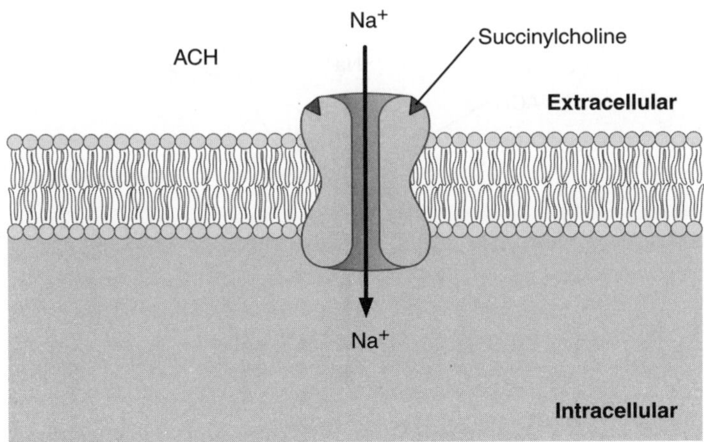

Figure 4–1. Actions of the depolarizing (noncompetitive) neuromuscular junction blocker succinylcholine on the skeletal muscle nicotinic receptor. Succinylcholine acts on skeletal muscle nicotinic receptors to produce initial depolarization followed by repolarization.

Thus, succinylcholine normally increases plasma K^+ level from 0.5 to 1.0 mEq. Thus in a patient with pre-existent hyperkalemia, the use of succinylcholine may place the patient at risk for cardiac arrhythmias. The succinylcholine-induced release of potassium is exaggerated in patients with lower motor neuron disease, third-degree burns, long-term immobility, Duchene muscular dystrophy, and rarely, intra-abdominal sepsis. In these clinical settings, its use can cause a hyperkalemic arrest. Succinylcholine has also been associated with painful myalgias in the postoperative period, and it is a potent trigger for malignant hyperthermia.

Succinylcholine is metabolized by plasma pseudocholinesterase. Genetics predispose some families to have either defective, or a deficient amount of pseudocholinesterase isoenzymes in plasma. In these individuals, the duration of action of succinylcholine may be prolonged, and can range from a couple of hours to many hours, depending on the enzymatic alterations. To ensure that pseudocholinesterase deficiency is diagnosed if present, patients are allowed to recover function following succinylcholine administration, before a nondepolarizing muscle relaxant is administered.

Succinylcholine has a rapid onset, and short duration making it an ideal agent for intubation. Because of its short duration of action, its use for the maintenance of relaxation would require administration by infusion, a practice rarely used today.

Nondepolarizing muscle relaxants represent the second class of NMBs, which compete with acetylcholine for the nicotinic receptor resulting in a competitive inhibition of blockade (Figure 4–2). While they act primarily at postsynaptic receptors, some, such as pancuronium, act at pre-junctional

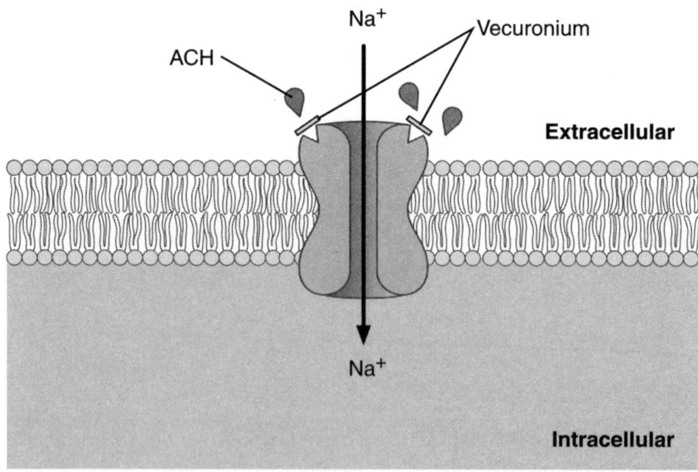

Figure 4–2. Actions of the competitive (nondepolarizing) neuromuscular junction blocker vecuronium on the skeletal muscle nicotinic receptor. Vecuronium competes with acetylcholine at these receptors.

receptors as well. The four nondepolarizing blockers in use today are distinguished by their duration of action and methods of excretion.

Three of the four competitive (nondepolarizing) agents have an intermediate duration of action (rocuronium, vecuronium, and cisatracurium). Rocuronium is distinguished from the other intermediate agents by its rapid onset of action which is similar to, but not quite as fast, as succinylcholine. One agent (pancuronium) is long-acting.

Rocuronium and vecuronium are largely metabolized (about 80%) and excreted by the hepatobiliary system. Thus, their duration of action may be prolonged in patients with severe liver disease. The main hepatic metabolite of vecuronium, 3-desacetyl-vecuronium, is an active metabolite excreted by the kidney. Thus, the duration of vecuronium's action is also prolonged in patients with end-stage renal failure. Pancuronium's clearance is about 80% renal, so its elimination may be delayed in patients with severe renal disease. Cisatracurium is independently cleared by Hoffman elimination (degradation in plasma at physiologic pH and temperature), so it is an ideal drug in patients with hepatic or renal failure.

Please refer to Table 4–1 for the clinical properties of the neuromuscular blockers.

Table 4–1 CLINICAL PROPERTIES OF NEUROMUSCULAR BLOCKERS

NEUROMUSCULAR BLOCKER	METABOLISM	EXCRETION	ONSET	DURATION
Succinylcholine	Plasma pseudo-cholinesterase	Insignificant	Rapid	Ultra-short
Cisatracurium	Hoffman elimination	Insignificant	Moderately rapid	Intermediate
Rocuronium	Insignificant	Biliary	Rapid	Intermediate
Vecuronium	Hepatic	Biliary Renal	Moderately rapid	Intermediate
Pancuronium	Liver	Renal	Moderately rapid	Long

Maintenance of Blockade: How Much is Enough?

The degree of neuromuscular blockade has been shown to correlate in a near-linear fashion with the height of the twitch derived from stimulation of the adductor pollicus longus muscle (which governs opposition of the thumb) at 2 Hz. This finding formed the basis for the Train-of-Four monitoring of muscle relaxation measured with a peripheral nerve stimulator. The Train of Four measures the response to four twitches administered over 2 seconds. If the anesthetist can feel the presence of four twitches, then the patient is 75% paralyzed or less. If he/she feels three twitches, then the patient can be up to 85% paralyzed. Two twitches indicate that the patient is 95% paralyzed, one twitch, 99%, and no twitches indicate that the patient is totally paralyzed, or more (meaning that there is an excess in muscle relaxant).

It is important to understand the implications of the two extremes of monitoring with the Train of Four. The first 75% or so of receptors paralyzed are not monitored. Thus, a patient can be paralyzed by 75% and still have all four twitches, similar to someone who is not paralyzed at all. At the other extreme, the absence of twitches gives no information as to the likely duration of the existing blockade. Thus, to measure the degree of relaxation between these two extremes, either one, two, or three twitches must be present. As the patient shows some evidence of recovery of neuromuscular function (three out of four twitches), the anesthetist can cautiously give more muscle relaxant intravenously. Generally the presence of one to three twitches is adequate for surgical relaxation.

Reversal of the Neuromuscular Blockade and Emergence

Nondepolarizing neuromuscular blockers are competitive antagonist acetylcholine at the neuromuscular junction. They are reversed by increasing the amount of acetylcholine relative to the NMB, using a peripheral anticholinesterase inhibitor, typically neostigmine, to reclaim the receptor from the blocker (Figure 4–3). Reversal of the neuromuscular blockade is possible if there is some evidence of spontaneous recovery at the neuromuscular junction, as detected by at least one out of four twitches.

However, neostigmine has some troublesome cholinergic side effects such as bradycardia, bronchospasm, and an increase in gut motility that reflect the stimulation of muscarinic receptors by increasing acetylcholine concentrations throughout the body (Figure 4–3). To reduce these untoward effects, glycopyrrolate, an anticholinergic agent, is administered concomitantly with the neostigmine.

It is important to note that clinical signs are the best indicators of an adequate reversal of neuromuscular blockade. The patient's ability to lift the head for 5 seconds, to protrude his or her tongue, and maintain an inspiratory pressure ≥ 21 cm H_2O are reliable signs of adequate reversal. The inability to sustain a prolonged muscle movement (such as extending the arm), and the

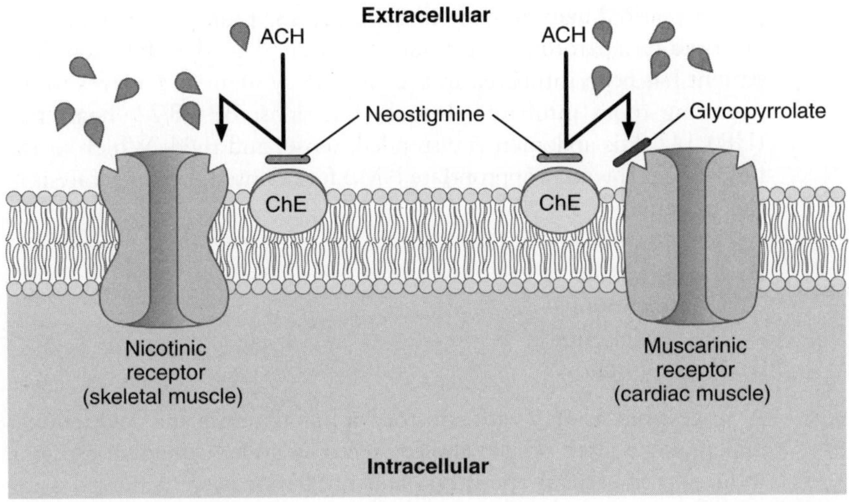

Figure 4–3. Actions of neostigmine and glycopyrrolate on nicotinic and muscarinic receptors. Competitive (nondepolarizing) neuromuscular junction blockers are reversed with neostigmine, which acts on the cholinesterase (ChE) enzyme to increase acetylcholine (ACH) throughout the body. An increase in acetylcholine is desired at the nicotinic receptors on skeletal muscle, but not at the cardiac muscarinic receptors. Accordingly, the antimuscarinic glycopyrrolate is coadministered with neostigmine to block ACH from stimulating the muscarinic receptors, but not blocking ACH from stimulating the skeletal muscle nicotinic receptors.

sensation that one is unable to breathe or handle secretions are signs of an inadequate reversal. Tidal volume respiratory mechanics and the Train-of-Four responses are not reliable indicators for adequate reversal.

Comprehension Questions

4.1. A 28-year-old man presents for shoulder surgery. The patient had a documented episode of malignant hyperthermia in a previous surgery under general anesthesia. Which of the following neuromuscular blockers is contraindicated in this patient?

A. Vecuronium
B. Rocuronium
C. Pancuronium
D. Succinylcholine
E. Cisatracurium

4.2. An 18-year-old man presents to the operating room for an emergency exploratory laparotomy for a gun-shot wound to the abdomen. The patient has been intubated in the emergency room and arrives to the operating room intubated. Initial vital signs: BP 68/22, heart rate (HR) 142. His abdomen is distended, tense, and rigid. Which of the following is the most appropriate NMB for maintenance of paralysis in this patient?

A. Vecuronium
B. Pancuronium
C. Cisatracurium
D. Succinylcholine
E. Rocuronium

4.3. A 36-year-old woman with a history of hiatal hernia and acid reflux is undergoing a laparoscopic cholecystectomy under general anesthesia. Induction of general anesthesia and intubation were achieved using propofol and succinylcholine. The patient did not recover from the neuromuscular blockade before the end of surgery; she had 0/4 twitches on the Train-of-four twitch response. She was transported to the recovery room intubated, mechanically ventilated, and sedated. Which of the following is the most likely cause of this patient's prolonged paralysis?

A. A prolonged effect of the intravenous anesthetic propofol
B. Atypical pseudocholinesterase enzyme
C. Pseudocholinesterase deficiency
D. Liver disease
E. Renal disease

ANSWERS

4.1. **D.** Malignant hyperthermia is a life-threatening hypermetabolic disorder that is triggered by succinylcholine and the volatile inhaled anesthetics (isoflurane, desflurane, and sevoflurane). All triggering agents are contraindicated in patients with a history of malignant hyperthermia.

4.2. **B.** Although any of these agents except succinylcholine can be used to maintain muscle relaxation in this clinical scenario, pancuronium might be the most appropriate. Pancuronium has a vagolytic effect leading to tachycardia, which is vital for this patient. With significant intra-abdominal blood loss and severe hypotension, the patient's cardiac output is dependent on the heart rate which should be maintained at high rates. For the same reason pancuronium may not be the most appropriate NMB in patients with severe angina where the tachycardia can produce myocardial ischemia due to increased myocardial work and decreased coronary blood flow.

4.3. **B.** Succinylcholine is metabolized in the plasma by pseudocholinesterase. Its effect does not usually last more than 10 minutes. In the rare condition of an atypical pseudocholinesterase enzyme, its paralytic effects may be prolonged for hours.

Clinical Pearls

- Neuromuscular blockers facilitate tracheal intubation and also provide muscle relaxation for certain types of surgery and for intubated ICU patients being mechanically ventilated.
- Vecuronium and rocuronium should be used with caution in patients with severe liver disease, as their clearance is 80% hepatobiliary.
- Pancuronium should be used with caution in the patient with severe renal disease, since its clearance is 80% renal.
- Succinylcholine may be used in the patient with renal disease, so long as the serum K^+ level is <5.5 mEq/L and there is no other contraindication to its use.
- Patients may experience recall if muscle relaxants are employed without concomitant anesthetic or sedative agents.

REFERENCES

Naguib M, Lien CA. Pharmacology of muscle relaxants and their antagonists. In: Miller RD, ed. *Miller's Anesthesia.* 6th ed. Philadelphia, PA: Churchill Livingstone; 2005: 481-572.

Pino RM, Ali HH. Monitoring and managing neuromuscular blockade. In: Longnecker DE, ed. *Anesthesiology*. New York, NY: McGraw-Hill Companies; 2008: 619-638.

Part 2. Anesthetic Principles and Equipment

Case 5

A 42-year-old woman is undergoing surgery for a bilateral tubal ligation. She has undergone endotracheal intubation. The medical student, who received a degree in physics in college, notices that the anesthesiologist is working with the Ambu bag to ventilate the patient. The student speculates about decreasing the work required by shortening the endotracheal tube (ETT).

- If the ETT is shortened by 25%, how would that affect the work of breathing?

ANSWER TO CASE 5: Application of Basic Science to Anesthesia

Summary: The patient has undergone endotracheal intubation.

- **Physiologic change:** Shortening the endotracheal tube by 25% would decrease the pressure required, and hence the work of breathing, by about one-third.

ANALYSIS

Objectives

1. Review principles of physics.
2. Understand how the above principles are applied to the practice of anesthesiology.

Considerations

Shortening the endotracheal tube would, indeed, theoretically reduce the work of breathing. However, during laparoscopy, the patient is paralyzed, and the work of breathing is assumed by the ventilator. Thus, from a practical perspective, it is rarely necessary to shorten the endotracheal tube.

APPROACH TO Basic Science in Anesthesia

Anesthesia practice involves application of basic science principles on a daily basis. These principles include fluid mechanics, physical properties of gases, combustion and fires, and electrical safety.

CLINICAL APPROACH

Fluid Mechanics

An understanding of basic fluid mechanics is important for the understanding of several processes managed by anesthesiologists in the operating room, such as gas flow and circulation. Most of the discussion that follows is derived from analysis of noncompressible newtonian fluids. But even though air and blood do not fall into this category, the concepts still apply.

The word "laminar" comes from the same root as the familiar "lamina" meaning "layers," and signifies that in this type of flow the layers do not mix. Laminar flow can be envisioned as flow down a straight, calm river. The water

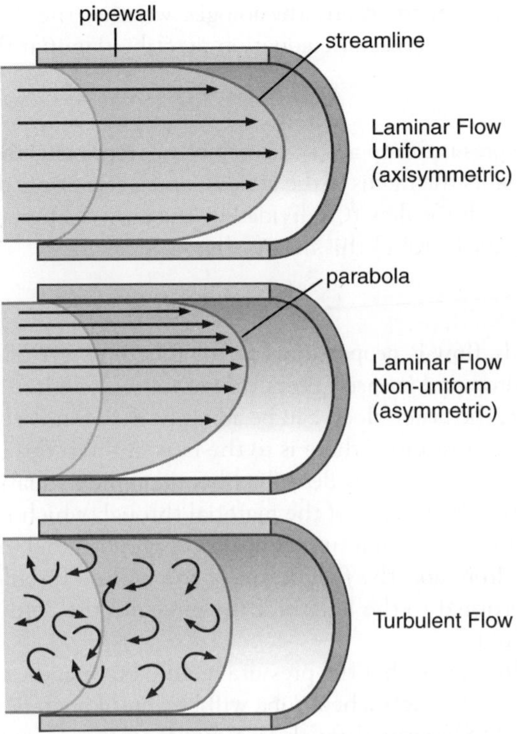

Figure 5–1. Types of flow are illustrated: axisymmetric laminar (top), asymmetric laminar (middle), and tubulent flow (bottom).

in the middle is flowing fastest and very little water is flowing at the sides; in fact, it can be described as a parabola. Turbulent flow, however, is more chaotic, and can be envisioned as the flow of the water as it flows over rocks or around a bend. The "lamina" of the water—and therefore the energy required to move them—are no longer all moving in the same direction (Figure 5–1).

What determines whether a flow is laminar or turbulent? The first factor to consider is the *properties of the fluid*, specifically the kinematic viscosity (ν) which is the ratio of the viscosity ( ) of the fluid to its density (ρ). Next to be considered are the *diameter of the conduit* (d) and the *linear velocity of the fluid* (v). The ratio of inertia force divided by the viscous force of the fluid is known as the Reynolds number. A dimensionless quantity, the Reynolds number is defined as:

$$\text{Reynolds number} = \mathrm{v}d/\mathrm{v}$$

Flow changes from laminar to turbulent at a Reynolds number of approximately 2300. It is apparent that for any given conduit and fluid, there will be a defined velocity at which the flow changes from laminar to turbulent. Turbulence will also occur wherever there is a sharp turn in the conduit, because the instantaneous velocity at that point increases.

Why does it matter to an anesthesiologist whether the flow is laminar or turbulent? The Hagen-Poiseuille equation describes laminar flow:

$$\Delta P = 8 \ \ v_{avg} L/r^2$$

where ΔP is the pressure drop across a conduit, v_{avg} represents the average linear velocity, r represents the radius of the conduit and L represents the length of the conduit. Since v_{avg} is the flow (Q) divided by the cross-sectional area, for a circular conduit (pipe or tube) this means that

$$Q = \Delta P \pi r^4/8 \ \ L$$

or in other words, **flow is proportional to the fourth power of the radius** for a given pressure drop and *inversely* proportional to the length of the tube. Thus, the larger an i.v., the faster blood can be administered. Similarly the longer the catheter, the more resistance there is to the flow of fluids through it.

Turbulent flow, however, is described by a complex equation which considers the frictional properties of the material through which the fluid is flowing. The equation tells us that turbulent flow is proportional to the *square root* of the pressure drop, and the *fifth* power of the radius. Turbulent flow is also inversely proportional to the length of the pipe and the density (*not* the viscosity) of the fluid.

Clinically, this means that the pressure required to breathe through a 6 mm ID (inner diameter) endotracheal tube will be approximately three times the pressure required to breathe through an 8 mm ID tube assuming laminar flow. For turbulent flow, the pressure required for the same breath will be approximately nine times as much. (In practice, such flow would typically be turbulent.) Shortening the endotracheal tube by 25% would decrease the pressure required, and hence the work of breathing, by about one-third. Similar comparisons can be made for the (usually laminar) flow through intravenous catheters and the (usually turbulent) flow through blood vessels.

Physical Properties of Gases

In addition to the fluid properties of a gas, static properties are also important. Although the gases we use in clinical practice are not "ideal gases," the qualitative properties of the ideal gas equation can still be applied:

$$PV = nRT$$

where P represents pressure, V represents volume, n represents number of moles, T represents absolute temperature, and R represents the ideal gas constant.

For example, for any amount of gas at a constant temperature, the product of pressure and volume will be a constant, so as pressure increases the volume decreases. Thus Boyle law can be represented:

$$PV = \mathrm{k} \quad \text{or} \quad P_1V_1 = P_2V_2$$

Similarly, at a given pressure, a rise in temperature will cause a gas to expand (Charles law.)

$$\frac{V}{T} = k \quad \text{or} \quad \frac{V_1}{T_1} = \frac{V_2}{T_2}$$

The concepts regarding pressure and partial pressure are also key to understanding many aspects of anesthetic gases. The pressure of a gas mixture (P_{total}) is the same as the atmospheric pressure to which the mixture is exposed in mm Hg (1 atm = 760 mm Hg). Moreover, the partial pressure of a gas in a mixture is the same as its proportion of molecules in the mixture (Dalton law).

$$P_{total} = P_1 + P_2 + \cdots P_n$$

For example, in a mixture of 21% oxygen in nitrogen at 760 mm Hg barometric pressure (1 atm of pressure), the partial pressure of oxygen is 160 mm Hg and the partial pressure of nitrogen is 600 mm Hg. The same mixture of air in a hyperbaric chamber at 1520 mm Hg (2 atm) would have a partial pressure of oxygen of 320 mm Hg.

At equilibrium, every liquid also has its own characteristic vapor pressure, which is exclusively a function of temperature. For example, the vapor pressure of isoflurane at 25°C is 295 mm Hg. So at room temperature (approximately 22°C), isoflurane exists primarily as a liquid, it must be heated slightly to enter the gaseous phase. And from the gas laws discussed earlier, it is easy to understand that the temperature must be constant in order to ensure the output of a specific, known quantity of isoflurane from the vaporizer.

At 1 atm, a saturated solution of isoflurane in air (such as found inside a vaporizer) would consist of 295 mm Hg partial pressure of isoflurane, 98 mm Hg partial pressure of oxygen, and 367 mm Hg partial pressure of nitrogen, or 38.8% isoflurane. In the same hyperbaric chamber at 2 atm, the mixture would consist of 295 mm Hg partial pressure of isoflurane, 257 mm Hg partial pressure of oxygen, and 968 mm Hg of nitrogen, or 19.4% isoflurane. Thus using the gas laws, the effect of varying atmospheric pressure on the output of a vaporizer calibrated at sea level can be understood. This has a clinical applicability when anesthetizing patients at high altitudes (even as in some parts of Colorado) or in a hyperbaric chamber.

Fires and Explosions

Despite the fact that highly flammable anesthetics are no longer used in the United States, fires and explosions in the operating room still occur. A fire requires three components: an oxidizer, a fuel, and a source of ignition.

Oxygen is not, in and of itself, flammable. But it is a potent, primary source of oxidation in an operating room. Nitrous oxide also supports combustion. In fact, several of the halogenated anesthetic agents are *more* flammable in nitrous oxide than in oxygen. Yet none approach the flammability of the older anesthetics, such as ether and cyclopropane.

Fuels abound in the operating room, especially on the operative field. Everything from tape to gauze to drapes will burn under the right conditions. Flammable gases present in the operating room include hydrogen and methane from the intestines (fires have been reported when electrocautery is used to open the bowel), as well as vapors from some skin-disinfection solutions. Alcohol-based disinfectants, which have pooled unnoticed around the surgical field, are especially flammable. (An explosion rather than a fire will occur if the flammable gas and the oxidizer are present in stoichiometric proportions.) The patient's tissues do not act as a fuel because of their high moisture content, but of course are at risk of thermal injury from adjacent flames.

Any heat source may act as a source of ignition if it generates enough energy. The most common ignition sources are the electrocautery and the laser. It should be noted that gases do not absorb laser energy, and therefore will not burn until the laser generates heat by contacting a solid such as tissue or any other object in the field. The energy of laser cautery is sufficient to ignite a fire either from the generation of heat or from the generation of a spark. Fires may occur when the laser beam contacts a surgical drape under which anesthetic gases are pooled (eg, patients receiving monitored anesthesia care with supplemental oxygen or a mask general anesthetic).

Head and neck surgery poses a special risk. Endotracheal tubes themselves are flammable. For surgery within the airway (eg, laser excision of a vocal cord lesion) specialized metallic tubes exist which will not burn. Alternatively, a regular endotracheal tube may be carefully wrapped with metallic tape, although the liability should an injury occur generally discourages this practice. The cuff of either of these tubes is still flammable. Many practitioners will therefore inflate the cuff with saline instead of air with the intent of immediately extinguishing any fire that may occur.

If an endotracheal tube is ignited, the most important goal is to minimize thermal injury. Before removing the burning tube from the patient, the oxygen source (anesthesia circuit) must be disconnected to prevent the tube from becoming a blowtorch injuring airway tissues on the way out. At the same time, if the fire is in the surgical field (eg, tracheostomy surgery), sterile saline should be poured on the fire to extinguish the flame, cool the surrounding tissues thereby minimizing thermal injury. Finally, the airway should be immediately re-intubated and not extubated until the full extent of airway injury and resultant edema can be assessed.

Electrical Safety

The risks of electricity in the operating room include macroshock, microshock, and electrical burns.

All electricity requires a "closed circuit" to flow. If the circuit is interrupted, the electricity flows to the ground (which acts as a huge sink for electrons). It flows through any pathway it can find, including an accidentally grounded patient or anesthesiologist. This is called a macroshock, which occurs when a grounded person makes contact with a live electrical wire.

Macroshock is prevented by the isolation of any equipment that will come in contact with the patient from the main electrical supply. Electrical isolation uses a transformer to convert electricity through a coil to a magnetic field, and then from the magnetic field to electricity again through a second coil, which has no connection to ground. (The metal cases of these pieces of equipment are grounded to prevent macroshock to personnel who may contact them.) Any short circuit between either side of the isolation transformer and ground will not result in the flow of current; however, the system would then be equivalent to a non-isolated, traditionally grounded one. Conversion of an isolated piece of equipment to a grounded piece of equipment is detected by the line isolation monitor in operating rooms. This monitor will alarm if any piece of equipment is inadvertently grounded and therefore no longer isolated.

Even tiny currents of electricity can be dangerous if they contact the myocardium, which can occur by the transmission of currents through pacemaker wires or saline-filled monitoring catheters. Again, since electricity takes the path of least resistance to either complete its circuit or flow to ground, the best way to avoid microshock, in addition to isolating the patient from the main power source, is to provide the current a path that takes it away from the heart. This is the purpose of the dispersive electrode of the electrocautery system—to complete the circuit of electricity back to the electrosurgical unit. (The electrode is often erroneously referred to as the "grounding pad" but its function is exactly the *opposite* of "grounding" the patient.) To minimize the current passing through or near the heart, the dispersive electrode should be placed as close as possible to the site of the surgery so that the current will travel minimally through the body. Ideally, the electrosurgical unit should have an alarm that will sound if the return current is interrupted for any reason.

The dispersive electrode has a relatively large surface area through which the electrical current can pass on its way back to the electrosurgical unit. (Remember that this is the same amount of electricity that is efficiently burning the tissue as it passes through the small tip of the cautery.) If the return to the unit passes through a smaller surface area, for example, if the dispersive electrode partially loses contact with the patient's skin, the skin under the electrode is at risk for a burn. In the same manner, if the patient were to be inadvertently grounded, say through his ECG electrodes, the current could preferentially pass through those very small electrodes on its way to ground and cause burns to the skin.

Comprehension Questions

5.1. A 63-year-old patient undergoing an open reduction internal fixation of a hip fracture requires a blood transfusion. After the fluid warmer is introduced into the i.v. circuit, the blood drips much more slowly than it previously had. Which of the following answers best accounts for this phenomenon?

A. The i.v. has infiltrated.
B. The diameter of the tubing in the blood warmer is smaller than the diameter of the intravenous tubing set.
C. The fluid warmer effectively adds length to the intravenous tubing set.
D. Blood is thicker than water.

5.2. The material used for a vaporizer should have which of the following qualities?

A. Low specific heat, low thermal conductivity
B. Low specific heat, high thermal conductivity
C. High specific heat, low thermal conductivity
D. High specific heat, high thermal conductivity

ANSWERS

5.1. **C.** The fluid warmer effectively adds length to the intravenous tubing set. While it is also possible that the i.v. has become infiltrated, the temporal association with the introduction of the blood warmer into the circuit suggests that the warmer is somehow related to the slowing of the infusion. Even if the diameter of the tubing in the blood warmer was smaller than the diameter of the i.v. set, the smallest diameter—and thus the "bottleneck" with respect to diameter is likely to be the i.v. catheter itself. Although blood is indeed more viscous than water, the blood ran faster prior to the induction of the fluid warmer.

5.2. **D.** High specific heat of the material will act as a heat source to replace the heat lost during vaporization, and high thermal conductivity will facilitate transfer of heat from the surroundings to replace the lost heat of vaporization as well, both helping to maintain the liquid at constant temperature and therefore maintain a constant vapor pressure. This is the reason that early vaporizers were constructed of copper ("copper kettle") or brass (Vernitrol vaporizer.)

Clinical Pearls

- Flow is proportional to the fourth power of the radius (r^4), and inversely proportional to the length of a tube.
- Even tiny currents of electricity can be dangerous if they contact the myocardium via pacemaker wires or saline-filled monitoring catheters.
- In case of fire, the goal is to minimize thermal injury to the patient. In the case of airway fire, this requires immediate disconnection of the patient from the oxygen source (before removal of the endotracheal tube.)

REFERENCES

Bird RB, Stewart WE, Lightfoot EN. *Transport Phenomena*. 2nd ed. New York, NY: John Wiley and Sons; 2007.

Davis PD, Kenny GNC. *Basic Physics and Measurement in Anesthesia*. 5th ed. Edinburgh, UK: Elsevier; 2003.

Lobato EB, Gravenstein N, Kirby RR, eds. *Complications in Anesthesiology*. 3rd ed. Philadelphia, PA: Lippincott, Williams & Wilkins; 2008.

Welty J, Wicks CE, Rorrer GL, Wilson RE. *Fundamentals of Momentum, Heat and Mass Transfer*. 5th ed. New York, NY: John Wiley and Sons; 2008.

Case 6

A 65-year-old man is undergoing a laparoscopic cholecystectomy. The case starts uneventfully, and the patient is paralyzed with a neuromuscular blocker, as is customarily used. After successful intubation, mechanical ventilation is attempted using the anesthesia machine's ventilator, but the tidal volume is not delivered.

➤ How could this situation have been prevented?

➤ What is your next step in the management of this patient?

ANSWERS TO CASE 6:
Basic Machine Checkout

Summary: General anesthesia has been successfully initiated on a 65-year-old man, who is undergoing cholecystectomy. The patient is paralyzed and intubated, but the anesthesia machine is not functioning and ventilation is not being provided.

- **How to have prevented this situation:** This situation could have been prevented if the anesthesia machine had been checked properly prior to the beginning of the case.
- **Next step in management:** Any time a patient is not breathing, or in this situation, is unable to breathe for himself, the basic life support algorithm of "airway, breathing, circulation" should be followed. The **airway** or endotracheal tube is already in place. "Breathing" or ventilation can be provided with an Ambu bag, which is always available in an operating room should it be needed. Anesthesia is maintained with intravenous medications.

ANALYSIS

Objectives

1. Understand the basic components of an anesthesia machine, and how these components must be checked to ensure its safe operation.
2. Describe the 2008 recommendations for preanesthesia checkout procedures, and understand which must be performed prior to the first case of the day, and which must also be performed prior to "to-follow" cases using the same machine during the same day.
3. Become familiar with the necessary auxiliary and backup equipment required when an anesthetic is administered.

Considerations

This patient is intubated, paralyzed, and the anesthesia machine is not operational. The situation could have been avoided by a basic machine checkout. In February 2008, the American Society of Anesthesiologists (ASA), through its Committee on Equipment and Facilities, set forth "recommendations for preanesthesia checkout procedures (2008)" which outline the necessary checks to be performed on anesthesia delivery equipment before every anesthetic, and the backup equipment which may be needed in the event of machine malfunction. The patient should be ventilated with an Ambu bag until an operational machine can be brought to the operating room.

APPROACH TO
Basic Machine Checkout

The anesthesia machine is broken down into **two main components**: the **circle system** (or breathing circuit), and the **machine proper.** The circle system is made up of the anesthesia circuit tubing (hoses from machine to the patient and back, not shown in Figure 6–1), unidirectional valves, a flow spirometer, an adjustable pressure-limiting valve, a scavenging system outflow site, a fresh-gas inlet site, a CO_2 absorber, an O_2 sensor, a ventilator, and reservoir bag (Figure 6–1). Flow spirometers are generally located on the machine side of the expiratory valve. The O_2 sensor is generally located on the inspiratory side to measure the concentration of oxygen inspired. In some situations, it may be located on the expiratory side, to measure the oxygen which has been exhaled.

The other component is the anesthesia machine proper, which receives gases, regulates the pressure and flow of those gases, allows addition of volatile anesthetics, and provides safety against an (accidental) hypoxic gas mixture. The anesthesia machine receives gas from internal pipes in the wall via wall connections which are gas specific. The oxygen, for example, is colored green and the gas plug-in will only attach to a (green) oxygen outlet. This is called the diameter index safety system (DISS). The gas mount on the anesthesia

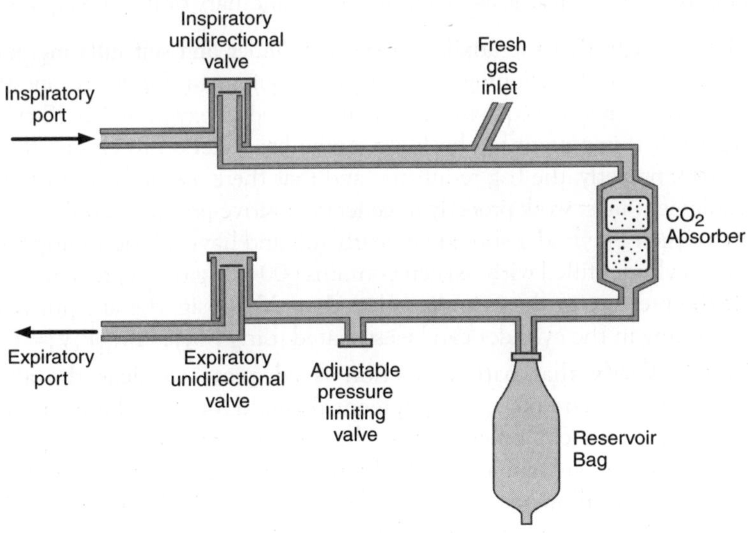

Figure 6–1. Inspiratory (IV) and expiratory (EV) unidirectional valves, respectively. Adjustable pressure limiting valve (APL), and fresh-gas inlet (FGI). The ventilator is not shown but it would bypass the APL and reservoir bag.

machine is specific to each gas as well. For example, the pin on the oxygen tank will only fit the oxygen specific yoke on the anesthesia machine or in the institution's basement (the source of piped gases). This is known as the pin index safety system. These systems combine to ensure that oxygen, instead of a hypoxic gas such as N_2 is delivered through conduits labeled for oxygen.

Gases for the anesthesia machine are either piped in from the wall are at a pressure of 50 psig, or received via an E-cylinder mounted on the machine containing a pressure regulator which reduces gas pressure to 45 to 50 psig. Gases pass through pressure sensors (further reducing the pressure), a vaporizer, and a flow meter before entering the circle system via the fresh-gas inflow. Since pressures of 45 to 55 psig would be damaging to the larynx and pulmonary parenchyma, additional pressure regulators ensure that only low-pressure gas enters the circle (breathing) system. Gases from the wall and from the E-cylinder mounted on the machine are connected in parallel to the anesthesia machine. But since the pressure is higher on the side coming from the wall, the E-cylinder remains as a backup in case the wall oxygen delivery system fails.

The American Society of Anesthesiologists has authored specific recommendations for preanesthesia checkout procedures of this complicated but vital device. The guidelines include **15 items** that should always be performed before the first case of the day (see Table 6–1). Once the full checkout has been performed, it is only necessary to perform 8 of the steps for subsequent cases (items #2, 4, 7, 11-15). The items are listed in the order with which they should be performed, and not necessarily organized according to the specific components of the anesthesia machine and its ancillary or backup equipment.

ITEM #1. Verify that the auxiliary oxygen cylinder and self-inflating devices are available and functioning. The backup equipment for every anesthetic includes hand-ventilation equipment (Ambu bag) and an oxygen source (E-cylinder of oxygen). It is important to check the Ambu bag function to be sure that the valves work properly, the bag re-inflates, and that there are no holes in the bag. The equipment must work properly to generate positive pressure ventilation.

The oxygen E-cylinder should be nearly full and have a functioning regulator. An E-cylinder filled with oxygen contains 600 L of gas at a pressure of 2000 psig. If the pressure in the cylinder is less than 2000 psig, the amount of oxygen remaining in the cylinder can be estimated using Boyle law: ($P_1V_1 = P_2V_2$).

ITEM #2. Verify that patient suction is adequate to clear the airway. Suction is an auxiliary piece of equipment required for safe administration of an anesthetic. This equipment can be lifesaving in the event of aspiration, and/or difficult airway management which may require the removal of secretions or blood to allow visualization of the vocal cords. It must be checked before administration of each anesthetic.

ITEM #3. Turn on the anesthesia delivery system and confirm that AC power is available. It is important to note that the machine is not running on its battery power, which is intended for emergency situations. Indeed, most anesthesiologists have been in the situation where the power goes off in the operating room during a procedure.

Table 6–1 THE AMERICAN SOCIETY OF ANESTHESIOLOGISTS' PREANESTHESIA CHECKOUT PROCEDURES

ITEM	PROCEDURE	PERSONNEL
#1	Verify auxiliary oxygen cylinder and self-inflating devices are available and functioning	Provider and technician
#2	Verify patient suction is adequate to clear the airway	Provider and technician
#3	Turn on anesthesia delivery system and confirm that AC power is available	Provider or technician
#4	Verify availability of required monitors, including alarms	Provider or technician
#5	Verify that pressure is adequate on the spare oxygen cylinder mounted on the anesthesia machine	Provider and technician
#6	Verify that the piped gas pressures are ≥ 50 psig	Provider and technician
#7	Verify that vaporizers are adequately filled and, if applicable, that the filler ports are tightly closed	Provider or technician
#8	Verify that there are no leaks in the gas supply lines between the flow meters and the common gas outlet (internal leak test)	Provider or technician
#9	Test scavenging system function	Provider or technician
#10	Calibrate, or verify calibration of, the oxygen monitor and check the low oxygen alarm	Provider or technician
#11	Verify carbon dioxide absorbent is not exhausted (Sodasorb)	Provider or technician
#12	Breathing system pressure and leak testing (circle system leak test)	Provider and technician
#13	Verify that gas flows properly through the breathing circuit during both inspiration and exhalation	Provider and technician
#14	Document completion of checkout procedures	Provider and technician
#15	Confirm ventilator settings and evaluate readiness to deliver anesthesia care—anesthesia pause	Provider

ITEM #4. Verify the availability of the required monitors and alarms. Monitors are critical to patient care and must be checked before an anesthetic is administered. Basic monitoring includes sphygmomanometer (measurement of blood pressure), 2-lead ECG, pulse oximetry, temperature, and capnography (which measures end-tidal CO_2). All equipment necessary for this monitoring must be present and functional. It is also important to be certain that alarms are set appropriately prior to the beginning of a case.

ITEM #5. Verify that the pressure is adequate on the spare oxygen cylinder mounted on the anesthesia machine.

ITEM #6. Verify that piped gas pressures are ≥ 50 psi. Next it is necessary to confirm the wall pressure is 50 psig and that the oxygen cylinder mounted to the anesthesia machine is full (2000 psig, 600 L). This confirms a sound connection to the wall, and the presence of a supply of oxygen in case of an emergency. Occasionally, the connections to the wall may imperfect, and the ancillary oxygen supply depleted—without knowledge of the anesthetist. These checks prevent this potentially hazardous situation.

ITEM #7. Verify that vaporizers are adequately filled. This prevents the vaporizer from being empty at a time when it would be hazardous to stop and refill it, such as during the induction of a patient with a difficult airway.

ITEM #8. Verify that there are no leaks in the gas supply lines between the flow meters and the common gas outlet. This is also known as the internal leak test. One way it is performed is by a negative pressure leak test. This involves placing a collapsed bulb on the fresh-gas outlet and seeing if it re-inflates with each vaporizer open. For many modern machines, the circle system leak test (described in the following paragraph) with each vaporizer open also identifies any internal leaks within the anesthesia machine via pressure backflow through the fresh-gas inflow. Each vaporizer should be filled if necessary, and the filler cap replaced tightly.

ITEM #9. Check the scavenging system's function. As gas is vented from the circle or breathing system, it enters a scavenging system to avoid operating room contamination. Scavenging systems are open (gas is removed constantly), or closed (waste gases are re-circulated). Open systems are most common since they do not have pressure valves. Scavenging systems are also either active or passive. An active system includes a vacuum in the system. Checking this system entails ensuring there are no kinks in the hoses, that the open system is not clogged (or the pressure valves are properly functioning), and that the vacuum is set properly. Most anesthesia machines have an indicator on or near the rear of the machine which indicates that the scavenger is working appropriately.

ITEM #10. Calibrate, or verify the calibration of the oxygen monitor and check the low oxygen alarm. The alarms signaling low oxygen are checked by disconnecting or turning off the oxygen sources (wall and tank), and an alarm will sound. The oxygen monitor's calibration is checked by observing that it accurately reflects 100% when pure oxygen is flushed through the circle, and then by removing the sensor to allow it to equilibrate to room air, and then observing a reading of 21% oxygen. The sensor must then be replaced into the breathing circuit, and the absence of a leak confirmed. *Failing to do so is one of the more common mistakes in the machine checkout procedure.*

ITEM #11. Verify carbon dioxide absorbent is not exhausted. The CO_2 absorber is checked to ensure that it is not more than 50% exhausted. When the absorber changes color, it needs to be replaced. The replacement of an absorber, without an appropriate seal, is also a common source of leaks.

ITEM #12. Breathing system pressure and leak testing. Part of the anesthesia equipment checkout includes checking the circle system. The circle system is checked to be sure there are no leaks by occluding the y-piece, building up 30 cm H_2O pressure and with no flow, and verifying the pressure does not decline. The last part of the circle system to check is the O_2 sensor which calibrated 100% oxygen and often room air.

ITEM # 13. Verify that gas flows properly through the breathing circuit during both inspiration and exhalation. The proper functioning of inspiratory and expiratory valves ensures unidirectional gas flow. These valves can be checked visually by observing their movement. A more rigorous evaluation involves attaching an extra breathing bag to the inspiratory port (the other breathing bag is attached at the standard position on the bag mount), and then pressurizing the breathing circle to 30 cm H_2O (Figure 6–2). If the adjustable pressure limiting valve is closed, the only way for gas to escape is retrograde through the expiratory valve. If no pressure decline is noted, then the adjustable pressure limiting valve is opened thus creating a pressure gradient retrograde across the inspiratory valve by the bag attached and inflated there. If that bag does not deflate, then the inspiratory valve is competent. To verify antegrade gas movement through the valves as well as ventilator function, a breathing bag is attached to the circuit at the elbow (similar to an "artificial lung") and the ventilator is turned on. The bag should inflate and deflate appropriately. During this step the ventilator can be set to the appropriate tidal volume and rate for the upcoming patient.

ITEM # 14. Document completion of checkout procedures.

ITEM #15. Confirm ventilator settings and evaluate readiness to deliver anesthesia care.

Anesthesia Pause. Documentation and confirmation of proper preparation in the form of a pause constitute the last two steps in the ASA machine checkout recommendations.

Modern anesthesia machines are very diverse and constantly changing. The ASA recommends that every anesthesia department adopt a checkout procedure for each specific machine used in its institution. Some machines have computerized machine checks. Even if these machine checks are utilized, manual checks are still added to ensure all the components of the ASA guidelines are met.

Ensuring a proper functioning machine will avoid situations like the one described where a patient is rendered unconscious and the machine malfunction is discovered. When the anesthesia machine fails, emergency equipment such as an Ambu bag is available, and the anesthetic can be readily converted

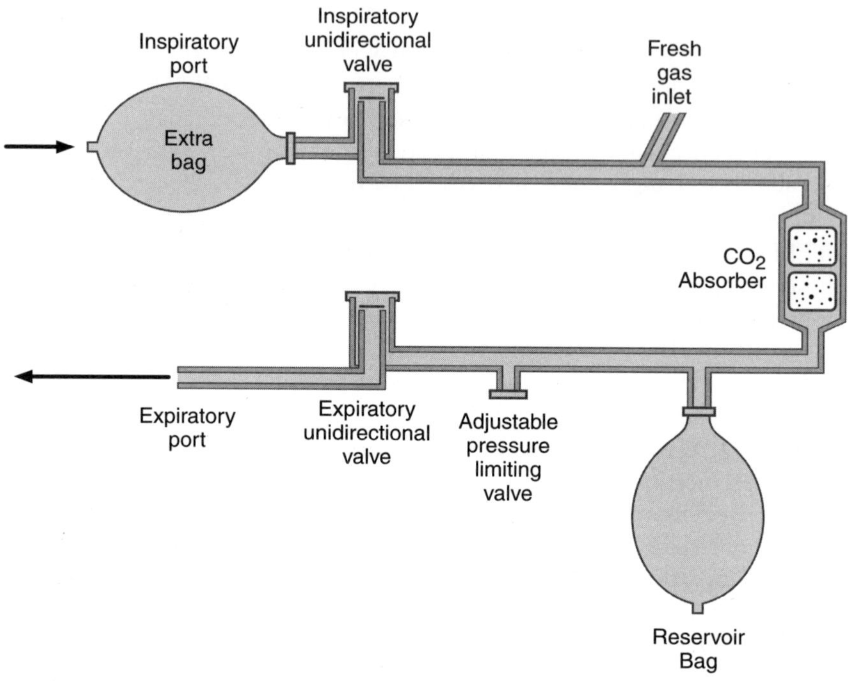

Figure 6–2. An extra bag attached at inspiratory port, and the system pressurized.

to an intravenous technique. If the surgical procedure has not yet begun then initial incision should be delayed until equipment issues are resolved.

Comprehension Questions

6.1. Which of the following guarantees that the hoses for oxygen and nitrous oxide will not be switched?
A. Diameter index safety system
B. Inspiratory unidirectional valve
C. Scavenging system
D. Flow spirometer

6.2. You are administering anesthesia in a location that does not have an oxygen supply line. The E-cylinder that you are using reads 500 psig. Your oxygen flows are 10 L/min. Approximately how long does it take for your E-cylinder to empty?
A. 5 minutes
B. 15 minutes
C. 50 minutes
D. 100 minutes

6.3. What is the purpose of the scavenging system?
A. To retrieve anesthetic gases for reuse and cost savings.
B. To retrieve exhaled gases for warming and humidification of inhaled gases.
C. To retrieve anesthetic gases and reduce operating room contamination.
D. To retrieve exhaled gases to use as carriers and reduce total fresh-gas flow.

ANSWERS

6.1. **A.** The diameter index safety system is used at the connection to wall gas supply lines. The pin index system is used at the yoke assembly on the anesthesia machine. Both of these systems are in place to ensure correct gas connections.

6.2. **B.** A full E-cylinder of oxygen contains 600 L of gas at a pressure of 2000 psig. Using Boyle law ($P_1V_1 = P_2V_2$) the volume of the partially depleted cylinder can be calculated, $V_2 = (P_1V_1)/P_2$ or $V_2 = (P_1/P_2) V_1$. There is a quarter tank left, and therefore a quarter of 600 L, or 150 L. At 10 L/min, this volume of gas would last 15 minutes.

6.3. **C.** The purpose of the scavenging system is to reduce the amount of anesthetic gas in the operating room. The National Institute of Occupational Safety and Health has set standards for anesthetic gas levels in the operating room. For example, there is to be no more than 2 ppm (parts per million) of a volatile anesthetic if used alone, and no more than 0.5 ppm of a volatile anesthetic when used in conjunction with nitrous oxide in the operating room. The maximum amount of nitrous oxide allowed in the operating room is 25 ppm (50 ppm in the dental office).

Clinical Pearls

- Routine check of anesthesia equipment is mandatory.
- Ambu bag and oxygen tent are essential equipment in case of machine failure.

REFERENCE

Design Guidelines for Effective Anesthesia Apparatus Checkout. www.asahq.org/clinical/FINALCheckoutDesignguidelines02-08-2008.pdf.

Part 3. The Patient Undergoing Anesthesia

Case 7

The surgeons have requested a brief general anesthetic for a dressing change to an open infected wound. They suggest that the procedure can be performed in the patient's bed on the hospital floor.

➤ Does this patient need special monitoring for this procedure?

ANSWER TO CASE 7: Introduction to Patient Monitoring

Summary: A patient undergoes a dressing change on the floor, and a brief anesthesia is required.

- This patient's monitoring must adhere to the standards for **basic monitoring** published by the American Society of Anesthesiologists. These standards are described in greater detail in the following discussion.

ANALYSIS

Objectives

1. Be familiar with the basic anesthetic monitoring parameters.
2. Be aware that monitoring the key parameters allows the anesthesiologist to assess clinical status and changes to patient condition.

APPROACH TO Patient Monitoring

Monitoring is an essential duty of an anesthesiologist. During administration of an anesthetic the anesthesiologist needs to be able to continuously monitor a patient's clinical status, rapidly detect changes in a patient's condition, assess responses to therapeutic interventions, and ensure proper equipment function at all times. The American Society of Anesthesiologists first established standards for **basic monitoring** in 1986, and these standards have formed the cornerstone of safe anesthetic care since that time.

Depending on the acuity and magnitude of the surgery additional monitoring may also be required; the decision to use more invasive monitoring is made by the anesthesiologist performing the case. In all instances, **vigilance is the most important action** required by the anesthesiologist and the provider should never consider monitors an adequate substitute for personal vigilance and participation.

CLINICAL APPROACH

Standards for Basic Anesthetic Monitoring

The first standard states that "anesthesia personnel shall be present in the room throughout the conduct of all general anesthetics, regional anesthetics, and monitored anesthesia care." This standard emphasizes the vital role of the anesthesiologist in the safe care of the patient.

The second standard states that "the patient's oxygenation, ventilation, circulation, and temperature shall be continually evaluated." These will be considered individually.

Oxygenation

During all anesthetics an assessment of blood oxygenation is required to ensure adequate oxygenation at all times. In addition, during a general anesthetic the oxygen concentration in the inspired gas must be measured, and there must be a low-oxygen concentration alarm in place.

The patient's blood oxygen saturation is determined by pulse oximetry. Pulse oximeters should be equipped with an audible pulse tone, and the pitch should change when the oxygenation drops, warning the anesthesiologist of a change in patient status. The pulse oximeter works by illuminating a tissue sample with two wavelengths of light: 660 nm red light and 940 nm infrared light. Plethysmography is used to differentiate the pulsatile arterial waveform from background tissue. As the pulse oximeter depends on both pulsatile flow and arterial color to determine saturation, any condition that affects detection of pulsatile flow (arrhythmias, patient movement, shivering, hypotension) or changes light absorption (intravascular dyes, dysfunctional hemoglobin) may falsely affect the oxygen saturation reading.

Oxygen sensors should be on the inspiratory limb of the anesthesia circuit to ensure recognition of a hypoxic mixture prior to the patient's inhalation. Polarographic analyzers are commonly used to determine oxygen concentration. Oxygen diffuses through a polymeric membrane and reacts with water to form hydroxide; this reaction produces a current change in proportion to the number of oxygen molecules present. Low-limit oxygen alarms alert the anesthesiologist when the inspired oxygen level falls below 21% or alternative parameters chosen for the case.

Ventilation

Ventilation must be monitored during all anesthetics. *This may be accomplished using qualitative clinical signs such as chest excursion and auscultation of breath sounds or quantitatively through continuous carbon dioxide monitoring of expired gas.*

Whenever an endotracheal tube/laryngeal mask airway is inserted, the placement must be confirmed by sustained presence of CO_2 for greater than three breaths. Although CO_2 production is in general associated with an endotracheal intubation, CO_2 can also be produced by the gastric bubble. Thus, confirming CO_2 for three breaths, as well as auscultating the stomach and chest are required to ensure tracheal intubation. The end-tidal CO_2 ($ETCO_2$) must also be monitored continuously until the removal of the endotracheal tube or LMA. During mechanical ventilation of a patient, an alarm must be present that will create a characteristic audible alert if the $ETCO_2$ is above or below a certain range and in the event of a circuit disconnect, which is determined by a drop in peak inspiratory pressure below a critical value.

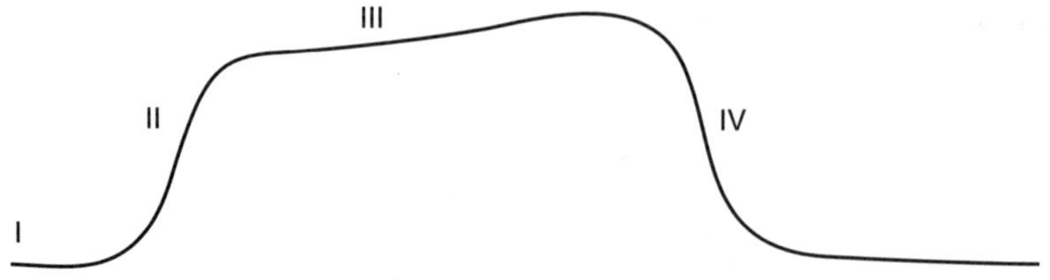

Figure 7–1. Normal capnograph where each phase represents the following: I-inspiratory baseline, II-expiratory upstroke, III-alveolar plateau, IV-inspiratory downstroke.

Monitors display a continuous waveform of inspiratory and expiratory carbon dioxide concentration over time; this is known as capnography (Please see Figure 7–1). This data can provide invaluable information such as a change in respiratory rate, dead space/perfusion, anesthesia circuit disconnect, and an estimate of arterial carbon dioxide concentration, $PaCO_2$. In healthy individuals undergoing general anesthesia, the difference between $PaCO_2$ and $ETCO_2$ is 5 to 7 mm Hg.

Circulation

The anesthetist continuously assesses circulation through observation of the patient, pulse, blood pressure, and continuous electrocardiography (ECG).

At least one lead of an ECG is displayed; this can provide valuable information about the patient's underlying cardiac rate and rhythm. If at least two leads are available, ST-segment analysis can detect myocardial ischemia. Myocardial ischemia leads to T-wave changes (flattening, inversion) followed by ST-segment changes (depression, elevation) and lastly by Q waves.

Heart rate and blood pressure must be checked at least every 5 minutes. In most instances the heart rate is determined using the pulse oximetry waveform or less commonly by direct palpation of the pulse. Noninvasive blood pressure can be detected by palpation, auscultation of Korotkoff sounds, and oscillotonometers. The oscillometric method is used most frequently in automated blood pressure readings; the cuff is inflated until oscillations are no longer seen (systolic blood pressure) and then deflated until maximal oscillations (mean arterial pressure). The diastolic blood pressure is actually a calculated value derived from the mean and systolic pressures. The upper arm is the most commonly used extremity for BP monitoring; regardless where the BP is monitored, it is important to ensure that the appropriate cuff size is applied. The cuff's width should be approximately 40% of the extremity's circumference and the length should be 60% of the circumference. A cuff that is too small can result in falsely high blood pressure measurements while a cuff that is too large can lead to falsely low measurements.

Temperature

Heat loss is common in surgery due to the exposed state of skin, operating room environment, and both general and regional anesthesia inhibiting thermoregulatory control. *Temperature monitoring is required to allow the anesthetist to detect changes in body temperature while the patient is anesthetized.* In most instances, temperature is measured by using electrical probes that change their electrical resistance depending on temperature changes.

Urine Output

Although not required as part of the American Society of Anesthesiologists standards for monitoring, urine output is measured in most anesthetics with a duration of more than 2 hours or where significant fluid shifts are anticipated. In some ways a "poor man's CVP," an adequate urine output of $^1/_2$ mL/kg suggests an adequate volume resuscitation and cardiac output. Measuring and recording urine output hourly, if not half hourly, can provide quite useful information in the absence of the monitoring of central venous pressure.

Invasive Monitoring

Depending on the type of surgery and comorbidities of the patient, more intense monitoring may be required to adequately care for the patient. The decision to use a particular invasive monitor involves balancing the benefits with the risks of insertion.

Arterial Line

In certain instances intermittent BP monitoring is not adequate and continuous invasive arterial blood pressure monitoring is indicated. For example, if wide swings in blood pressure are expected such as during a carotid endarterectomy or aortic aneurysm repair, or if tight control of BP is necessary during an intracranial or cardiac case. At times an arterial line is needed to closely monitor arterial blood gases and laboratory studies. The blood pressure is monitored by transducing a small catheter placed directly into a peripheral artery. The most common site is the radial artery, but the brachial, axillary, femoral, and dorsalis pedis arteries can also be cannulated. The blood pressure transducer attached to the catheter converts the transmitted arterial pulsatile force into a change in voltage. The arterial BP trace is continuously monitored.

Invasive arterial pressure monitoring is dependent upon an appropriate zeroing of the transducer, and that the transducer is positioned properly at the level of the right atrium. Mechanical pitfalls include a potential damping of the signal (such as from bubbles entrained in tubing), or an under damping or amplification of the signal (observed, eg, when an excessive length of tubing is used). Complications of the arterial cannulation include hematoma, thrombosis, embolism, infection, aneurysm formation, nerve damage, and distal ischemia.

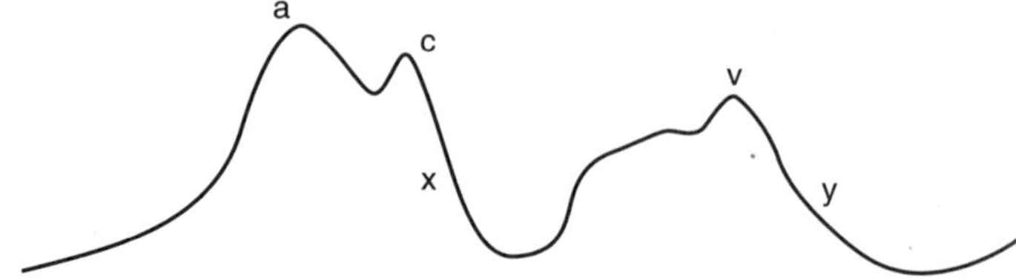

Figure 7–2. Normal CVP tracing where a wave-right atrial contraction, c wave-bulging of tricuspid valve in right atrium, x descent-atrial relaxation, v wave-rise in right atrial pressure before tricuspid valve opens, and y descent-right atrial emptying into right ventricle.

Central Venous Line

Most often central venous pressure (CVP) monitoring is used to estimate volume status by measuring the right atrial pressure, which provides an estimate of right ventricular preload. The CVP tracing (see Figure 7–2) depends on many factors: heart rate, arrhythmias, tricuspid valve function, and right ventricular compliance. Assuming no cardiopulmonary disease, the CVP is often used as a marker of left ventricular preload. The most common site of insertion is the right internal jugular vein, but the left internal jugular vein, subclavian veins, and external jugular veins can also be utilized. Complications of placement include arterial puncture, nerve injury, pneumothorax, air embolism, sepsis from catheter infection, thrombophlebitis, and venous thrombosis.

Pulmonary Artery Monitoring

A pulmonary artery (PA) catheter is a 110-cm plastic tube; the tip is placed in the pulmonary artery by "floating" the balloon through a large vein (internal jugular, subclavian, external jugular) → right atrium → tricuspid valve → right ventricle → pulmonary artery. Catheter location is indicated by the pressure waveform from the distal end of the catheter (see the following discussion). The PA catheter can measure cardiac output, mixed venous oxygen saturation, PA, and right atrial pressures as well as calculating systemic vascular resistance, pulmonary vascular resistance, and stroke index. The pulmonary artery occlusive pressure (PAOP) is measured when the distal balloon is inflated in the pulmonary artery; this is used as an estimate for left ventricular end-diastolic pressure. There is a static column of fluid between the tip of the catheter and left atrium.

The indications for the use of PA monitoring include poor left ventricular function, valvular heart disease, recent myocardial infarction, adult respiratory distress syndrome, massive trauma, and major vascular surgery. Complications of PA monitoring include those listed earlier for CVP monitor as well as dysrhythmias (ventricular tachycardia or fibrillation, right bundle branch block, complete heart block), pulmonary artery rupture, pulmonary infarction, and valvular or endocardial vegetations.

Echocardiography

Echocardiography uses a piezoelectric crystal to emit ultrasound waves; these ultrasound waves penetrate tissue and then bounce back to the crystal giving information about velocity, distance, and density. Echocardiography has revolutionized perioperative cardiac monitoring by enabling the clinician to determine stroke volume, cardiac valve function, presence of intracardiac air, ventricular preload, and possible myocardial ischemia through the detection of wall motion abnormalities.

Category 1 indications (supported by the strongest evidence or expert opinion) include heart valve repair, congenital heart surgery, hypertrophic obstructive cardiomyopathy repair, thoracic aortic aneurysm/dissection repair, pericardial window procedures, unstable patients with unexplained hemodynamic disturbances, suspected valvular disease, or thromboembolic disease. Complications of TEE (transesophageal echocardiogram) use include esophageal trauma, dysrhythmias, hemodynamic instability, lip/dental injuries, hoarseness, and dysphagia.

Monitoring of Neurological Function

Awareness is an uncommon but dreaded complication of general anesthesia; it has been estimated to occur in 1 to 2 out of 1,000 general anesthetics. The typical signs of "light" anesthesia rely on signs of sympathetic stimulation such as an increase in heart rate and blood pressure, presumably in response to the sensation of surgical pain. Despite the availability of monitors to determine these hemodynamic parameters, it is difficult to accurately quantify a patient's anesthetic depth consistently. The bispectral index or BIS monitor has been developed to monitor the patient's level of consciousness.

The bispectral index, also known as the BIS monitor, is one measure of anesthetic depth which is derived from a reduction of the EEG. Selected EEG signals are reduced to a number, between 1 and 100 (the algorithm is currently under patent). A reading of 100 represents the awake state and numbers between 45 to 60 are considered optimal for general anesthesia. While certainly a useful monitor, there is still controversy as to what level is required to ensure amnesia, and the BIS is not perfect. Although controversial, this monitor has not been added to the list of required monitors by the American Society of Anesthesiologists.

Certain surgeries may place important neural structures at risk (spine, brainstem, intra-cerebral surgery.) These neural pathways can be stimulated with evoked potentials (small electrical signals) in order to assess functionality. Somatosensory evoked potentials (SSEPs) monitor the integrity of the dorsal columns of the spinal cord by placing stimulating electrodes near the median or ulnar nerves of the arms and posterior tibial nerves of the legs. The electrical signal is applied to the peripheral nerve and travels to the dorsal root ganglia → posterior columns of the spinal cord → dorsal column nuclei → medial lemniscus → opposite thalamus → frontoparietal sensorimotor cortex. Anesthetic agents such as volatile anesthetics, nitrous oxide, and barbiturates can decrease the amplitude and increase latency of SSEPs similarly to ischemia's effects making it difficult to determine a clear etiology. Motor evoked potentials (MEPs) monitor the functionality of the corticospinal tracts; a stimulating electrode is placed on the scalp and the recording electrode is placed on the contracting muscle. MEPs are more sensitive to anesthetic agents and more difficult to obtain limiting their accuracy and clinical use.

CONCLUSION

Continuous monitoring of the patient is a key part of the anesthesiologist's responsibility during surgery. Basic monitoring requirements include the minimal acceptable standards for patients. The complexity of additional monitoring is determined by the type of surgery and the patients; however there is no monitor that can replace the required vigilance of the anesthesiologist.

Comprehension Questions

7.1. Which of the following is the most important skill of an anesthesiologist?
   A. Caring for patients through the acquisition of knowledge
   B. Technical facility with invasive lines
   C. Vigilance
   D. An understanding that mastering anesthesiology is not only a science, but also an art

7.2. For any anesthetics, the basic standards of monitoring include a continuous evaluation of all but which one of the following?
   A. Oxygenation
   B. Ventilation
   C. Circulation
   D. Hematocrit
   E. Temperature

ANSWERS

7.1. **C.** While each of the answers is true for the anesthesiologist, the most important attribute of an anesthesiologist is vigilance.

7.2. **D.** The basic monitoring standards of the American Society of Anesthesiologists states that "the patient's oxygenation, ventilation, circulation, and temperature shall be continually evaluated." D, continuous monitoring of the hematocrit, is not necessary and even during cases associated with a massive blood loss, is rarely accomplished.

Clinical Pearls

- Simply adhering to the basic monitoring standards adopted by the American Society of Anesthesiologists has been found to reduce anesthetic mortality.
- CO_2 can also be contained in a gastric "bubble." Hence, it is important to confirm endotracheal intubation by observing the end-tidal CO_2 for three breaths, and auscultating the chest.
- An appropriately sized blood pressure cuff is necessary to accurately measure blood pressure using a noninvasive technique.

REFERENCES

American Society of Anesthesiologists. (last amended Oct. 25, 2005). *Standards for Basic Monitoring*, 1986.

American Society of Anesthesiologists. (last amended Oct. 18, 2006). *Statement on Transesophageal Echocardiography*, 2001.

Barash P, Cullen B, Stoelting R. *Clinical Anesthesia.* 5th ed. Philadelphia, PA: Lippincott Williams & Wilkins; 2005.

Miller R, Stoelting R. *Basics of Anesthesia.* 5th ed. New York, NY: Churchill Livingstone; 2006.

Murray M, Morgan E, Mikhail M. *Clinical Anesthesiology.* 4th ed. New York, NY: McGraw Hill Medical; 2005.

Pickering T, et al. American Heart Association's recommendations for blood pressure monitoring in humans and experimental animals. *Hypertension.* 2005;45:142-161.

Case 8

A 54-year-old man is undergoing a laparotomy and colon resection for carcinoma. The anesthesiologist is attempting to calculate the fluid replacement.

➤ What are the components that must be considered when calculating the volume of fluid that should be replaced?

ANSWER TO CASE 8: Management of Fluid and Electrolytes

Summary: A 54-year-old man is undergoing bowel surgery, for which the volume of fluid replacement is being calculated.

➤ **Factors affecting volume of fluid to be replaced:** Preoperative fluid deficits, insensitive fluid losses, intraoperative blood loss, and urine output

ANALYSIS

Objectives

1. Review the distribution of infused fluids within the various bodily compartments.
2. Acquaint the student with methods of calculating the fluid replacement in the intraoperative period.
3. Allow the student to become familiar with the advantages and disadvantages of crystalloids and colloids.

Considerations

Patients undergoing intestinal surgery are well known to require more fluid replacement than might otherwise be expected. This patient will no doubt have preoperative fluid deficits, because he has not been eating or drinking, and has also undergone a bowel prep. Intraoperatively, the patient will lose blood, and there is also likely to be a significant insensitive loss from the intestines exposed to air. Fluids—crystalloids or blood products—will be required to ensure the preservation of renal and cardiovascular function, maintaining urine output at normal levels.

APPROACH TO The Management of Fluids and Electrolytes

Many factors make fluid management in the perioperative setting different from any other situation. Preoperative fasting, insensible fluid losses, blood loss from the surgical site, postoperative dietary restrictions, and nasogastric tube drainage require the use of replacement fluids. Such fluids include crystalloids, colloids, and blood products. Administration of fluids is guided by the nature of the bodily fluid loss, and the patient's disease process.

Fluid Compartments

Total body water constitutes approximately 70% of lean body weight, although this percentage varies with the deposition of adipose tissue. Total body water is distributed between the extracellular and intracellular compartments.

Intracellular fluid is the fluid contained within cells and comprises approximately two-thirds (30 L) of total body water. (Please see Figure 8–1.)

Extracellular fluid is further compartmentalized into intravascular fluid and extravascular fluid, and comprises about one-third (15 L) of total body water.

Intravascular fluid consists of plasma (3 L), plus blood cells (2 L), which together constitutes circulating blood volume (5 L).

Extravascular fluid (12 L) is mostly found in tissues adjacent to the microvascular circulation, and is called the "functional compartment." In contrast, the "nonfunctional" fluid compartment is ill defined, and devoid of fluid in the normal physiologic state. However, fluid can distribute into this "third" space postoperatively. Common examples of "third-spacing" include the bowel, peritoneal cavity, and traumatized tissues.

During normal circumstances, the lymphatic system removes the excess interstitial water and returns it to the intravascular compartment, maintaining the equilibrium and preventing intravascular depletion. In the perioperative setting, this mechanism may be depressed due to processes such as inflammation, rendering the body unable to redistribute the interstitial fluid and effectively causing edema.

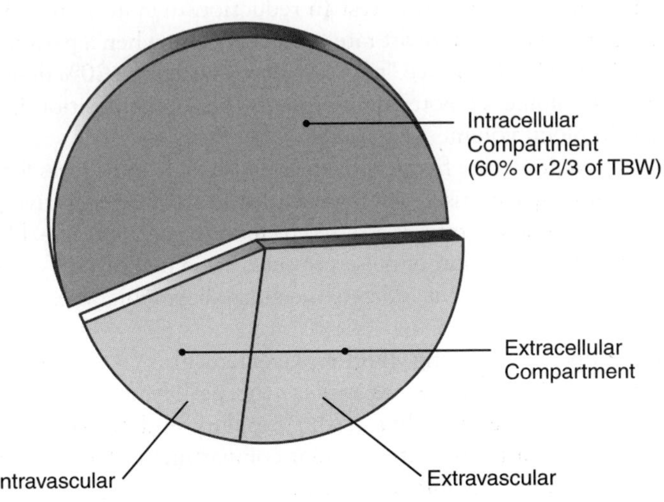

Figure 8–1. Relationship and distribution of bodily fluid spaces.

Distribution of Infused Fluids

The prediction of plasma volume expansion in response to a fluid administration (assumes that the body fluid spaces are static).

Plasma volume increment = volume infused plasma volume/distribution volume. Rearranging this equation facilitates an estimation of the amount of fluid that needs to be administered.

Volume infused = desired plasma volume increment distribution volume/plasma volume.

For example, to get 2 L increment in plasma volume:

2 45(TBW)/3 = 30 L D5W, or 2 15(ECF)/3 = 10 L crystalloid, or 2 3(PV)/3 = 2 L of colloid will be required.

The primary goal of any fluid management regimen is to maintain adequate tissue perfusion. Fluid shifts during the perioperative period, and the physiological responses to surgical stress have significant implications for perioperative fluid prescribing.

The homeostasis of total body water balance is maintained with intake and losses of 2.5 to 3 L/d. Intake from ingested fluid (1300 mL), solid food (800 mL) and metabolic waste (400 mL) is balanced by insensible losses of 0.5 mL/kg/h (850 mL) from skin and lungs, plus urine (1500 mL) and feces (100 mL). The insensible losses are typically replaced by oral intake, lacking in presurgical fasting patient. Therefore, the perioperative fluid replacement has to take this "(NPO) loss" into account.

Still, many patients arrive in the operating room volume-depleted from preoperative fasting and/or the use of bowel preps. A patient's volume status may be assessed by the conventional clinical signs of oliguria, hypotension, tachycardia, and a positive "tilt" test (a reduction in systolic blood pressure > 20 mm Hg and increase in heart rate > 20 beats/min when a patient assumes an upright position). A positive "tilt" test signals at least a 20% deficit in circulating blood volume. Hypotension while in the supine position indicates a 30% deficit in blood volume. (Please see Table 8–1.)

Intraoperative losses are frequently underestimated, and excess losses, both surgical and third-space losses, often persist into early postoperative period.

Intraoperative volume status is assessed by monitoring heart rate, blood pressure, the respiratory variation of pulse pressure, urine output (≥ $^{1}/_{2}$ cc/kg/min), central venous pressure and if indicated, echocardiographic assessment of the heart.

In the perioperative setting, fluid replacement also takes into consideration the insensible fluid losses, as well as the perioperative stress response which increases the permeability of the capillary endothelium and causes movement of water into the extravascular compartment. The stress response also causes retention of sodium and water.

Table 8–1 SIGNS OF PREOPERATIVE HYPOVOLEMIA

Hypotension
Tachycardia
Oliguria
Supine hypotension
Positive tilt test
Increased BUN/Creatinine (>10:1)
Increasing urinary osmolality (>450 mOsm/L)
Decreased urinary sodium (<10 mEq/L)
Increase in urine specific gravity (>1.010)
Metabolic alkalosis (mild hypovolemia)
Metabolic acidosis (severe hypovolemia)
Increasing serial hematocrits

Fluid Replacement Therapy

There are many ways of calculating the fluid replacement in the intraoperative period all of which take into consideration the preoperative fluid deficits, intraoperative blood loss, and urine output.

Pre-existing Fluid Deficits

Patients undergoing surgery often have 6 to 8 hours of fasting and the deficit can be estimated by multiplying the maintenance rate by the duration of fast. Patient's preprocedural volume status may vary due to factors such as vomiting, diarrhea, ileus, fever, burns, ascites, effusions, hemorrhage, bowel preparations, or diuretics.

Maintenance Requirements

Two simple formulas are often used to estimate maintenance fluid requirements:

WEIGHT (kg)	mL/kg/h	mL/kg/d
1-10	4	100
11-20	2	50
>20	1	20

For example, a 70-kg adult will require (10 4) + (10 2) + (50 1) = 110 mL/h of maintenance. To calculate the deficit, this amount is multiplied by the hours of fasting. The deficit is infused over 3 hours, half in the first hour and the rest over the next 2 hours.

The hourly fluid replacement will also include the maintenance and losses.

Daily requirements for sodium and potassium are approximately 2 mmol/kg and 1 mmol/kg, respectively. Therefore a healthy 70-kg adult requires about 2500 mL of water containing 30 mEq/L of Na and 15 to 20 mEq/L of K. Intraoperatively, fluids containing sodium-free water Na <30 mEq/L are rarely used because of the need to replace isotonic losses and the risk of postoperative hyponatremia.

Surgical Volume Losses

3 cc crystalloid = 1 cc blood

1 cc colloid = 1 cc blood

The redistributive and evaporative losses are proportionate to the degree of tissue trauma on the surgical field. This can be estimated by the following values:

- **4 mL/kg/h for minimal trauma to the tissues (arthroscopy, hand surgery, etc.)**
- **6 mL/kg/h for moderate tissue trauma without significant bowel exposure (cholecystectomy, hysterectomy, etc.)**
- **8 mL/kg/h for severe tissue trauma (aortic aneurysm repair, Harrington rod spinal fusion, most bowel surgery)**

When a significant amount of fluid is required for a more major surgery, fluids may be titrated to physiologically relevant biometric end points such as urine output, central venous pressure, wedge pressure, pulse pressure variation, venous oxygen saturation, or left ventricular end-diastolic volume measured dynamically in the intraoperative setting. However, calculations which permit a periodic estimation of appropriate fluid administration are an invaluable addition to the physiologic end points.

The Choice of Fluids: Crystalloid vs Colloids

Despite a decade's long debate, systematic reviews show no difference in pulmonary edema, mortality, or length of hospital stay following preferential administration of crystalloids or colloids.

Crystalloids are solutions typically containing glucose or saline, and are useful for the replacement of insensible losses. They are nontoxic, nonallergenic, and inexpensive. However, their ability to remain within the intravascular space is limited, leading to a propensity to cause interstitial edema in large quantities due to dilution of plasma proteins and thus plasma oncotic pressure. The most commonly used crystalloids are normal saline and lactated Ringer solution. Rarely, large amounts of 0.9% or normal saline can lead to hyperchloremic metabolic acidosis, whereas large quantities of lactated Ringer may result in metabolic alkalosis due to increased production of bicarbonate from the metabolism of lactate.

Colloids are homogenous noncrystalline substances consisting of large molecules dissolved in a solute. They are more likely to remain in the intravascular space and therefore serve as effective volume expanders. Hypersensitivity reactions, including anaphylaxis, have been reported with all colloids.

Coagulation abnormalities are seen with the synthetic colloids. Dextrans produce a dose-related reduction in platelet aggregation and adhesiveness, whereas hydroxyethyl starch can lead to a reduction in factor VIII and von Willebrand factor, impairing platelet function and prolonging partial thromboplastin time. Coagulation and bleeding times are not usually prolonged after 1 L of colloid infusion.

The types of colloids in clinical use today include:

Albumin, purified from human plasma pasteurized at 60°C for 10 hours. Albumin is available as 5% or 25% solution and has a plasma half-life of 16 hours, and is by far the most expensive colloid available today.

Hydroxyethyl starch is composed of amylopectin linked with hydroxyethyl groups in a glucose moiety, resulting in a polymer similar to glycogen. Examples are 6% Hespan and Hextend. Their half-life is 17 days.

Dextran is a biosynthesized commercially from sucrose by the bacterium *Leuconostoc mesenteroides*. Dextran 40 and Dextran 70 differ based on molecular weight. Dextran 40 is thought to improve blood flow in microcirculation, presumably by decreasing blood viscosity. Dextran 1 (also known as Promit) may be administered before dextran 40 or 70 to prevent severe anaphylaxis.

CONCLUSIONS

Perioperative fluid management is a complicated and controversial topic, with an ongoing debate regarding the type and amount of intraoperative fluid to be administered. Currently, there is a trend toward limiting fluid administration in the intraoperative setting, especially crystalloids, due to their inability to stay in the intravascular space for long periods of time. Colloid administration is not without risk, as allergic reactions and coagulopathies are not uncommon. The bottom line for fluid administration: biometric end points guide fluid replacement with the goal of maintaining adequate tissue perfusion.

Comprehension Questions

8.1. A patient suffering a stab wound to the abdomen arrives in the operating room for an emergency exploratory laparotomy. His BP is 70/40, and his HR is 118. Which of the following fluid regimens are appropriate for his fluid resuscitation?

A. Normal saline, at a ratio of 3 mL per estimated 1 mL of blood lost
B. Blood at a ratio of 3 mL blood administered to 1 mL of blood lost
C. Hetastarch (Hespan) in a ratio of 3 mL per estimated 1 mL of blood lost
D. D5W in a ratio of 3 mL of D5W to 1 mL of blood lost

8.2. A 70-kg college freshman is undergoing an arthroscopy of the knee as an 8 AM case. Does he need fluids intraoperatively? If so, what type of fluids, and at what rate?

A. Crystalloids, 10 mL/kg/h maintenance
B. Crystalloids, 1 mL/kg/h maintenance
C. Crystalloids, approximately 1,000 mL for NPO losses
D. Crystalloids, approximately 1,600 mL for NPO losses

8.3. The surgery of the freshman mentioned is delayed until 3 PM in order to accommodate an emergency. Does he need fluids intraoperatively? If so, what type of fluids, and at what rate?

A. Crystalloids, 10 mL/kg/h maintenance
B. Crystalloids, 1 mL/kg/h maintenance
C. Crystalloids, approximately 1,000 mL for NPO losses
D. Crystalloids, approximately 1,600 mL for NPO losses

ANSWERS

8.1. **A.** Normal saline, at a ratio of 3 mL per estimated 1 mL of blood lost, or blood at a ratio of 1 mL blood administered to 1 mL of blood lost are appropriate resuscitation regiments. Since hetastarch is a colloid, it would be administered in a ratio of 1 mL of hetastarch per 1 mL of blood lost. D5W is not an appropriate resuscitative fluid for hemorrhage secondary to trauma.

8.2. **C.** If the patient has been NPO for 8 hours and weighs 70 kg, he should receive approximately 1000 mL of crystalloids to replace his NPO losses. Since an arthroscopy is a minimally invasive procedure, maintenance fluids should be administered at a rate of 4 mL/kg/h.

8.3. **D.** If the patient's surgery is delayed and he has been NPO for some 15 hours, he should receive approximately 1,600 mL of crystalloids to replace his NPO losses. Since an arthroscopy is a minimally invasive procedure, maintenance fluids should also be administered at a rate of 4 mL/kg/h.

Clinical Pearls

- Factors affecting fluid management in the perioperative setting include preoperative fasting, insensible fluid losses, blood loss from the surgical site, postoperative dietary restrictions, and nasogastric tube drainage.
- There is little evidence to support the advantages or disadvantages of crystalloids over colloids, or vice versa.
- The bottom line for fluid administration: biometric end points guide fluid replacement with the goal of maintaining adequate tissue perfusion.

REFERENCES

Barash PG, Cullen BF, Stoelting RK. *Clinical Anesthesia.* 6th ed. Philadelphia, PA: Lippincott, Williams and Wilkins, 2009.

Chappell D, Jacob M. A rational approach to perioperative fluid management. *Anesthesiology.* 2008;109: 723-740.

Grocott MPW, Mythen MG, Gan TJ. Perioperative fluid management and clinical outcomes in adults. Review article. *Anesthesia and Analgesia.* 2005;100: 1093-1106.

Miller RD. *Anesthesia.* 5th ed. Vol 1. 2000.

Rassam SS, Counsell DJ. Perioperative electrolyte and fluid balance. Continuing Education. In *Anesthesia Critical care and Pain.* 2005;5: 157-160.

Roberts I, Alderson P, Bunn F, et al. Colloids versus crystalloids for fluid resuscitation in critically ill patients. *Cochrane Database Syst Rev.* 2004;4:CD 000567.

Case 9

A 45-year-old man is undergoing a preoperative evaluation for a laparoscopic cholecystectomy due to acute cholecystitis. He has a history of rheumatoid arthritis for 10 years. After the evaluation, the anesthesiologist determines that the patient is ASA status 3.

➤ What does ASA status 3 mean?

➤ What is the focus of the anesthesia evaluation of the arthritis?

ANSWERS TO CASE 9: Preoperative Evaluation

Summary: A 45-year-old man is undergoing preoperative evaluation and is determined to be ASA 3. He had a prior MI 6 months ago.

- **Meaning of ASA 3:** Patients with systemic disease with functional limitations
- **Relevance of the arthritis:** The impact on the patient's functional capacity and mobility, as well as any potential difficulties with the airway that may occur

ANALYSIS

Objectives

1. Understand the goals of the pre-anesthetic evaluation.
2. Review the components of a basic preoperative examination.
3. Understand which tests are required prior to surgery and why.

Considerations

The preoperative evaluation is a vital step that must be completed prior to the administration of anesthesia. It is performed to reduce the patient's risk of morbidity and mortality when undergoing surgery, and to promote efficiency and reduce costs by minimizing delays and cancellations in the operating room on the day of surgery. (Please see Table 9–1.) In contrast to the history performed by a primary care provider during which chronic conditions are documented carefully, the anesthesia preoperative evaluation focuses on the current functional status of the patient and how their chronic diseases may limit the patient's functionality. For example, the relevance of this patient's arthritis to the anesthesiologist is mostly the impact on the patient's functional capacity and mobility, as well as any potential difficulties with the airway that may occur, as opposed to the long-term prognosis of a patient's chronic condition. It is also important to determine whether the arthritis impairs the patient's ability to open his mouth or extend his neck, both of which are important to ensure a successful intubation.

APPROACH TO Preoperative Evaluation

When patients undergo surgery or any type of procedure that requires anesthesia, they are exposed to both the risk of surgery as well as the risk of anesthesia.

Table 9–1 THE GOALS OF PREOPERATIVE ASSESSMENT

1. To obtain a history of the patient's medical condition and relevant anesthesia history, and to complete a physical examination targeting the airway and relevant systems such as the cardiopulmonary status of the patient.
2. To recommend further testing or consultation as needed to optimize the patient for the anesthesia and surgery.
3. To obtain informed consent from the patient or health care proxy.
4. To allay anxiety and educate patients and their families about anesthesia.
5. To implement risk reduction strategies as appropriate.

During the course of the preoperative evaluation, the anesthesiologist must accurately assess the risk to the patient and formulate a safe and appropriate anesthetic plan. The attendant anesthetic risks must be balanced against the potential benefit the patient will derive from the procedure. For example, in fragile individuals with multiple comorbidities, the risk of general anesthesia involving airway manipulation and hemodynamic fluctuations may be significant. In this situation, the anesthesiologist must use the preoperative evaluation to assess the patient's underlying condition and recommend further testing or interventions, and optimizing the patient's medical condition prior to the operation.

History and Physical Examination

The preoperative evaluation begins with a thorough history and physical examination. The history should include a brief description of the type and extent of the surgery planned as well as the urgency of the situation. Other relevant aspects of the surgery include the indication for surgery and the history of the current condition. An elective surgery may present significantly different challenges compared to an emergency procedure, when there may be little time to optimize the patient's condition. For example, in an elderly patient with abdominal pain and vomiting, it will be important to assess the patient's current hydration, including how long the patient has been ill. This history may influence recommendations for additional laboratory testing and the anesthetic plan. In contrast, the orthopedic history of the healthy young male scheduled for an elective knee arthroscopy, or anterior cruciate ligament (ACL) repair is unlikely to warrant additional testing.

In all patients, current and past medical problems should be listed along with an indication of severity, treatment, and stability of these conditions. This is particularly relevant for cardiopulmonary diseases such as congestive heart failure, and for chronic obstructive pulmonary diseases (COPD) that are associated with an increased postoperative risk for complications.

An accurate medication history is an important part of the preoperative evaluation and all medications need to be carefully documented. This includes prescription medications, over-the-counter medications, and herbs, and vitamins and supplements. When patients, especially the elderly, are on multiple medications, they should be instructed to bring all medications or a detailed list with them to the preoperative visit to help ensure documentation of these medications.

A list of allergies including the response and severity of the allergic reaction should also be described. Previous surgeries and anesthetic experiences are important and can be useful in helping understand how a patient may respond to their upcoming surgery. The use of tobacco, alcohol, and illicit drugs are part of the routine evaluation, as are questions about a patient's family history of adverse reactions to anesthesia such as malignant hyperthermia or pseudocholinesterase deficiency. A review of systems may uncover symptoms that may suggest previously undiagnosed conditions and positive findings may warrant the anesthesiologist to modify the anesthetic plan. For example, if the patient has symptoms consistent with gastroesophageal reflux disease, the anesthetic plan should include a rapid sequence induction.

The preoperative evaluation is also an opportunity to evaluate the patient's physiologic reserve. It is particularly important to assess the functional capacity of the patient since this might determine whether the patient will need further cardio-respiratory evaluation prior to surgery. In every patient, past anesthetic records should be reviewed if available, and ordered if unavailable and likely to affect formation of the anesthetic plan. This is especially important if the patient has a history of a difficult airway or is a poor historian.

At a minimum, the patient's physical examination should include vital signs, height and weight, an airway examination, and auscultation of the heart and lungs. For the anesthesiologist, the airway examination is a vital component of the examination, for failure to secure an airway during the procedure may result in catastrophic consequences. The components of an airway examination include determining the Mallampati classification of the oral cavity (please see Case 10), the degree of neck flexion, head extension, thyromental distance, and dental status. Other factors such as body habitus and heavy facial hair may also affect the anesthesiologist's ability to mask and intubate the patient. If a difficult intubation is anticipated, the option of an awake fiberoptic intubation should be discussed with the patient. If applicable, other methods of anesthesia besides general anesthesia should also be considered at this time.

Preoperative Testing

After a thorough history and physical examination has been performed, the anesthesiologist will determine whether or not laboratory testing is needed. Depending on the surgical procedure and the health status of the patient, a history and physical examination may be sufficient. For example, a healthy patient undergoing a noninvasive surgical procedure such as a hernia repair or knee arthroscopy is unlikely to need any further workup.

Diagnostic tests can aid in the risk assessment for anesthesia and surgery, guide interventions to optimize medical conditions, and provide baseline results for perioperative management. However, screening tests can yield false positive results that may result in further morbidity in patients without a medical indication due to an unnecessary follow up. Pre-anesthetic testing should only be performed when indicated by the patient's underlying medical condition. Indications for common tests are described in Table 9–2.

Table 9–2 PREOPERATIVE TESTING

Hematocrit (Hct)	Hct should be ordered if there is likelihood of unexpected or symptomatic anemia, or significant blood loss is anticipated. If significant blood loss is possible, a type and screen or crossmatch is also indicated.
Coagulation studies (PT, PTT, INR)	Coagulation studies should be ordered if patient's history suggests a coagulation disorder (such as hemophilia, von Willebrand disease), liver disease, malnutrition or malabsorption, or if the patient is on anticoagulants.
Chemistries (electrolytes, BUN, creatinine, glucose)	Chemistries should be ordered if patient has known kidney disease, has risk factors for renal dysfunction (eg, age >55, diabetes, vascular disease, lupus), is on diuretics, or will be exposed to radiographic dye. Liver function tests are generally not required, although a low albumin has been associated with increased morbidity and mortality in ill patients, and may be requested to establish a baseline.
ECG	An electrocardiogram is one of the only tests that may be ordered based on both the medical history and age. In general the incidence of cardiac disease rises steadily with age and baseline. ECGs are often ordered for males over 45 years and females 55 years in age. An ECG should also be ordered for patients with cardiac disease or symptoms of cardiac disease.
Chest x-ray (CXR)	Routine screening chest x-rays are not recommended before surgery. A CXR is only indicated in patients who have clinical evidence of active pulmonary disease (eg, pneumonia, pulmonary edema, a mediastinal mass) or are undergoing an intrathoracic procedure.

Cardiac Assessment in Non-Cardiac Surgery

Cardiac complications are the most significant adverse events in the perioperative period. The preoperative evaluation should be used to identify patients with modifiable conditions or those at a high risk for perioperative cardiac events. The guidelines for cardiac evaluation before non-cardiac surgery by the American College of Cardiology and American Heart Association (ACC/AHA) are the national standards of care and are organized in a stepwise approach.

STEP 1. Determine the urgency of the proposed surgery. If the patient needs emergent surgery, the focus is on perioperative surveillance and risk reduction measures such as serial ECGs, cardiac enzymes, adequate pain control, and beta blockers to control heart rate.

STEP 2. Determine if the patient has an active cardiac condition such as an acute MI, unstable or severe angina, decompensated heart failure, severe valvular disease, or significant arrhythmias (eg, ventricular tachycardia and rapid atrial fibrillation). For these patients, surgery should be postponed except for life-saving emergencies.

STEP 3. Determine the severity of the proposed surgery. The ACC/AHA categorizes surgical procedures into three categories: low-, intermediate-, and high risk. Low-risk surgeries include endoscopic procedures, breast and superficial surgeries, and most ambulatory procedures. Intermediate-risk surgeries include most orthopedic and intraperitoneal surgeries. High-risk surgeries include aortic or vascular surgeries. Patients with no active cardiac conditions who need low-risk surgery do not need further cardiac testing.

STEP 4. Assess the patient's functional capacity. A common way to assess a patient's functional status is by estimating a patient's exercise tolerance in metabolic equivalents or METs. Asymptomatic patients who have a functional status greater than 4 METs, which is roughly equivalent to walking up two flights of stairs, can proceed with surgery without any additional cardiac workup.

In patients with poor or indeterminate functional capacity who are scheduled for vascular, intermediate, or high-risk procedures, five clinical predictors: ischemic heart disease, heart failure, cerebrovascular disease, diabetes and renal insufficiency are important comorbidities. The number of clinical predictors determines the recommendations for cardiac testing. Patients with no clinical predictors may proceed to surgery. Patients with three or more of the clinical predictors would most likely benefit from further cardiac testing. Other risk factors for coronary artery disease such as smoking, hypercholesterolemia, age, and hypertension have not been shown to predict perioperative cardiac morbidity.

If the patient has a pacemaker or automatic implantable cardioverter defibrillator (AICD), a consult with the device manufacturer, cardiologist, or electrophysiology service may be desirable. Patients with pacemakers and AICDs are at risk for adverse events for unexpected activation and/or firing due to electric interference from devices such as electrocautery during surgery.

NPO Status

To avoid the risk of pulmonary aspiration, patients should receive NPO instructions prior to the surgery. The ASA task force on preoperative fasting currently recommends a fasting of solids and nonhuman milk to exceed 6 hours prior to any procedure requiring general anesthesia, regional anesthesia, or sedation/analgesia. Fasting rules have been liberalized at most centers to allow clear liquids (water, carbonated beverages, sports drinks, coffee or tea without milk) up to 2 hours before surgery in patients who are not at risk of delayed gastric emptying. To avoid confusion, patients should receive a written copy of all instructions. Some institutions may adhere to stricter guidelines such as NPO after midnight except for sips of clear liquids when taking medications, or allowing clear liquids up to 4 hours before surgery for surgery scheduled late in the day.

For pediatric patients, clear liquids may be taken up to 2 hours before surgery. Breast milk is allowed until 4 hours before surgery; formula or nonhuman milk should be held for 6 hours preoperatively.

Preoperative Medications

During the preoperative evaluation, the patient's current medication regimen should be reviewed, and any potential interactions of these medications with drugs administered in the perioperative period must be considered. Depending on the nature of the procedure and the patient's comorbidities, some medications may have beneficial effects on the surgery and some may have detrimental effects. Some of the commonly encountered medications are:

1. Cardiac and antihypertensive medications: In general, all antihypertensive medications should be continued through the morning of surgery. Stopping beta blockers or alpha-2 agonists (clonidine) may result in rebound hypertension. Angiotensin-converting enzyme (ACE) inhibitors and angiotensin receptor blockers have been associated with prolonged and resistant hypotension after induction of anesthesia. Currently, whether or not these drugs should be held prior to surgery is controversial within the anesthesiology community, and practice varies widely. Diuretics can be held on the morning of surgery provided they have not been prescribed for congestive failure. Patients with cardiovascular disease taking statin drugs, beta blockers, digoxin, antiarrhythmics, and antiplatelet agents should continue taking these medications because discontinuation can have detrimental effects.
2. Aspirin, antiplatelet agents such as clopidogrel, low-molecular-weight heparin, and warfarin: The decision to discontinue these medications, in general, depends on the surgeon's preference and the type of surgery. Anticoagulation

or antiplatelet therapy may limit the choice of anesthetic to general or sedation, as a spinal or epidural is relatively contraindicated.

Whenever a decision is made to hold these agents, it is important to carefully weigh the risks and potential benefits, and to involve the patient's cardiologist or primary care physicians. There may be an increased risk of vascular events if chronic aspirin or antiplatelet medications are stopped perioperatively. In general, for high-risk patients such as those with cardiac or vascular disease, renal insufficiency, and diabetes, aspirin should not be stopped for procedures with minimal bleeding such as cataract surgery or endoscopies. If there is concern over significant blood loss such as may occur in intracranial surgery, stopping aspirin for 3 to 4 days prior to surgery should be sufficient.

For patients with recently placed coronary stents (< 1 year), aspirin and clopidogrel should not be stopped unless absolutely contraindicated, and then, only with the coordination of the patient's cardiologist. Premature discontinuation of antiplatelet therapy may result in stent thrombosis, MI, and/or death. If a patient can stop warfarin safely, it should be held for at least four doses to allow the INR (international normalized ratio) to normalize (<1.5). If the INR remains elevated on the day of surgery, fresh frozen plasma (FFP) and vitamin K can be given to reverse anticoagulation. Low-molecular-weight heparin should be held for at least 12 to 24 hours before surgery or neuraxial anesthesia to minimize the risk of surgical bleeding and epidural or spinal hematomas.

3. Antiseizure, antipsychotics, narcotics, and medications for asthma and heartburn should be continued on the day of surgery.
4. Herbs and non-vitamin supplements should be stopped 1 week prior to surgery since they may interact with perioperative medications and some may cause increased risk of bleeding.

ASA Status

After the patient has been fully evaluated, the anesthesiologist assigns a physical status to the patient based on his or her medical condition. The American Society of Anesthesiologist (ASA) Physical Status Classification System ranks patients for risk of adverse events during a surgical procedure. (See Table 9–3) This assignment is based on the physical condition of the patient, and is independent of the surgical procedure. The grading system ranks patients from ASA 1, denoting a normal and healthy patient, to ASA 5, signifying a moribund patient who is not expected to survive without the operation. Intraoperative adverse events are encountered more frequently in patients with a poor physical status, greater or equal to ASA 3, especially in emergency situations. Some examples of patients that have a poor physical status who are at high risk for anesthesia and surgery include patients with active heart disease (CHF, aortic stenosis), chronic renal disease, end-stage liver disease, and patients scheduled for surgery who are already in the intensive care unit.

Table 9–3 ASA PHYSICAL STATUS CLASSIFICATION

ASA 1	Normal healthy patient
ASA 2	Patients with mild systemic disease with no functional limitations
ASA 3	Patients with systemic disease with functional limitations
ASA 4	Patients with severe systemic disease that is a constant threat to life
ASA 5	Moribund patients who are not expected to survive without intervention.
"E"	The suffix "E" is attached to the ASA classification for all emergent procedures, that is, ASA 3E

Informed Consent

Most patients are anxious and apprehensive before surgery. The preoperative visit is an opportunity for the patient to discuss the anesthetic plan and express his or her concerns before the surgery. In order to obtain informed consent, the patient should receive a fair and reasonable account of the proposed procedures and the inherent risks. Risks that are reasonably likely to occur with the anesthetic should be mentioned, for example, nausea/vomiting, sore throat with a general anesthetic, or subdural puncture headache following placement of a spinal or epidural. The discussion should be informative and reassuring, answering all the patient's questions. This discussion should also be documented appropriately in the medical chart.

In summary, the preoperative evaluation consists of a history, physical examination, relevant laboratory tests, and consultations which allow the anesthesiologist to assess the patient's physical status and optimize his or her medical condition preoperatively. Using this information, an appropriate anesthetic plan is formed by the anesthesiologist, the patient is educated about anesthesia, and informed consent is obtained. Successful preoperative assessment and management of the patient in the preoperative period may result in decreased perioperative morbidity and mortality, as well as an improved efficiency in the operating room.

Comprehension Questions

9.1. The hospital has asked its anesthesia department to reduce the resources utilized in the pre-op clinic. To comply, the department agrees to reduce the number of patients by agreeing that the anesthesiologists will evaluate which patient(s) in the pre-op holding area on the morning of surgery?

A. An ASA II patient undergoing a thoracotomy for lymphoma.
B. An ASA II patient undergoing a hemipelvectomy for tumor resection.
C. An ASA III patient undergoing a carpal tunnel release.
D. An ASA IV patient undergoing a laparoscopic cholecystectomy.

9.2. Which of the following are the benefits of preoperative testing?

A. Inducing anxiety by informing the patient about his or her risks of surgery
B. Allowing for the generation of additional revenue from routine laboratory tests
C. Increasing cancellations on the day of surgery
D. Reducing the ordering of unnecessary laboratory tests

ANSWERS

9.1. **C.** Healthy patients undergoing minor or even moderately complex surgical procedures may, in general, be evaluated by the anesthesiologist on the morning of surgery (unless the institution has a policy to the contrary). Healthy patients undergoing a complex or high-risk surgical procedure (A, B) need to be evaluated prior to the morning of surgery, to be certain that their condition is optimized.

Patients with moderate or significant comorbidities (ASA III or IV) and who are undergoing minor low-risk surgical procedures may be evaluated on the morning of surgery if their medical condition is stable (C). Patients with significant comorbidities who are undergoing a complex or high-risk surgical procedure need to be evaluated prior to the morning of surgery.

9.2. **D.** Preoperative evaluation allays a patient's anxiety, and allows for the optimization of his or her medical condition prior to surgery. Since the lab tests in the preoperative clinic are usually prescribed by protocol, the preoperative clinic actually reduces the ordering of unnecessary tests prior to surgery. The preoperative evaluation of complex patients or patients undergoing complex or high-risk procedures has been shown to reduce cancellations on the day of surgery.

Clinical Pearls

- The preoperative evaluation is a vital step as the information provided can reduce the patient's perioperative risk, as well as promote operating room efficiency by minimizing delays and cancellations on the day of surgery. Also, the preoperative evaluation is a valuable means to ease a patient's preoperative anxiety.
- Preoperative laboratory studies can aid in risk assessment, and guide optimization of medical treatment as well as provide baseline values that guide intraoperative treatments. Only appropriate laboratory studies should be ordered, based on the patient's medical condition and type of surgery.
- The ACC/AHA guidelines on preoperative cardiac evaluation consider the type of surgery as well as the patient's active cardiac conditions and functional capacity to assess a patient's cardiac risk for surgery and need for additional testing.

REFERENCES

Barash PG, Cullen BF, Stoelting RK. *Clinical Anesthesia*. 5th ed. Philadelphia, PA: Lippincott, Williams and Wilkins; 2006.

Practice advisory for the perioperative management of patients with cardiac rhythm management devices: Pacemakers and implantable cardioverter-defibrillators. *Anesthesiology*. 2005;103:186-198.

Sweitzer BJ. ACC/AHA 2007 guidelines on perioperative cardiovascular evaluation and care for noncardiac surgery. ASA *newsletter*. 2008; 72.

Sweitzer BJ. *Preoperative Assessment and Management*. 2nd ed. Philadelphia, PA: Lippincott, Williams and Wilkins; 2008.

SECTION III

Clinical Cases

Part 1. Introductory Cases

Case 10

A 52-year-old man has had progressive knee pain with swelling, and a Baker cyst just behind his right knee. Recently, the pain has increased in intensity, and has kept him from sleeping at night. His orthopedic surgeon has tentatively diagnosed a torn meniscus, and recommended an arthroscopy as an outpatient. The patient has had no major illnesses other than the typical childhood diseases. He has had no previous operations or anesthetics, nor a family history of problems with anesthesia. He has no allergies to medications, does not smoke, and consumes alcohol occasionally at social events. His laboratory results and physical examination by an internist were all normal. He has had nothing to eat or drink since he went to bed last night. On examination, the patient weighs 160 lb and is 5 ft, 8 in tall. His neck appears to be supple and mobile. He opens his mouth without difficulty, and with his head extended and tongue protruding, his uvula is completely visible.

- ➤ How are a patient's general medical condition, and his risk for difficult airway management classified?
- ➤ In which stage of anesthesia is the patient most vulnerable, and why?
- ➤ Which components of a pre-anesthetic evaluation are often not included in a patient's typical history and physical examination?

ANSWERS TO CASE 10:
Anesthesia for the "Healthy" Patient

Summary: A 52-year-old healthy patient with persistent and increasing knee pain is scheduled for an outpatient arthroscopy. His uvula is completely visible.

- A patient's **ASA Physical Status Classification**, noted as ASA I-IV, categorizes patients according to their comorbidities. **The Mallampati airway classification** describes the amount of a patient's uvula visible when a patient extends his neck and protrudes his tongue, and is one predictor of the risk of difficult airway management.
- **Patients are most vulnerable in Stage II** of anesthesia, since they are hyperexcitable to external stimuli, and have lost both their airway reflexes and autonomic stability.
- **An anesthetic evaluation prior to surgery** should include the patient's history regarding their response to previous anesthetics, NPO status, presence or absence of gastric reflux, difficulty or ease of airway management, history or family history of malignant hyperthermia or pseudocholinesterase deficiency, an examination of the oral cavity, airway and neck mobility, and the ease of i.v. access.

ANALYSIS

Objectives

1. Introduce the learner to fundamental terminology and processes used by anesthesiologists.
2. Emphasize the anesthesiology-specific components of the pre-anesthetic evaluation which are in addition to typical routine physical examination.
3. Introduce the learner to common categorizations of patients according to their comorbidities using the American Society of Anesthesiologists (ASA) Physical Status Classification, and to their risk for difficult airway management using the Mallampati classification of airways.
4. Familiarize the learner with the stages of anesthesia and their physiologic sequela.

Considerations

A commonly-used method of describing the complexity of a patient's medical condition is the American Society of Anesthesiologists' (ASA) Physical Status Classification (Please see Table 10–1). This classification is a useful indicator of surgical mortality. (Please see Figure 10–1.) Since this patient

Table 10–1 ITEMS IN PRE-ANESTHESIA EVALUATION IN ADDITION TO A ROUTINE PHYSICAL EXAMINATION

- Response to previous anesthetics including difficulty or ease of airway management, postoperative intubation, tracheotomy, malignant hyperthermia, or pseudocholinesterase deficiency
- NPO status
- Presence or absence of gastric reflux
- Medications on the day of surgery (particularly bronchodilators)
- Examination of the airway and neck mobility
- Ease of i.v. access

(Please also see the fundamental information regarding the preoperative evaluation)

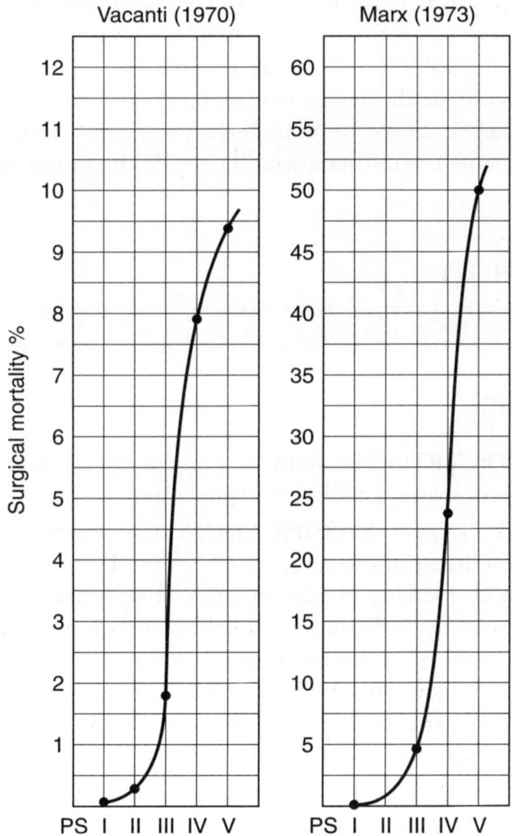

Figure 10–1. ASA Physical Status Classification correlates with surgical mortality in two studies. *(Reproduced from ASA Newsletter 2002;66(9) [Mark J. Lema, editor]. http://www.asahq.org/Newsletters/2002/9_02/vent_0902.htm. Reprinted with permission of the American Society of Anesthesiologists, 520 N. Northwest Highway, Park Ridge, Illinois 60068-2573.)*

Table 10–2 MALLAMPATI CLASSIFICATIONS

Mallampati class 1	The uvula is entirely visible	Easy intubation
Mallampati class 2	The uvula is partially visible	Intubation may be challenging
Mallampati class 3	The uvula is not visible	Intubation likely to be difficult

has no medical comorbidities, he is classified as an "ASA Class 1." He has not had anything to eat or drink since midnight, so he can be considered as "NPO." The potential ease or difficulty of intubation is often addressed using the Mallampati airway classification. In this particular patient, the uvula is completely visible when the patient's head is extended and his tongue protruded (Please see Table 10–2). Thus, this patient is anticipated to pose little or no difficulty with airway management and his airway is classed as Mallampati Class 1. Since he is undergoing a quick procedure such as an arthroscopy, a general anesthetic would provide the fastest recovery with few complications.

APPROACH TO
The "Healthy" Patient: ASA I, Mallampati Class I

DEFINITIONS

AIRWAY PROTECTION: The ability to prevent the aspiration of gastric contents into the lungs which could cause pneumonia.

ASA PHYSICAL STATUS CLASSIFICATION: Addresses the extent of a patient's medical comorbidities prior to surgery as ASA I to IV. Comorbidities are often associated with an increase in postoperative complications. Both comorbidities and complications influence the likelihood that this ambulatory patient could be discharged on the day of surgery, versus needing to remain in the hospital. For an emergency case, an "E" is added. The ASA classifications are also commonly used by other specialties. (Please see Table 10–3.)

DEPTH OF ANESTHESIA: The level of a patient's progression from consciousness to unconsciousness following the administration of anesthesia. Depth is indicated by the stages of anesthesia. (Please see Table 10–4.)

MALLAMPATI CLASSIFICATION: One of the factors predicting the difficulty of airway management and the placement of an endotracheal tube. It refers to the amount of the uvula visible when a patient's head is extended and his or her tongue protruded. (Please see Table 10–2.)

Table 10–3 ASA CLASSIFICATIONS

ASA I	**No systemic disease**	
ASA II	**Mild systemic disease**	Smoking, controlled hypertension, etc.
ASA III	**Major systemic disease**	Stable coronary artery disease, reactive airway disease, mild renal or hepatic impairment, etc.
ASA IV	**Severe systemic disease**	Unstable coronary artery disease, chronic renal failure, severe COPD, etc., or a combination
ASA V	**Imminent death**	Ruptured aortic, aneurysm, etc.

E is added to the above to signify an emergency case.

CLINICAL APPROACH

The preparation for any surgical procedure includes an history, a physical examination, and laboratory tests which are appropriate when considering the patient's age, medical problems, and the type of procedure. In addition to the typical presurgical "work up," an anesthetic evaluation is also important prior to the administration of anesthesia—whether general, regional anesthesia, or monitored anesthesia care (local infiltration with monitoring and sedation by an anesthesia provider). The pre-anesthesia evaluation addresses factors such as the patient's NPO status, the presence or absence of gastric reflux, his or her response to previous anesthetics, a reconciliation of medications taken on the day of surgery, and any pertinent family history including direct queries regarding malignant hyperthermia

Table 10–4 PHASES AND STAGES OF ANESTHESIA

PHASES OF ANESTHESIA	STAGES OF ANESTHESIA
Induction	**I.** Analgesia. Patient is awake and responsive. **II.** Hyper-excitable, delirium, movement, autonomic instability, loss of airway protection, significant risk of complications. Protective airway reflexes lost.
Maintenance	**III.** Return of autonomic stability, preservation of vital functions. Stage III is separated into 4 planes. Planes 2 and 3 are **surgical anesthesia.** **IV.** Depression of vital functions, autonomic instability **V.** Cardiac arrest
Emergence from anesthesia	**Stage III, Stage II, then Stage I.** Stage II also happens at emergence.

or pseudocholinesterase deficiency. In addition to the routine history and physical, this information is necessary to allow the formulation of a safe and effective anesthetic plan. (Please also see the chapter on preoperative evaluation).

Additional items on the physical examination include a careful evaluation of the patient's airway anatomy and neck mobility, and the ease of i.v. access. In particular, the airway examination, including the "fingers breadth" of mouth opening, hyomental distance, and Mallampati classification, provide information regarding the potential difficulty or ease of intubation. The patient's NPO status, and presence or absence of gastric reflux or of a syndrome that significantly increases gastric volume may signal the need for a rapid sequence induction (Please see Case 11), and similarly influences the anesthetic plan.

The anesthetic plan should allow for a rapid return of mental function, and especially in the case of outpatients, recovery of psychomotor skills prior to discharge, as well as to minimize complications. Patients must be able to walk (if they could walk prior to the procedure), be medically stable, and free of pain, and nausea or vomiting prior to discharge from the hospital.

The temporal progression of an anesthetic can be separated into several phases: the beginning is typically referred to as induction, the middle, as maintenance, and the end, emergence. The depth of anesthesia, or progression to and from unconsciousness, is referred to as the stages of anesthesia. (Please see Table 10–4). Stage I lasts from full consciousness until a patient closes his eyes. Stage II begins when the patient closes his eyes. It is characterized by a hyperexcitability to external stimuli which may include vocalization and movement, the loss of protective airway reflexes, and autonomic instability. Stage II ends when patients regain autonomic stability. It is during this stage that patients are most vulnerable. Stage III is the stage of surgical anesthesia. It is divided into four planes; planes 3 and 4 are optimal for surgery.

Prior to the induction of anesthesia, monitors are placed including a blood pressure cuff, an electrocardiogram, a pulse oximeter, a capnograph (which monitors end-tidal CO_2, detecting any deficit in ventilation or metabolism or elimination of CO_2), and an oxygen analyzer in the breathing circuit (which confirms the continuous flow of oxygen).

Anesthesia is most frequently *induced* using an intravenous anesthetic such as propofol, etomidate, or sodium thiopental. Patients perceive intravenous anesthetics as a pleasant way to go to sleep, and these agents rapidly render the patient into Stage III of anesthesia, quickly traversing the troublesome Stage II.

Once anesthesia is induced and patients enter Stages II or III, the oral and pharyngeal muscles lose tone and the patient's airway often begins to obstruct. The airway can be managed by tilting the head back and moving the jaw forward at the angle of the mandible until the airway is patent. An oral airway may be helpful in preventing the tongue from obstructing the pharynx, or it may not be necessary. Induction can also be accomplished with inhalational anesthetics, and with the newer agents, can be quite pleasant. However, patients do not traverse Stage II as rapidly, and are thus vulnerable to aspiration and difficult airway management for that short period of time.

Table 10–5 INDICATIONS FOR TRACHEAL INTUBATION

- Airway access
- Airway protection
- Need for muscle relaxation (paralysis)
- Length of procedure (> 2 hours)
- Need for mechanical ventilation

Anesthesia is typically *maintained* with an inhalation agent such as desflurane or sevoflurane, or with an intravenous infusion of propofol. Oxygen and inhalation anesthetics are administered with a mask or through airway device such as a laryngeal mask airway (LMA) or an endotracheal tube. It should be noted that after a period of 2 hours, pressure on nerves from a mask may cause nerve palsies involving small branches of the facial nerves, particularly in the peri-oral region, potentially yielding hyperesthesia or analgesia on the face. The laryngeal mask airway can similarly cause pressure on the recurrent laryngeal nerves, leading to (usually transient) vocal cord paralysis.

Unlike a mask or laryngeal mask airway, the placement of an endotracheal tube usually requires paralyzing a patient with a neuromuscular blocker. Since paralysis removes the patient's ability to breathe, and since intubation requires the mechanical instrumentation of the pharynx and trachea (which can lead to complications), intubation is only performed when there is an indication. (Please see Table 10–5.)

The maintenance of anesthesia is often supplemented with an opiate to reduce pain during and after surgery. This in turn facilitates a reduction in the amount of anesthetic that is required. This patient, for example, would receive desflurane as the inhalation agent, O_2, and a small amount of fentanyl added near the end of the procedure to minimize postoperative pain.

As wound closure begins, the anesthetic agent is discontinued. *Emergence* begins, and the patient is allowed to awaken. He traverses the stages of anesthesia in reverse order, including Stage II. In fact, Stage II is more likely to be observed at emergence than induction, because at induction, patients receive an intravenous induction agent and pass rapidly (and almost imperceptibly) through Stage II.

CLINICAL SUMMARY

This healthy man undergoing an arthroscopy will be monitored with a blood pressure cuff, electrocardiogram, pulse oximeter, end-tidal CO_2 monitor (capnograph), and a circuit oxygen analyzer. His anesthetic will be induced with propofol, a laryngeal mask placed, and his anesthetic maintained with desflurane including a small amount of opiate at the end of the case. Once he awakens and can respond to commands (meaning that he has successfully traversed Stage II), the laryngeal mask will be removed.

Comprehension Questions

10.1. A 32-year-old woman is scheduled for a laparoscopic tubal ligation. A surgical admission history and physical, and pre-anesthesia evaluation are performed. The patient's personal and family history of problems with anesthesia (ie, malignant hyperthermia or pseudocholinesterase deficiency), her NPO status, the presence or absence of gastric reflux, and medications taken on the day of surgery are elicited. Which of the following should also be included in her preoperative management?

A. An abdominal examination, noting any tenderness and/or rebound.
B. An electrocardiogram and chest x-ray.
C. An airway examination including the degree of mouth opening and neck range of motion.
D. A prescription for postoperative analgesics.

10.2. A 63-year-old man presents for an elective laparoscopic cholecystectomy. He is obese, has angina unpredictably and at rest, and chronic obstructive pulmonary disease (COPD). Which of the following would be his ASA classification?

A. ASA I
B. ASA II
C. ASA III
D. ASA IV
E. ASA V

10.3. With his neck extended, mouth open, and tongue protruded, the patient's uvula is not visible. His airway should be classed as which of the following?

A. Mallampati 1
B. Mallampati 2
C. Mallampati 3

10.4. As this patient awakens from a general anesthetic for an arthroscopy, he coughs, moves his arm, squirms on the table, and phonates when touched by the surgeon. He does not open his eyes or squeeze his hand on command. Which of the following is most accurate?

A. Movement and phonation indicate that the patient is "awake."
B. The patient is emerging from anesthesia. Since he can phonate, he can protect his airway.
C. Stage II is the stage at which the risk of complications is greatest.
D. This stage of anesthesia is observed more frequently at induction than emergence.

ANSWERS

10.1. **C.** An anesthetic evaluation includes an airway examination addressing the patient's degree of mouth opening typically expressed in "fingers breadths," and neck range of motion including flexion and extension, and side-to-side motions. An electrocardiogram is not necessary for young, healthy patients, and a chest x-ray is only necessary as medically indicated.

10.2. **D.** The patient is obese, with angina unpredictably and at rest, and COPD. His angina at rest represents a systemic disease which is unstable, and which could be life threatening. In addition, he also has another comorbidity, COPD. His classification is ASA IV. Because this is a scheduled case, no "E" is added after the "IV."

10.3. **C.** Since this patient's uvula is not visible, his airway is classed as Mallampati 3, suggesting a difficult intubation.

10.4. **C.** During Stage II of anesthesia, patients are hyperexcitable to external stimuli, and may phonate, move, manifest autonomic instability including arrhythmias, and cannot protect their airways. This is the stage at which the risk of complications is greatest. Because of the rapidity with which patients receiving intravenous induction agents pass through Stage II, this stage of anesthesia is observed more frequently at emergence than induction. The patient's ability to phonate is not related to his ability to protect his airway.

Clinical Pearls

- The pre-anesthetic evaluation determines the anesthetic plan.
- Difficult intubations may often be predicted.
- The excitement stage of anesthesia (Stage II) happens at induction and emergence.
- Intubation requires an indication.

REFERENCES

Miller RD, ed. *Anesthesia*, 6th ed. Philadelphia, PA: Elsevier Churchill Livingstone; 2005.

Case 11

A 27-year-old woman presents to the emergency department complaining of abdominal pain, nausea, and vomiting. Her pain began in the peri-umbilical region and has now migrated toward the right lower quadrant of the abdomen. Her serum HCG is negative. A surgery consult is obtained, and based on her history, physical, and findings suggestive of acute appendicitis seen on abdominal CT scan, she is scheduled for emergency appendectomy. The patient is otherwise healthy and takes no regular medications. Her surgical history includes a tonsillectomy at age 10, and a dilatation and curettage (D&C) at age 25. She has not had problems with previous anesthetics.

➤ What would you include in your preoperative evaluation of this patient?

➤ What medications will you use for induction and maintenance of anesthesia?

➤ How will you manage postoperative pain in this patient?

ANSWERS TO CASE 11:
Anesthesia for Emergency Appendectomy

Summary: A healthy woman presents with acute appendicitis. The urgent nature of the surgery precludes any delay due to risk of rupture and subsequent peritonitis.

- **Preoperative evaluation:** Complete history and physical examination, and time of last ingestion of food or contrast. Because of her age and healthy status, no laboratory tests are required.
- **Medications used for induction and maintenance of anesthesia:** Combination of a narcotic, an inhalational agent, and a muscle relaxant. The patient will receive general anesthesia, with a rapid sequence induction to minimize the chances of aspiration. The choice of induction agent will not significantly impact her hemodynamic status, as the patient is neither hypovolemic nor hypotensive.
- **How to manage postoperative pain:** Postoperative pain is managed with intravenous narcotics. Other postoperative issues that may present are nausea, vomiting, and ileus.

ANALYSIS

Objectives

1. Consider the elements of the preoperative evaluation and optimization prior to emergency abdominal surgery (airway examination, comorbidities, hemodynamic status, perforated vs. nonperforated appendicitis, NPO guidelines, and other testing as indicated by the patient's comorbidities).
2. Understand the techniques used in patients with "full stomachs" including rapid sequence induction and aspiration prophylaxis.
3. Consideration implication of surgical procedure on anesthesia: full stomach precautions and rapid sequence induction, laparoscopic versus open appendectomy, fluid management, premedication, prophylaxis for postoperative nausea and vomiting, postoperative pain control.

Considerations

Several special considerations are warranted in this healthy, young woman scheduled for an emergency surgical procedure. Appendectomy is a minor surgical procedure with a low probability of significant blood loss, so an adequately running peripheral intravenous suffices for intravenous access.

A physical examination and review of the patient's vital signs can help determine the patient's volume status and hemodynamic stability. Volume-depleted patients should receive resuscitative fluids before proceeding with anesthesia. Many patients presenting with acute appendicitis are febrile and tachycardic at baseline, so a "tilt test" may be helpful to determine degree of intravascular depletion.

Since the patient is of reproductive age, it is important to inquire about the possibility of pregnancy. Many institutions routinely perform pregnancy tests in women of reproductive age undergoing surgery; others inquire, and a pregnancy test may be performed if the history indicates such a possibility.

The anesthetic plan in this patient is general anesthesia with endotracheal intubation, controlled mechanical ventilation, and standard monitoring. Since the procedure is an emergency, the patient is unlikely to have fasted as she would have before a scheduled surgical procedure. Moreover, pain in and of itself reduces gastric emptying. Thus she is said to have a "full stomach," and will thus require precautions to prevent the aspiration of gastric contents. In the operating room, the standard monitors are applied, and the patient is preoxygenated (≥ 3 minutes). Anesthesia is induced with propofol 1.5 to 2.5 mg/kg. Cricoid pressure (Sellick maneuver) is applied by an assistant to reduce the risk of passive regurgitation of gastric contents. Succinylcholine 1 to 2 mg/kg is administered for paralysis, and the patient is intubated.

Patients are typically paralyzed for abdominal surgery in order to facilitate exposure of the surgical field, and minimize trauma to the abdominal muscles. Once the patient recovers from the short-acting neuromuscular blocker, succinylcholine, she is treated with a longer-acting, nondepolarizing blocker, vecuronium.

Two potential postoperative problems are optimally addressed preemptively, and prior to emergence. First, morphine 0.1 mg/kg is administered during the case as an adjuvant to anesthesia and for postoperative pain relief. Second, young women are most likely to experience postoperative nausea and vomiting. Ondansetron, 4 mg, is given in the last 15 minutes of case to reduce the incidence of this unpleasant complication.

At the end of the surgery, the patient's muscle relaxation is reversed with neostigmine 0.05 mg/kg and glycopyrrolate 0.01 mg/kg. Before she is fully responsive, the normal airway reflexes are absent, and she is unable to protect her airway from the aspiration of stomach contents. She is extubated once she is alert, following commands, and shows good strength. Following extubation, the patient is transferred to the post-anesthesia care unit (PACU) for postoperative care.

APPROACH TO
Anesthesia for Emergency Appendectomy

DEFINITIONS

PREOXYGENATION: Since room air is only 21% oxygen, and since the patient will be paralyzed and apneic during intubation, it is desirable for the patient to have additional oxygen reserves. This is accomplished by asking her to breathe 100% oxygen for 3 minutes prior to induction. Alternatively, six large breaths of 100% oxygen have been shown to be equally effective.

In addition to inspiring oxygen, "denitrogenation" also occurs as the nitrogen in plasma, which reflects the nitrogen concentration in room air, seeks equilibrium, and diffuses out across the alveolus. This process of denitrogenation is actually as important as the inspiration of oxygenation in preventing alveolar hypoxia and hypoxemia. The rationale for preoxygenation is that in the event that a patient cannot be ventilated or intubated, he or she will have adequate oxygen in reserve to survive long enough to awaken and resume breathing.

RAPID SEQUENCE INDUCTION (RSI): A technique of rapid induction and intubation used to minimize the risk of aspiration. It involves preoxygenation by mask, the administration of an intravenous induction agent immediately followed by a rapid acting neuromuscular blocking drug, and the use of cricoid pressure. Mask ventilation before endotracheal intubation is avoided to prevent insufflation of gas into the patient's stomach.

CRICOID PRESSURE (SELLICK MANEUVER): Cricoid pressure is the posterior displacement of the cricoid cartilage against the vertebral body in attempt to occlude the esophagus. It is applied by an assistant before the loss of consciousness (and protective airway reflexes), and is released only after correct placement of the endotracheal tube has been confirmed.

SUCCINYLCHOLINE: A depolarizing neuromuscular blocker often used for rapid sequence induction because of its rapid onset (usually <60 seconds). Potential side effects include myalgias, bradycardia and arrhythmias, hyperkalemia in certain patients (recent burn injury, upper and lower motor neuron disease, prolonged bed rest, muscular dystrophies, and closed head injuries). Succinylcholine can trigger malignant hyperthermia in susceptible patients.

MALIGNANT HYPERTHERMIA (MH): A potentially lethal hypermetabolic syndrome that occurs in susceptible patients after exposure to a triggering anesthetic agent. The presenting signs include tachycardia, acidosis, hypercarbia, sustained muscle contraction, hypoxemia, and hyperthermia. Common triggering agents include succinylcholine, and volatile anesthetics including halothane, enflurane, desflurane, sevoflurane, and isoflurane.

POSTOPERATIVE NAUSEA AND VOMITING (PONV): A common side effect seen in patients undergoing general anesthesia. Risk factors include prior history of postoperative nausea, motion sickness, major abdominal surgery, nonsmoker, female gender, and use of opioids.

CLINICAL APPROACH

Aspiration

The American Society of Anesthesiologists has described and standardized guidelines for fasting or "NPO (nothing by mouth) Guidelines" for patients prior to elective surgery. The guidelines require an abstinence from clear liquids for 2 hours, and from milk or a light meal for 6 hours. But the patients undergoing emergency surgery are in a different category. Pain, trauma, and abdominal emergencies are associated with a delay in gastric emptying, thus increasing the risk of these patients for the aspiration of gastric contents. Certain diseases, such as diabetes delay gastric transit time and may also pose an aspiration risk. Other conditions associated with increased aspiration risk are ileus, obesity, pregnancy, hiatal hernia, scleroderma, and altered mental status which occurs following stroke.

The risk of aspiration with anesthesia is 5 events per 10,000 anesthetics. Since the mortality from aspiration is significant and varies from 3% to 70%, **all patients presenting for emergency surgery should be treated as though they have a full stomach.** Early studies showed that the risk of aspiration and the resulting damage to the respiratory mucosa increase with a gastric volume of more than 25 mL and pH less than 2.5. So some practitioners attempt to reduce the volume and increase the pH of the gastric contents. Nonparticulate antacids such as sodium citrate decrease the acidity, but increase gastric volume. Histamine receptor antagonists such as ranitidine decrease the secretion of gastric acid, but do not affect the acidity of the contents already present in the stomach (thus reducing the value of their administration just prior to an anesthetic). Metoclopramide stimulates gastric emptying, and increases the lower esophageal sphincter tone. Anticholinergic drugs like glycopyrrolate decrease the gastric secretions, but also decrease the lower esophageal sphincter tone, an undesirable trait in the presence of a full stomach. However, none of these drugs have been shown to alter the incidence of aspiration, and none of them are approved by the Food and Drug Administration for aspiration prophylaxis.

The use of a nasogastric tube to decompress the stomach is common, but controversial, as it does not guarantee gastric emptying. Somewhat paradoxically, a nasogastric tube may actually be detrimental by mechanically decreasing tone of the upper and lower esophageal sphincters, and acting as a "wick" to facilitate the movement of gastric contents into the pharynx.

Patients presenting for abdominal emergencies can also present with ileus. Factors predisposing for ileus include narcotics, antacids, anticoagulants, phenothiazines, ganglionic blockers, metabolic derangements like hyponatremia, hypokalemia, hypomagnesemia, sepsis, infection, and inflammation. Ileus can also persist in the postoperative period as well. Small bowel function commonly recovers within a day and gastric motility within 1 to 2 days. However, colonic motility can take up to 5 days. Thus even though patients status post abdominal surgery may have been fasted, they still require attention to the risk of aspiration if an additional operation is required.

Preoperative Optimization: Resuscitation of Blood Volume

Patients presenting with an acute abdomen are often quite dehydrated as a result of vomiting and loss of fluids into the intestine. This may be reflected as tachycardia, oliguria, altered sensorium, decrease in skin turgor, dry mucus membranes, and orthostatic hypotension. It may also manifest as increased variation of pulse pressure with respiration, if not outright tachycardia. An elevated hematocrit is suggestive of dehydration, and serum electrolytes may be abnormal since severe vomiting can lead to metabolic alkalosis due to loss of gastric acid. Patients should receive adequate and appropriate volume resuscitation prior to the induction of anesthesia to prevent significant hypotension due to vasodilation caused by some anesthetic drugs, as well as the removal of the patient's endogenous sympathetic responses to pain once anesthesia is induced.

The anesthetic options for an open appendectomy are general anesthesia or central neuraxial anesthesia. The usual practice is general anesthesia, using a rapid sequence induction and tracheal intubation. Previously known as a "crash" induction, the rapid sequence induction is not without hazard. Complications include failure to ventilate due to closure of the vocal cords, cricoid ring fracture, esophageal rupture, and profound hypotension. It involves the application of cricoid pressure to minimize the risk of aspiration. First described by Sellick in 1961, it is designed to cause temporary occlusion of the upper end of the esophagus by posterior pressure of the cricoid cartilage ring against the cervical vertebra. Active vomiting, cervical spine injury, and tracheal injury are contraindications to the use of cricoid pressure.

Propofol is most frequently used as the induction agent of choice due to its rapid onset, short duration of action, and smooth and pleasing emergence. However, propofol causes vasodilation, so its use presupposes that the patient is well hydrated and not demonstrating signs of hypovolemia. The typical dose of propofol is 1.5 to 2.5 mg/kg for induction, although the individual dose requirement varies markedly. In patients in whom hypotension is a concern, ketamine (1 mg/kg i.v.) or etomidate (0.1-0.4 mg/kg i.v.) are suitable alternatives. Because of its rapid onset, succinylcholine (1-1.5 mg/kg i.v.) is the neuromuscular blocking drug of choice in rapid sequence inductions. Its short duration allows the paralyzed patient, who can neither be ventilated nor intubated, to resume breathing promptly, thus lessening the likelihood of morbidity when compared to the longer-acting neuromuscular agents.

Once intubation is accomplished and proper endotracheal tube placement is confirmed, cricoid pressure can be released. If intubation is unsuccessful, cricoid pressure should be maintained continuously during subsequent intubation attempts and during mask ventilation.

Another possible approach is neuraxial anesthesia (such as spinal). Indeed, spinal may be preferred in pregnant patients in order to minimize the systemic concentrations of general anesthetics. However, the sensory level required for a routine appendectomy is T4, which is quite high.

An open appendectomy is a short procedure, hence the anesthetic agents used should have a short half-life to facilitate quick emergence. Desflurane and sevoflurane have low blood-gas partition coefficients, thus low solubility in blood, and are suitable for short procedures. The role of nitrous oxide in the maintenance of anesthesia is controversial due to its effect on bowel distention and postoperative nausea and vomiting. Muscle relaxants are required for adequate surgical visualization. In general, intermediate-acting nondepolarizing agents are used in appropriate doses.

It is important to ensure that the patient is awake and following commands prior to extubation. If a patient can follow commands, then his or her laryngeal reflexes, which enable the larynx to close during vomiting, are likely to be intact. Conversely, patients who are unable to follow commands are also unlikely to be able to protect their own airways.

If a patient vomits, the head of the bed should be dropped ten degrees and the pharynx suctioned. Intact laryngeal reflexes enable the patient to clear secretions and protect their airway. Respiratory criteria for extubation include adequate tidal volumes, a normal respiratory rate, and the ability to cough and breathe deeply. A sustained head lift lasting 5 seconds typically predicts that the muscle relaxants have been successfully reversed.

Postoperative Complications

Nausea and vomiting are troublesome complications of anesthesia, especially in young women. The etiology of postoperative nausea and vomiting is multifactorial. The vomiting centre is located in the area postrema of the brainstem and receives vagal afferents from the gastrointestinal tract. Selective serotonin receptor antagonists like ondansetron, dolasetron, and granisetron have proven to be effective in alleviating postoperative nausea and vomiting with minimal side effects when administered just prior to the end of a case. Other classes of drugs including anticholinergics, dopamine antagonists and antihistamines may also be utilized, but have significant side effects. Clonidine, dexamethasone, and acupuncture have also been found to be effective. Combination of therapies for the prevention of postoperative nausea and vomiting provides maximal benefit.

The management of postoperative pain should begin in the operating room. The goal is to minimize any potential sensitization of the spinal cord and brain propagated by tissue injury and pain stimuli. One method of the preemptive analgesia involves central neuraxial blockade. However, if a general anesthetic is used, local field block in the area of the incision is effective as well. Opioids are most widely used to control postoperative pain but have significant side effects like ileus, respiratory depression, nausea, and vomiting. Nonsteroidal anti-inflammatory drugs (NSAIDs) may also be used for postoperative pain control in these patients.

Comprehension Questions

11.1. During a rapid sequence induction, when would it be appropriate to release cricoid pressure?
   A. When the patient becomes unconscious.
   B. After the induction agent has been given but before the neuromuscular blocking drug is given.
   C. After proper placement of the endotracheal tube has been confirmed.
   D. Cricoid pressure is not indicated in this instance.

11.2. Which of the following is the most significant risk factor for postoperative nausea and vomiting?
   A. Female gender
   B. Surgery on the breast
   C. Smoking
   D. Nonsteroidal anti-inflammatory agents given during surgery
   E. Age over 60 years

11.3. Which of the following is the major advantage of spinal anesthetic in the pregnant patient?
   A. A peripheral neuraxial block minimizes central sensitization to pain.
   B. The level of a spinal anesthesia necessary for an appendectomy is quite low.
   C. Spinals rarely cause headaches in pregnant patients.
   D. A spinal anesthetic allows for anesthesia without significant plasma concentrations of the anesthetic.

ANSWERS

11.1. **C.** Cricoid pressure or Sellick's maneuver is intended to occlude the esophagus to prevent passive regurgitation of gastric contents into the airway. It should be maintained throughout the induction sequence until proper endotracheal tube placement has been confirmed or until successful intubation occurs and during mask ventilation, if needed. Cricoid pressure is indicated in this case.

11.2. **A.** Postoperative nausea and vomiting is most common in women, young people, and patients who have received opioids during surgery. Surprisingly, perhaps the one advantage of smoking (option C) is that smokers tend to have less postoperative nausea and vomiting than nonsmokers. Similarly, the incidence of postoperative nausea and vomiting is lower in the geriatric population.

11.3. **D.** The major advantage of spinal anesthetic in the pregnant patient is that a spinal anesthetic allows for anesthesia without significant plasma concentrations of the anesthetic. While a peripheral block may minimize central sensitization to pain, it is hardly adequate as an anesthetic for an appendectomy. The level of a spinal anesthesia necessary for an appendectomy is T4, which is quiet high. And, a common complication of spinal anesthesia is "spinal headache."

Clinical Pearls

- An appendectomy is a surgical emergency.
- A rapid sequence induction is generally used for patients undergoing anesthesia for emergency surgery, as this is thought to reduce the risk of pulmonary aspiration of gastric contents.
- The patient's hemodynamic status should be taken into account when choosing an induction agent. Patients who appear to be septic or volume depleted should have appropriate volume resuscitation before the induction of anesthesia.
- Adequate pain control prior to emergence and in the postoperative period has many advantages and is the hallmark of an appropriate anesthetic plan.

REFERENCES

Fengler BT. Should etomidate be used for rapid-sequence intubation induction in critically ill septic patients? *Am J of Emerge Med.* 2008;26:229-232.

Hurford WE, Bailin MT, Davison JK, et al., eds. *Clinical Anesthesia Procedures of the Massachusetts General Hospital.* 6th ed. Philadelphia, PA: Lippincott Williams & Wilkins; 2002:174-175, 293, 573-574.

Jackson WL. Should we use etomidate as an induction agent for endotracheal intubation in patients with septic shock?: A critical appraisal. *Chest.* 2005; 127:1031-1038.

Jaffe RA, Samuels SI, eds. *Anesthesiologist's Manual of Surgical Procedures.* 3rd ed. Philadelphia, PA: Lippincott Williams & Wilkins; 2004:407-410, 472-474.

Lejus C, et al. Randomized, single blinded trial of laparoscopic versus open appendectomy in children: effects on postoperative analgesia. *Anesthesiology.* 1996;84:801-806.

Mazurek AJ, et al. Rocuronium versus succinylcholine: are they equally effective during rapid sequence induction of anesthesia? *Anesthesia and Analgesia.* 1998;87:1259-1262.

Miller RD, et al eds. *Miller's Anesthesia.* 6th ed. Philadelphia, PA: Elsevier Churchill Livingstone; 2005:1635, 1647, 2456, 2599-2600.

Sluga M, et al. Rocuronium versus succinylcholine for rapid sequence induction of anesthesia and endotracheal intubation: a prospective, randomized trial in emergent cases. *Anesthesia and Analgesia.* 2005;101:1356-1361.

Stoelting RK, Miller RD, eds. *Basics of Anesthesia.* 5th ed. Philadelphia, PA: Elsevier Churchill Livingstone; 2007:180, 575, 581.

Case 12

An 88-year-old man slipped on the kitchen floor yesterday and fractured his right hip. He is scheduled for an open reduction and internal fixation (ORIF) of the fracture. His past medical history includes coronary artery disease with remote coronary stent placement, congestive heart failure, and hypertension. He is not aware of angina, and states that he sleeps on one pillow at night. However, on interview, he is noted to be mildly confused. He is oriented to time and place, but thinks the year is 1974. He has a sedentary lifestyle, and leaves his apartment only to go to his physician's office, and the pharmacy. His housekeeper performs most of his daily chores, including grocery shopping. The patient's medications include metoprolol, clopidogrel, aspirin, lisinopril, and simvastatin. He took NSAIDs as needed for arthritic pain prior to the fall. The patient has no known drug allergies.

The physical examination reveals an elderly, cachectic male 5 ft 8 in tall, weighing 145 lb. His vital signs include a blood pressure of 135/67 mm Hg, heart rate of 66, and respiratory rate of 16 with an oxygen saturation of 98% on room air. He has a mild limitation of mouth opening, and on airway examination, his airway is a Mallampati class 1. His heart is regular and slow, and his lungs are clear. Laboratory values include a hemoglobin of 9.8 g/dL, a platelet count of 221,000, an international normalized ratio (INR) of 1.1, potassium of 4.1 mEq/L, and blood urea nitrogen (BUN) of 35, and a creatinine of 1.2 mg/dL. His ECG is notable for left ventricular hypertrophy, and his chest x-ray is normal.

- ➤ What are the preoperative concerns for this patient?
- ➤ What are the anesthetic options?

ANSWERS TO CASE 12:

Anesthesia for Elderly Patient with Hip Fracture

Summary: This is an elderly patient with revascularized coronary artery disease who presents for ORIF of a right hip fracture.

- **Preoperative considerations** for this patient include understanding why he fell (did he trip, have a stroke, an arrhythmia, etc.), the status of his mental function and ischemic heart disease including the possibility of stent thrombosis, his NPO status prior to coming to the operating room, the intraoperative possibility of massive blood loss, volume depletion, and coagulopathy.
- **Anesthetic options:** This patient can have this procedure done under general or regional anesthesia in the form of epidural, spinal, or combined spinal epidural block. Given the dual platelet therapy, general anesthesia is probably a safer option. There is increased risk of epidural hematoma with neuraxial anesthesia.

ANALYSIS

Objectives

1. Discuss the preoperative evaluation of an elderly patient.
2. Identify some of the choices of anesthetic technique for hip surgery.
3. List the benefits and risks of regional anesthesia and general anesthesia in the geriatric population.

Considerations

The primary issues for this patient are his confusion, his anemia, and the history of coronary artery disease and stent placement. It is not uncommon for elderly patients to become confused, particularly as their environment changes and they experience pain. However, since the fracture occurred as the result of a fall, it is always important to keep in mind that the "fall" may in fact have represented another type of event. Similarly, a fall also carries the potential for other occult injuries, including a subdural hematoma. Since a hip fracture is not an urgent emergency, these possibilities will usually have been carefully considered prior to a patient's coming to the operating room. Nevertheless, they are important possibilities to keep in mind while caring for these fragile patients.

It is also not uncommon for patients to loose a unit of blood silently into a hip fracture before coming to the operating room. Thus, it is important to ascertain the patient's volume status prior to induction of general anesthesia or placement of a regional anesthetic. Blood should be available prior to surgery, and a large bore intravenous line placed and connected to a fluid warmer. Arterial pressure monitoring in this patient allows for beat-to-beat BP monitoring as well as enable frequent hemoglobin and blood gas assessment.

In the presence of coronary artery disease, the risk of intraoperative and postoperative myocardial ischemia increase during periods of intense stimulation such as during induction, intubation, awakening, and in the presence of postoperative pain. Both general and regional anesthesia can be safely achieved. However, given the presence of both clopidogrel and quite possibly an NSAID, regional anesthesia loses favor as the risk of bleeding outweighs the benefits of a regional technique.

APPROACH TO Anesthesia for Elderly Patient with Hip Fracture

Older individuals often present a multitude of issues which influence the choice of anesthetic to be provided. The aging process affects many of the body's vital functions, many, relevant to the administration of an anesthetic. However, there is significant variability in the relationship between chronological age and physiological age.

Aging reduces the requirement for and clearance of a variety of drugs. This is particularly an issue with respect to the sedative hypnotics, probably resulting from a combination of mechanisms such as a lower volume of distribution, fewer neurons, and an enhanced drug susceptibility. Sedative hypnotic drugs in the context of an anesthetic include anxiolytics, and the induction agents for general anesthesia. These drugs should be administered judiciously and in small doses, if at all.

Aging affects the cardiovascular system by decreasing the responsiveness of beta receptors. Hence, the maximum heart generated by the heart's compensatory mechanisms is reduced with age. An elderly patient may or may not become tachycardic in the presence of fever. Similarly, tachycardia may or may not occur in the presence of hypovolemia. This has two potential consequences: first, acute hypovolemia may be missed; and second, arterial pressure may be more labile since it is one of the few remaining compensatory mechanisms. In addition, arteriosclerosis and coronary artery disease may necessitate that mean arterial pressure be maintained to preserve coronary perfusion.

Pulmonary reserve also declines with age. In particular, aging is associated with decreased vital capacity (VC) and increased residual volume (RV), an increased air trapping and V/Q mismatch (especially when supine), a reduction in the resting arterial O_2 tension (PaO_2), a decreased ventilatory response to hypoxia or hypercarbia, and a reduced ability to cough or clear secretions. These alterations in respiratory physiology can directly affect the ability to ventilate and oxygenate a patient during surgery, and may necessitate a delay in extubation.

Hepatic and renal function also declines with age, often leading to a reduced elimination of drugs. A patient's ability to handle a glucose load also significantly declines with age.

The Preoperative Evaluation: Special Items in Elderly Patients

The goal of the anesthetic is to assess and optimize the patient's condition as much as possible prior to the procedure. If possible, it is desirable to note the patient's functional status prior to the illness—both physically and mentally. Any evidence of central nervous system dysfunction and/or residual from previous illnesses such as stroke should be carefully documented, since these conditions could evolve during the course of the current hospitalization.

If a patient has coronary artery disease, it is especially important to take a clear history as to whether or not chest pain is occurring, whether it is stable and has been assessed, or whether the pain represents a new and thus acute event. The functional capacity, such as ability to walk two flights of stairs (equivalent to 4 METS) or more vigorous activity (ie, any type of sports) will generally indicates an adequate cardiac reserve for a surgical procedure of low or intermediate cardiac risk. But if the chest pain has been present and escalating in requirements for sublingual nitroglycerin, then there may be active ischemia and further assessment of myocardial function should be performed. Other symptoms such as bilateral swelling of the ankles, palpitations, and gastric distress may also suggest myocardial dysfunction.

Patients should also be asked about bruising (increased or more noticeable or lack of recovery from), epistaxis, or bleeding from the gums while brushing teeth as history directed questions which point to bleeding abnormalities. Family or medical history questions which indicate bleeding or clotting disorders such as sickle cell disease, factor deficiencies (ie, factor 5, factor 7, factor 9...), von Willebrand disease, and platelet abnormalities, should guide one away from regional anesthesia techniques.

Medications must also be carefully reconciled with the patient or his or her caregiver. This includes not only what medications have been prescribed, but whether they have actually been taken (perhaps in excess, or perhaps not at all).

The Anesthetic Plan

The patient's physical condition and the surgical procedure dictate the anesthetic plan. General anesthesia typically involves an intravenous induction, paralysis, subsequent intubation, and maintenance with opiates and volatile agents. In some individuals, securing the airway is advantageous to prevent aspiration and allow for the administration of 100% oxygen. General anesthesia may also be more desirable if the anticipated surgical time is beyond the duration of the regional block, or if the procedure is sufficiently long that the patient cannot lie still even with sedation in a prolonged supine position.

Regional techniques are advantageous because of the reduced need for systemic medications which may alter the patient's sensorium or cause hypotension and myocardial depression. Indeed, regional anesthetics such as spinal are the anesthetics of choice for reduction of a hip fracture. An epidural has the added advantage of offering surgical anesthesia and postoperative pain relief. Any hemodynamic changes from a regional-induced sympathectomy can be easily controlled with vasopressors. The disadvantages of regional anesthetics in the elderly include difficulty in placing the block, particularly in situations such as a fractured hip, where it can be most painful to turn a patient on his or her side or ask them to sit for block placement. Additional risks are rare, but serious, and include epidural hematoma, seizure, and neural injury, and rarely, cardiac arrest. The incidence of spinal headache decreases with age, and rarely presents in the geriatric population.

In an anticoagulated patient, regional anesthesia is relatively contraindicated. The American Society of Regional Anesthesia (ASRA) consensus statements for oral anticoagulants states that medications must be discontinued for a minimum of 7 days prior to neuraxial anesthesia in most cases. On history and physical examination, questions as to medications which are being actively used for anticoagulation should be elicited, that is, warfarin, low-molecular-weight heparins, recent administration of thrombin inhibitors, platelet inhibiting agents, or fibrinolytics. Unfractionated heparin, administered subcutaneously more than 1 hour from needle placement, has not been associated with any significant comorbidity or mortality. Concomitant use of aspirin and/or use of herbal medications such as ginkgo, ginseng, and garlic have also been noted to have increased risk for bleeding abnormalities.

Age is the number one factor to be considered in the incidence of postoperative delirium. Sedative hypnotics such as the benzodiazepines, barbiturates and inhaled agents, or perhaps general anesthesia itself likely contribute to this syndrome. In addition, the combination of pain, and new surroundings may well contribute to postoperative delirium as well. Postoperative cognitive dysfunction, sometimes lasting for weeks, sometimes months, and sometimes forever is a recently recognized phenomenon which occurs most frequently in elderly patients. The etiologies of this syndrome are as of yet unknown. However, one hypothesis relates postoperative cognitive dysfunction to "deep" general anesthesia, and some general anesthetics have been shown to cause neuronal cell death in vitro.

The social situation of elderly patients who have recently undergone surgery deserves special mention. The geriatric patient is susceptible to loss of "routine" items of daily living, such as missing dentures and glasses. These items may be exceedingly difficult to replace in the patient recovering from surgery, and their loss may perpetuate postoperative delirium. The home environment, and whether a patient can care for himself is also a consideration prior to discharge from the hospital, particularly for ambulatory procedures where patients are discharged on the same day as the operation.

Comprehension Questions

12.1. Which of the following is the most concerning symptom/sign suggestive of impaired cardiac function?

A. Ability to perform daily activities such as normal hygienic maintenance, but unable to ambulate up/down two flights of stairs
B. Inactivity
C. New onset of shortness of breath with lying flat
D. Chest pain which improves on treatment with omeprazole

12.2. Regional anesthesia for a total knee replacement is advantageous because of which of the following?

A. It decreases postoperative nausea and emesis by reducing opioid required for pain relief.
B. It increases total surgical blood loss.
C. It increases the risk of deep vein thrombosis (DVT).
D. It is very useful in patients with atrial fibrillation who are anticoagulated.

12.3. Which of the following is increased in elderly patients compared with their younger counterparts?

A. Vital capacity
B. Air trapping
C. Resting arterial oxygen tension (PaO_2)
D. Ventilatory response to hypoxia or hypercarbia

ANSWERS

12.1. **C.** New onset of shortness of breath raises suspicion of an acute change in the patient's cardiovascular status. Assessment of cardiac function in the preoperative patient with cardiac disease includes assessment of exercise tolerance. The ability to climb two flights of stairs demonstrates a metabolic equivalent (MET) of 4. Studies have demonstrated that a MET = 4 is reasonable for intermediate risk surgical procedure. While functional status is a good indicator of cardiac function, geriatric patients may be inactive for other reasons as well. That's why a careful history and physical examination are important.

Chest pain which responds to omeprazole (D) is most likely to represent gastric reflux.

12.2. **A.** Regional anesthesia provides preemptive and superior analgesia when compared to parenteral therapy. Parenteral narcotics also have side effects such as somnolence and a decreased arousability. Neuraxial blockade actually reduces surgical blood loss. Neuraxial blockade also causes sympathectomy, which reduces the incidence of DVT by decreasing the thrombogenicity. Regional anesthesia is contraindicated in patients who are anticoagulated.

12.3. **B.** The propensity for air trapping is increased with age. In contrast, the vital capacity (A), arterial oxygen tension (C), and ventilatory response to hypoxia or hypocarbia are decreased with age.

Clinical Pearls

- Regional anesthesiology should be considered for as the primary anesthetic for repair of a hip fracture.
- Regional anesthesia is relatively contraindicated in patients who are anticoagulated and/or receiving antiplatelet therapy.
- Administering anesthesia in the geriatric population must be guided by the physiologic changes that accompany the aging process, and which affect almost every major organ system.
- Postoperative cognitive dysfunction is a major consideration in choosing an anesthetic technique for the elderly.

REFERENCES

Belmar CJ, Barth P, Lonner JH, Lotke PA. Total knee arthroplasty in patients 90 years of age and older. [Journal Article. Research Support, Non-U.S. Gov't] *Journal of Arthroplasty*. Dec. 1999;14(8):911-914.

Eagle, Kim A MD et al. ACC/AHA Guideline update for perioperative cardiovascular evaluation for noncardiac surgery. *Anesthesia & Analgesia*. 2002;94: 1052-1064: Updated in 2007.

Modig J, Borg T, Karlstrom G, et al. Thromboembolism after total hip replacement: Role of epidural and general anesthesia. *Anesthesia and Analgesia*. 1983;62:174-180.

Rowlingson, John C, Hanson, Peter B. Neuraxial anesthesia and low-molecular-weight heparin prophylaxis in major orthopedic surgery in the wake of the latest American Society of Regional Anesthesia Guidelines. [Miscellaneous] *Anesthesia and Analgesia*. May 2005;100(5):1482-1488.

Yeager M, Glass D, Neff R, et al. Epidural anesthesia and analgesia in high risk surgical patients. *Anesthesiology*. 1987;66:723-724.

Case 13

A 37-year-old woman presents for weight loss surgery. She is 5 ft 3 in and 245 lb, yielding a BMI (body mass index) of 43.4 kg/m^2. She has tried for many years to lose weight through diet and exercise without success. She has a history of hypertension treated with lisinopril, type II diabetes mellitus controlled with metformin, gastroesophageal reflux disease (GERD) well-controlled with omeprazole, and her husband states that she snores at night. She has no allergies, no family history of problems with anesthesia, and has never had surgery before. After discussion with her surgeon, she is electing to have a laparoscopic gastric banding procedure.

- ➤ What additional history would be helpful in the management of this patient?
- ➤ What preoperative testing should be done?
- ➤ How will you manage her airway?
- ➤ How can her postoperative pain be safely and effectively controlled?

ANSWERS TO CASE 13: Anesthesia and the Obese Patient

Summary: A morbidly obese 37-year-old woman with hypertension, type II diabetes mellitus, GERD, and possible obstructive sleep apnea (OSA) presents for weight loss surgery via laparoscopic gastric banding.

- **Additional history:** A detailed history with an emphasis on evaluating her functional capacity and other comorbid conditions.
- **Preoperative testing:** Cardiac testing such as echocardiography may be indicated to look for heart failure. Polysomnography (sleep study) may be indicated to document the presence or absence of sleep apnea and initiate CPAP therapy.
- **Airway management:** A cautious approach to induction and intubation is essential. Patient positioning and adequate preoxygenation are critical, as obese patients do not tolerate prolonged periods of apnea. Airway rescue devices such as a laryngeal mask airway and additional personnel should be readily available.
- **Postoperative pain control:** Maintain patient comfort without causing oversedation and respiratory depression.

ANALYSIS

Objectives

1. Understand the special considerations for the preoperative evaluation of obese patients.
2. Become familiar with the alterations in physiology and pharmacodynamics in obesity.
3. Outline the anesthetic considerations specific for the obese patient.

Considerations

This patient has several comorbid conditions related to her obesity. Her hypertension, type II diabetes, and GERD may all improve after weight loss surgery. It is important to find out in her preoperative assessment whether or not these conditions are controlled. Also, this patient may have OSA, especially since she has a history of snoring. It would be beneficial to screen for OSA using polysomnography prior to her surgery.

APPROACH TO Anesthesia and the Obese Patient

DEFINITIONS

GERD: Gastroesophageal reflux disease.
OBESITY: Body mass index (BMI) > 30 kg/m^2
MORBID OBESITY: Body mass index (BMI) > 40 kg/m^2
OBSTRUCTIVE SLEEP APNEA (OSA): Condition characterized by repeated episodes of upper airway obstruction during sleep, causing oxyhemoglobin desaturation and awakening.
OBESITY-HYPOVENTILATION SYNDROME (OHS): The syndrome of obesity, chronic daytime hypercapnia, alveolar hypoventilation leading to hypoxemia, polycythemia, hypersomnolence, and right ventricular failure. OHS is also associated with alterations in the central nervous system, and in particular, the ventilatory response to CO_2.
POLYSOMNOGRAPHY: A formal test or "sleep study," in which a patient is continuously monitored as they sleep and specific physiologic variables are recorded. These variables include EEG, eye movements, ECG, muscle movements (EMG), respiration, and leg movements. Information gathered from this test can be used to diagnose OSA and provide appropriate settings for treatment with CPAP.
CPAP: Continuous positive airway pressure. This treatment is provided via a face mask to treat OSA. It works by forcing air through nasal or oral passages at pressures high enough to overcome upper airway obstruction, effectively stenting open the patient's airway.

CLINICAL APPROACH

Preoperative Evaluation

Morbidly obese patients often have a number of comorbid conditions, including cardiovascular disease, type II diabetes, hypertension, GERD, OSA, dyslipidemia, chronic back or joint pain, and headaches, which may or may not be medically controlled. Functional capacity should be carefully assessed (ie, exercise tolerance and overall activity level), since obese patients may develop congestive failure and/or pulmonary hypertension. Either of these conditions is associated with an increase in the risk of surgery. A social history should also be obtained, especially regarding tobacco use. Obese patients who are current smokers should be strongly encouraged to quit smoking at least 6 weeks prior to surgery.

On examination, special attention should be paid to the patient's height and weight (which determines BMI), the airway, the heart and chest, and the extremities. A thorough airway examination should include Mallampati classification; assessment of mouth opening, hyomental distance, neck circumference and extension, and the evaluation of dentition. In addition to auscultation of the heart and lungs, chest physiognomy should also be examined in obese patients. Excess chest wall adipose or soft tissue, and large breasts (especially in female patients), adds additional weight to the chest wall thus restricting chest compliance. Restrictive respiratory mechanics are not unusual results in pulmonary function testing. Since obese patients may have congestive failure, the extremities should be examined for overall shape and evidence of edema.

Basic laboratory tests that are recommended within 6 months of weight loss surgery include: hematocrit, blood glucose, creatinine, and blood urea nitrogen. Additional lab tests, such as electrolytes, thyroid function tests, or coagulation studies may be indicated based on the patient's other comorbidities. In 20% to 30% of obese patients, liver function tests may be elevated due to fatty liver, but this usually does not have any clinically significant effect on drug metabolism.

In patients with a very high BMI (> 50 kg/m^2), a baseline arterial blood gas (ABG) may be useful to detect OHS. Screening for obstructive sleep apnea is similarly important in morbidly obese patients. Studies estimate that more than 70% of patients presenting for weight loss surgery may have OSA. Because they are prone to upper airway obstruction, patients with OSA may be more difficult to mask ventilate. Morbidly obese patients also have higher rates of difficult intubation and postoperative respiratory failure. Pulmonary function testing is likely to demonstrate a restrictive breathing pattern. However, given the marginal respiratory mechanics associated with obesity, any potential reversible obstructive defect should be diagnosed and treated preoperatively.

OSA, if present, can significantly affect a patient's overall cardiovascular health. The frequent episodes of apnea during sleep lead to repeated oxyhemoglobin desaturation and awakening during the night. Consequently, these patients have an increased baseline sympathetic tone, which is thought to contribute to higher rates of hypertension, arrhythmias, acute coronary events, congestive failure, and sudden death. Patients at high risk for OSA should have a formal polysomnography study prior to their surgery. Starting these patients on CPAP as soon as possible can reduce hypoxic pulmonary vasoconstriction, and may help decrease their overall cardiovascular risk. Patients should be instructed to bring their CPAP devices with them on the day of surgery for use in the recovery room and throughout their hospital stay.

Intraoperative Course

A careful approach to induction and intubation is essential in morbidly obese patients. Patients should be placed in the appropriate "sniffing" position in order to facilitate intubation. When obese patients lie flat, excess soft tissue and breast tissue may slide up toward their neck, interfering with mask ventilation and intubation. An intubating "wedge," additional padding, or blankets may be placed under the patients' shoulders. Elevating the shoulders creates a "ramp," allowing excess tissue to fall caudally, away from the patient's airway.

The oxygen saturation declines quite rapidly in obese patients during periods of apnea. This is due in part to the decreased functional residual capacity in obese patients, as well as their increased cardiac output and oxygen consumption due to their large body mass. Time must be taken for adequate "preoxygenation" prior to induction. Breathing 100% oxygen for 3 to 4 minutes prior to induction accomplishes two things. First, the partial pressure of oxygen is increased in blood. But second, and more importantly, hypoxemia is attenuated because "denitrogenation" has also occurred. Seventy-nine percent of room air is nitrogen. Since the N_2 in room air equilibrates with plasma across the alveolus, N_2 is also the predominant gas in blood. When pure oxygen is inspired, N_2 in blood again seeks equilibrium across the alveolus, so N_2 is expired. But during this process, N_2 can quickly become the predominant gas in the alveolus, leading to alveolar hypoxia. The breathing of 100% oxygen allows safe "washout" of N_2 from the blood stream by allowing the alveolus to be filled predominantly with oxygen and thus attenuating any hypoxemia that may occur with apnea at induction. In addition, the functional residual capacity (FRC) may fall below FRC, leading to alveolar collapse with ventilation/perfusion mismatch. The use of CPAP during preoxygenation and induction increases FRC, and extends the length of time until clinically significant oxygen desaturation occurs, also known as the "safe apnea period". In obese patients, *the importance of a long (3-5 minutes) period of preoxygenation cannot be underestimated.*

Ventilation by mask may be difficult in obese patients, and particularly in patients with OSA because the excess soft tissue in the oropharynx can make patients prone to upper airway obstruction. Airway management can be optimized by carefully positioning the patient as previously described, placing head straps in position prior to starting the case, and having an appropriately-sized laryngeal mask airway available for rescue if needed. In patients with particularly difficult airways, a four-handed ventilation technique, where one anesthetist elevates the mandible and holds the mask, and another manages the bag and valve, may be required.

Most obese patients can be intubated via direct laryngoscopy. If difficult airway management is anticipated, the safest approach is to initially use a special intubating device such as a fiberoptic laryngoscope (used awake, with topical spray for the most extreme cases), or a Wu or Glide scope, or a videolaryngoscope such as the McGrath or Glidescope. In patients with severe GERD, rapid sequence induction may be indicated. Rescue airway devices, such as an Eschmann stylet (bougie), LMA or intubating LMA, and fiberoptic or video laryngoscopes, should always be readily available in the OR, in case an unanticipated difficult airway is encountered. Additional anesthesia personnel and members of the nursing and surgical teams should also be nearby and ready to provide assistance in the event of a difficult intubation.

It is particularly important to comprehensively document the ease of, and techniques used for ventilation and intubation. Knowing that a patient's airway can be easily managed by mask can save him or her from the need for an awake intubation. Similarly, understanding which laryngoscope blades, head positions, etc. were successful or unsuccessful allows the anesthetist to approach management of the airway in the most expeditious manner.

In the absence of significant medical comorbidities, standard monitors are sufficient for an obese patient having a laparoscopic gastric banding procedure. Morbidly obese patients frequently have a conical shape to their arms, which may make it difficult to get an adequate fit from a noninvasive blood pressure cuff. In these cases, the cuff may need to be placed on the forearm or calf, or an arterial line may need to be placed to facilitate the measurement of blood pressure.

The anesthetic for laparoscopic gastric banding is maintained using a balanced technique of inhaled anesthetic gas, muscle relaxation, and low-dose opioids. As stated previously, morbidly obese patients frequently have a restrictive pattern of respiratory mechanics due to the excess weight restricting the chest wall and extra adipose tissue that accumulates around the ribs and under the diaphragm. Peak inspiratory pressures are typically elevated in morbidly obese patients. As the surgeons insufflate the abdominal cavity during laparoscopy, inspiratory pressures become even higher. It is important to provide adequate muscle relaxation to facilitate mechanical ventilation and to maximize the surgical workspace. The addition of positive end-expiratory pressure (PEEP) may also help improve oxygenation and ventilation in morbidly obese patients.

Inhaled anesthetic agents that have lower tissue/blood partition coefficients will achieve induction and recovery at faster rates than more soluble agents. Sevoflurane and desflurane have lower solubility coefficients than isoflurane, and will therefore have faster rates of tissue "wash-in" and "wash-out" than isoflurane. These less soluble agents are preferred in morbidly obese patients because they allow for more rapid recovery from anesthesia, which is important to ensure that obese patients are fully awake prior to extubation. Returning the patient to the 30 degree reverse Trendelenburg position will help facilitate return of adequate spontaneous ventilation. Neuromuscular blockade should be completely reversed, and patients should be alert and following commands prior to removal of the endotracheal tube. Inadequate strength could lead to loss of a patent airway and the need for re-intubation. Prior to extubation, preparations should be made to ensure that the patient can be ventilated and re-intubated if necessary.

When dosing medications, it is important to consider the class of drug when deciding whether total body weight (TBW), lean body mass, or ideal body weight is most appropriate to be used when calculating drug dosage.

The pharmacodynamics and pharmacokinetics of many drugs are altered by obesity, but specific data regarding specific drug dosing is limited. Obese patients have a higher TBW, but they also have more adipose tissue, which is poorly perfused when compared to muscle. Though counterintuitive, this relatively poor perfusion actually somewhat reduces the volume of distribution (V_d) of a lipid soluble agent. When dosed based on TBW, opioids may achieve higher blood levels than anticipated, especially when infusions are used. A conservative approach would be to dose lipid soluble medications according to a patient's lean body mass (ideal body weight + 20%), and titrate to effect. Neuromuscular blocking agents should be dosed according to lean body mass. Obese patients typically have an increase in pseudocholinesterase activity. Since pseudocholinesterase metabolizes succinylcholine, succinylcholine should be dosed according to TBW to facilitate ideal conditions for intubation .

Postoperative Care

Morbidly obese patients are at risk for complications in the postoperative period, and should be closely monitored. Obese patients, especially those with OSA, may become apneic with the administration of narcotics. Postoperative pain control should be tailored to provide patient comfort, without excessively sedating the obese patient. **Opioids dosed according to lean body mass and delivered via PCA (patient-controlled analgesia) are a good option.** Non-opioid adjuvants should also be considered, as these may reduce the opioid requirement while allowing for preservation of respiratory drive. Such adjunctive therapies include NSAIDs, ketamine, alpha agonists such as dexmedetomidine, and infiltration of the wound with local anesthetic. If an open gastric banding had been performed, an epidural for postoperative pain control would be an appropriate pain-management strategy.

Patients with CPAP machines should be encouraged to bring their devices with them to the hospital on the day of surgery. CPAP can be used in the recovery room and throughout the hospital stay. Even those patients without a prior diagnosis of OSA, but in whom OSA is suspected, will likely benefit from CPAP use and the care of a respiratory therapist in the PACU. ASA guidelines recommend that patients with OSA be monitored by continuous pulse oximetry until their room air saturation is 90% or greater during sleep. For this reason, obese patients may need to remain in the PACU for several hours or overnight for monitoring.

Management of the morbidly obese patient undergoing minor, ambulatory surgery under general anesthesia remains quite controversial within the anesthesia community today. Postoperative deaths have been reported, and no studies have demonstrated conclusively the predictive factors for morbidity and postoperative mortality. Whether morbidly obese patients should receive their care in a free-standing ambulatory surgery center, and whether they should remain in a monitored bed overnight following a general anesthetic varies widely across institutions, and to date, no consensus has been reached.

Comprehension Questions

13.1. Which of the following is an important test for patients with suspected OSA prior to weight loss surgery?
A. Complete blood count (CBC)
B. Electrolytes
C. Chest x-ray
D. Polysomnography
E. Exercise stress test

13.2. Morbidly obese patients have which of the following alterations in respiratory physiology?
A. Reduced FRC
B. Reduced peak inspiratory pressures
C. Increased lung volumes
D. Increased chest wall compliance

13.3. Which of the following medications should be dosed according to total body weight (TBW), instead of lean body mass in morbidly obese patients?
A. Morphine PCA
B. Vecuronium
C. Succinylcholine
D. Pancuronium

ANSWERS

13.1. **D.** A formal sleep study, or polysomnography, is an important test for patients with suspected OSA. In this test, a patient is continuously monitored as they sleep and variables such as EEG, eye movements, ECG, muscle movements (EMG), respiration, and leg movements are recorded. Using this information, OSA can be diagnosed and recommendations can be made for appropriate settings for treatment with CPAP.

13.2. **A.** Morbidly obese patients have restrictive pulmonary mechanics, and therefore have a reduced FRC in addition to decreased chest wall compliance due to an excess of soft tissue on the chest wall and fat between the ribs and under the diaphragm. The reduced FRC contributes to a rapid decline in the oxygen saturation following induction.

13.3. **C.** Succinylcholine should be dosed according to total body weight (TBW), not lean body mass. Morbidly obese patients have elevated activity of pseudocholinesterase, the enzyme responsible for the metabolism of succinylcholine. Thus, dosing by total body weight is necessary to ensure complete relaxation prior to intubation. Morphine by PCA, vecuronium, and pancuronium should be dosed according to lean body mass.

Clinical Pearls

- Obstructive sleep apnea is extremely common in morbidly obese patients, and can increase the risk for difficult ventilation, intubation, and postoperative respiratory failure. Treatment for OSA should be initiated early, prior to surgery if possible.
- Pulmonary function and physiology are altered in morbidly obese patients. They desaturate quickly during periods of apnea, so adequate preoxygenation is essential prior to intubation. Rescue airway devices and additional anesthesia personnel should always be immediately available to help with difficult airway management.
- Obesity modifies both the pharmacokinetics and pharmacodynamics of anesthetic agents. Some agents should be dosed according to total body weight, and others, lean body mass. Insoluble inhalation anesthetics facilitate a more rapid recovery from anesthesia, and are thus favored in obese patients.
- Given the high incidence of OSA and adverse outcomes amongst morbidly obese patients, appropriate precautions must be taken when discharging patients from the post-anesthesia recovery unit.

REFERENCES

Benumof JL. Obstructive sleep apnea in the adult obese patient: implications for airway management. *J Clin Anesth*. 2001;13:144-156.

Frey WC, Pilcher J. Obstructive sleep-related breathing disorders in patients evaluated for bariatric surgery. *Obes Surg*. 2003;13:676-683.

Jones S. Anesthesia for bariatric surgery. In: *Harvard Anesthesia Review and Update*. 2008 [CME course syllabus].

O'Keeffe T, Patterson EJ. Evidence supporting routine polysomnography before bariatric surgery. *Obes Surg*. 2004;14:23-26.

Schumann R, Jones S, Ortiz, VE, et al. Best practice recommendations for anesthetic perioperative care and pain management in weight loss surgery. *Obes Res*. 2005;13:254-266.

Schumann R, Jones SB, Cooper B, et al. Update on best practice recommendations for anesthetic perioperative care and pain management in weight loss surgery 2004–2007. *Obes Res. 2009;17:889-894*.

Siyam M, Benhamou D. Difficult endotracheal intubation in patients with sleep apnea syndrome. *Anesth and Analg*. 2002;95:1098-1102.

Case 14

A 72-year-old man has had pain and drainage from several non-healing ulcers on the toes and ball of his right foot. He was treated initially with careful dressing changes, antibiotics, and weight-bearing restrictions. However, the drainage became frankly purulent and gangrenous changes developed. His vascular surgeon determined that no additional revascularization of the lower extremity was likely to help heal these wounds, so he scheduled the patient for a transmetatarsal amputation of the right foot today.

The patient's medical history is significant for coronary artery disease (CAD), evidenced by several myocardial infarctions with a coronary artery bypass grafting for revascularization. On recent catheterization, his cardiologist notes no additional treatment is indicated and that he should be managed medically. He also has type II diabetes mellitus, poorly compensated congestive heart failure (CHF), a 40-pack-year smoking history, chronic obstructive pulmonary disease, and paroxysmal atrial fibrillation. In addition to insulin, he takes carvedilol, simvastatin, lisinopril, warfarin (held for 5 days), a baby aspirin, and an albuterol/ipratropium inhaler. On examination, the patient weighs 190 lb and is 5 ft, 7 in tall. He has poor dentition limited mouth opening of approximately 1.5 cm. Auscultation of his heart reveals a slow, regular heart rate. His lungs are coarse with diminished breath sounds in the bases and a prolonged expiratory phase. His labs are significant for an INR of 1.3 and a hematocrit of 28. The patient states that he does not want a general anesthetic.

- What type of anesthetic options could be considered for this procedure?
- Which spinal nerves provide the innervation of the lower extremity?
- What are the risks of neuraxial anesthesia in an anticoagulated patient?

ANSWERS TO CASE 14:

Anesthesia for Lower Extremity Surgery (Peripheral Nerve Block)

Summary: A 72-year-old man with a gangrenous forefoot presents for transmetatarsal amputation. His past medical history is remarkable for diabetes mellitus, CAD, CHF, and COPD. His laboratory results are significant for INR of 1.3 and Hct of 28. He desires avoiding general anesthesia.

- **Anesthetic options:** Subarachnoid block (spinal), popliteal (sciatic) and saphenous nerve block, or ankle block.
- **Lower extremity innervation:** The lumbosacral spinal nerves from L2 to S3 provide the source of the innervation of the lower extremity. (Please see Figure 14–1.)
- **Risks of neuraxial anesthesia in an anticoagulated patient:** Local bleeding from the puncture site, and in the case of spinal, an epidural hematoma with or without neurological injury.

ANALYSIS

Objectives

1. Understand the regional anesthetic choices for transmetatarsal amputation.
2. Describe the innervation of the lower extremity.
3. Recognize the risks of neuraxial anesthesia in an anticoagulated patient.

Considerations

In this case, our 72-year-old patient asks to avoid general anesthesia, leaving us with the options of neuraxial (spinal or epidural) anesthesia, or a peripheral nerve block. Both peripheral nerve blocks and central neuraxial anesthetics minimize effects on pulmonary function, and generally have fewer hemodynamic alterations than general anesthesia.

A spinal anesthetic is typically performed by a single injection of a local anesthetic into the subarachnoid space. It provides excellent anesthesia over low thoracic, lumbar, and sacral dermatomes. In this patient's case, a subarachnoid block would be the preferable choice of neuraxial anesthesia, due to the better coverage of sacral nerves and the relatively brief (< 2 hours) duration for the procedure. A spinal also provides an intense block in the entire lower extremity, allowing the surgeon more flexibility particularly if the extent of the patient's ischemic tissue is uncertain. This patient had been treated with warfarin for his atrial fibrillation, but the warfarin was stopped 5 days prior to surgery and his coagulation parameters had returned to normal.

A peripheral nerve block such as an ankle block is also an excellent choice for this patient, and is associated with fewer propensities for hemodynamic changes and a less time in the recovery room than a spinal. However, peripheral nerve blocks require several injections, and are less well tolerated by some patients.

APPROACH TO
Anesthesia For Lower Extremity Surgery (Peripheral Nerve Block)

CLINICAL APPROACH

Neuraxial anesthesia refers to an anesthetic placed in the epidural or subarachnoid space, or (in the case of obstetric anesthesia) both. The anesthetic can be injected in a single injection, or by continuous infusion. Subarachnoid anesthesia is typically performed as a single injection, and can provide excellent anesthesia over low thoracic, lumbar, and sacral dermatomes. Its advantages include an arguably easier technical approach, the use of a smaller needle, thus a lower risk of bleeding complications (ASRA 2003 Consensus Statement), good coverage of sacral dermatomes for gynecological, urologic, and podiatric procedures, and dense anesthesia. Disadvantages include inability to easily re-dose the anesthetic and difficulty in controlling block height except by drug choice considering drug dosage, volume, and baricity (the anesthetic's density relative to CSF).

A profound vasodilatation accompanies the sympathectomy that results from neuraxial blockade. The result is often marked hypotension from reduced cardiac filling, from slowing of heart rate from a decreased stretch of the right atrium and great veins, and in blocks above T2 to T4, blockade of the cardio accelerator fibers. If performing a central neuraxial technique, vasopressors should be prepared in advance to counteract the vasodilation in the event that it is needed.

Epidural anesthesia is typically performed as a continuous technique and can provide good anesthetic coverage of thoracic and lumbar dermatomes. It can be associated with similar hemodynamic changes to spinal, though since the onset of an epidural is somewhat slower, so are the hemodynamic changes somewhat more profound. The advantages of an epidural include the ability to titrate block coverage by intermittent injection of local anesthetic until the desired location is adequately anesthetized, and easy re-dosing of the anesthetic in the event of a very long procedure. Disadvantages include the potential for inadequate density of blockade (not "numb" enough), patchy or incomplete blockade, and poor coverage of sacral dermatomes, even with large volumes of local anesthetic.

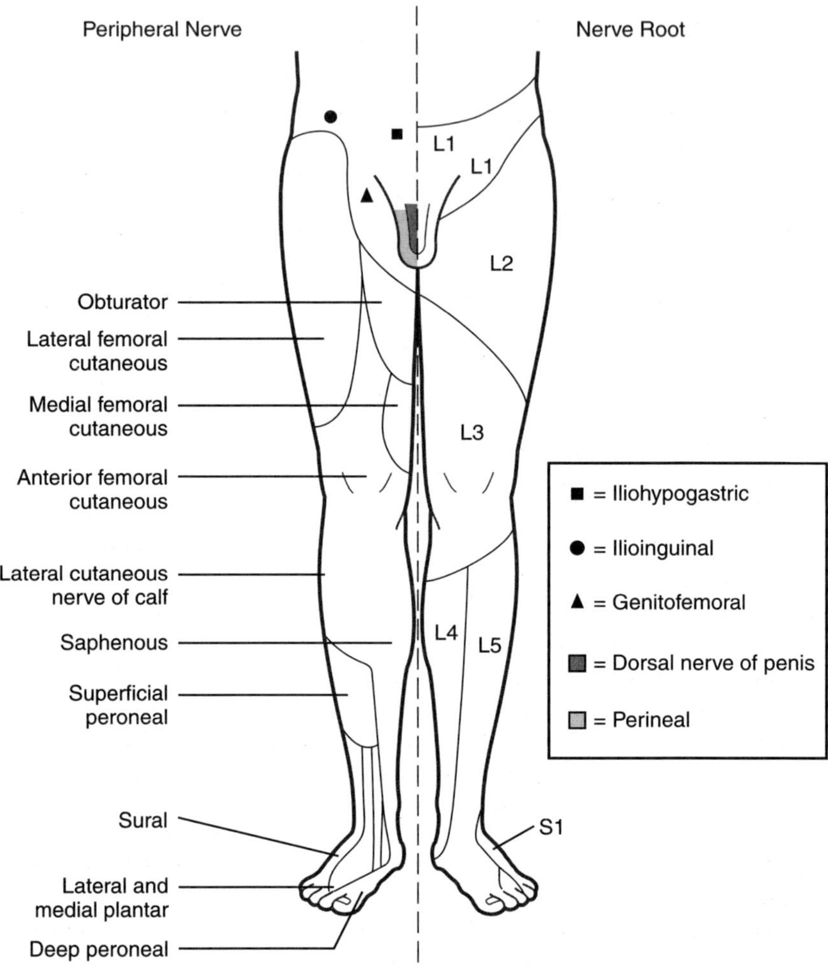

Figure 14–1. Innervation of the lower extremity. *(Redrawn from: Morgan GE, Mikkail MS, Murray MJ.* Clinical Anesthesiology, *4th edition. http://www.accessmedicine.com. Copyright © The McGraw-Hill Companies, Inc. All rights reserved.)*

Like neuraxial anesthetics, peripheral nerve blocks may be divided in several ways as well. Anesthetics may be placed selectively at nerve roots, in the distribution of large collections of trunks, such as the lumbar plexus (psoas block), at large conducting nerves such as the sciatic or femoral nerves, or at individual nerves such as the deep peroneal nerve as a portion of an ankle block.

Innervation of the Lower Extremity

The innervation of the lower extremity begins with the lumbar and sacral spinal nerve roots from L2 to S3. The upper portion of these nerves, from L2

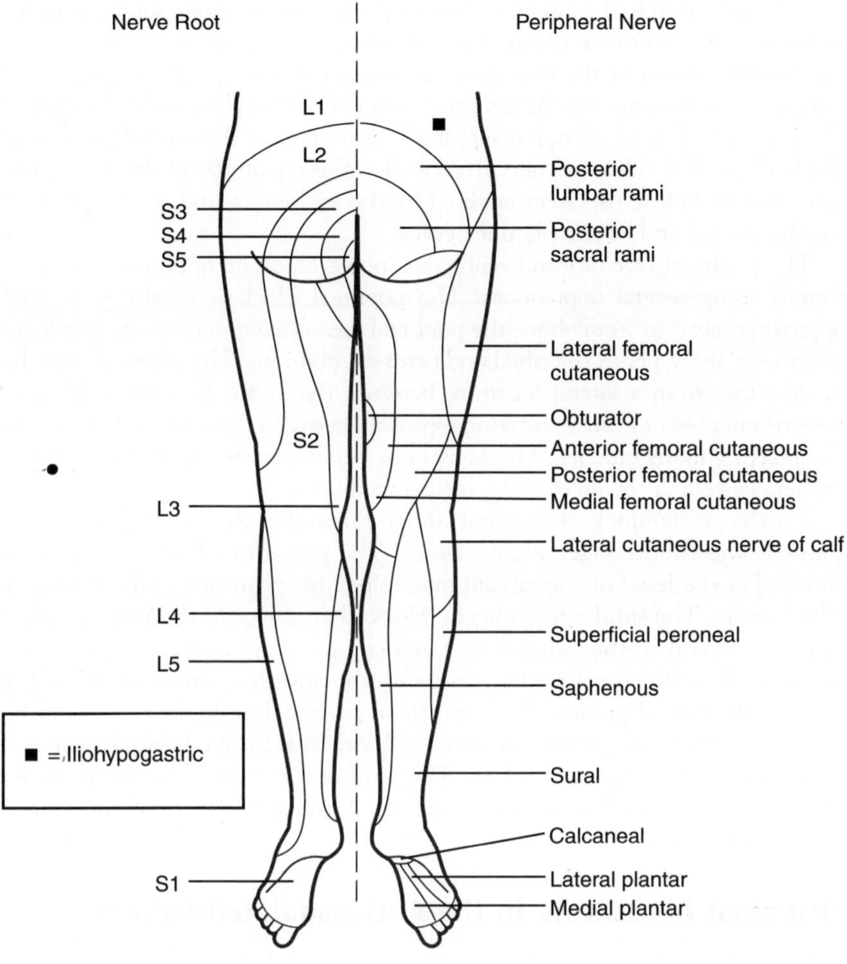

Figure 14–1. (*Continued*)

to L4, forms the lumbar plexus. The lumbar plexus supplies innervation to the anterior and medial thigh and medial leg via branches of the lateral femoral cutaneous nerve (L2-L3), the femoral nerve (L2-L4), and the obturator nerve (L2-L4). The femoral nerve supplies the saphenous nerve below the knee and is responsible for sensation along the medial portion of the leg ankle, and the very posterior medial portion of the foot.

The lower group of spinal nerves, from L4 to S3, form the tibial and peroneal divisions of the sciatic nerve. In addition, sensation over the posterior portion of the thigh is supplied by the posterior cutaneous nerve of the thigh, which is formed separately from the S1 to S3 roots. The peroneal division provides sensation to the lateral portion of the leg via the lateral sural cutaneous nerve and the superficial peroneal nerve. The posterior portion of the leg and the lateral portion of the heel and foot (lateral calcaneal and lateral dorsal cutaneous nerves) are supplied via the sural nerve which is another branch of the peroneal. The tibial nerve supplies sensation over the medial portion of the heel (medial calcaneal nerve), as well as the remainder of the sole of the foot (not including the areas covered by the saphenous and sural branches) via the medial and lateral plantar nerves.

The popliteal (sciatic) and saphenous nerve blockade option may be performed using several approaches. The popliteal block is usually performed approximately 6 to 7 cm above the popliteal crease, in attempt to deposit local anesthetic around both the tibial and peroneal divisions. The approach may be made either from a lateral location, between the vastus lateralis and biceps femoris muscles, or from a posterior approach, between the semitendinosus and the biceps femoris muscles. The saphenous nerve may be blocked around the saphenous vein at the level of the medial malleolus.

For the ankle block, it is important to remember that 5 separate nerves must be anesthetized (see Figure 14–2.) The posterior tibial nerve may be blocked at the level of the medial malleolus, just posterior to the posterior tibial artery. The sural nerve may be blocked posterior to the lateral malleolus and lateral to the calcaneus. The deep peroneal nerve is approached just lateral to the anterior tibial artery on the anterior portion of the ankle deep to the fascial planes. The superficial peroneal nerve branches can be blocked with a subcutaneous ring of local anesthesia from the lateral malleolus to the anterior tibia. The saphenous nerve should then be blocked as described in the description of the popliteal and saphenous combination block.

Neuraxial Anesthesia in the Anticoagulated Patient

The risks of neuraxial anesthesia are not trivial, and the potential for bleeding, infection, and neurologic injury must all be considered. In particular, the increasingly common use of anticoagulants in outpatient therapy, including warfarin, low-molecular-weight heparin, and antiplatelet medications such as clopidogrel, raises the issue of the risk of spinal hematoma from neuraxial anesthetics. Guidance for the safety of performing these blocks comes from the American Society of Regional Anesthesia. There are, however, significant limitations to the evidence-based nature of their recommendations due to the very low incidence of spinal hematoma. The group's consensus depended upon anecdotal case reports, and the understanding of individual drug pharmacology.

This patient had been maintained on warfarin because of his history of atrial fibrillation until 5 days prior to surgery, and a PT/INR was checked. It is important to remember that PT/INR primarily reflects factor VII, and may *overestimate* the adequacy of coagulation after discontinuing warfarin therapy. PT/INR should

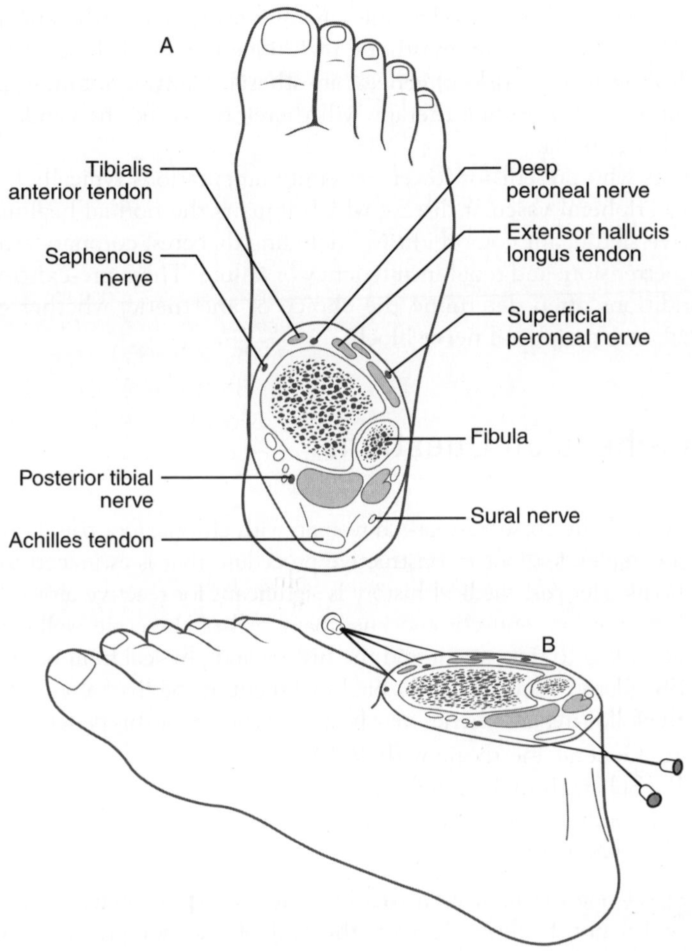

Figure 14–2. Anatomy and approaches to the nerves constituting an ankle block. *(Redrawn from: Morgan GE Jr, Mikhail MS, Murray MJ, eds. Clinical Anesthesiology, 4th ed. New York, NY: McGraw-Hill, 2006:352.)*

be back in the normal range (< 1.5) prior to any neuraxial anesthetic. In the case of other anticoagulants, the ASRA consensus guidelines should be used for reference regarding a time line for discontinuation of medications and testing.

The suitability of patients on antiplatelet drugs for neuraxial anesthesia is a topic of common discussion. Patients receiving thienopyridine medications for anticoagulation pose obvious risks of bleeding in the epidural or subarachnoid space. And patients who have undergone implantation of drug-eluting coronary stents are recommended to continue thienopyridine therapy uninterrupted for 12 months after implantation. On the other hand, these are often the very patients for whom a regional technique would be desirable, in order to minimize any hemodynamic changes associated with general anesthesia. Thus, the choice of anesthetic technique requires balancing the risks of bleeding against the risks of general anesthesia. Many, if not most, patients who require thienopyridine therapy will therefore not be the candidates for neuraxial anesthesia.

Patients who present for lower extremity amputations typically have significant peripheral vascular disease which impairs the normal healing. They often have significant comorbidities, including diabetes, coronary artery disease, hypertension, and renal insufficiency or failure. These pre-existing medical conditions often determine the choice of anesthetic, whether general, neuraxial, or a peripheral nerve block.

Comprehension Questions

14.1. A morbidly obese 55-year-old woman with chronic foot pain presents for a complex forefoot reconstructive procedure that is estimated to take 2 hours. Her past medical history is significant for reactive airway disease, hypertension, and chronic knee pain. All of these are well-controlled according to the patient and the history and physical from her internist. She plans to stay in the hospital overnight as she lives alone. Which of the following anesthetics may be a poor choice for this patient?

A. General anesthesia with an LMA
B. Subarachnoid (spinal) anesthesia
C. Popliteal and saphenous nerve blocks
D. Epidural anesthesia

14.2. A 49-year-old man with treatment-refractory coronary artery disease and a non-healing ulcer on the ball of his foot presents for transmetatarsal amputation. You plan an ankle block for this anesthetic. Which of the following nerves may be omitted in this anesthetic?

A. Deep and superficial peroneal nerves
B. Saphenous nerve
C. Sural and posterior tibial nerve
D. Greater tarsal nerve

14.3. Which of the following medications may be continued prior to performing a neuraxial anesthetic?

A. Aspirin
B. Warfarin
C. Clopidogrel
D. Low-molecular-weight heparin

ANSWERS

14.1. **D.** Epidural anesthetics are often chosen for lower extremity surgery as they provide relatively rapid anesthesia, ease of re-dosing, and the potential use postoperatively for analgesia. However, in this patient, the operation will involve some of the sacral dermatomes, which are often poorly anesthetized compared to the lumbar and low thoracic dermatomes. The other three options would be better choices for this operation.

14.2. **D.** The "greater tarsal nerve" does not need to be anesthetized for this procedure. All of the other listed nerves must be anesthetized. The ankle block is a fundamental skill of all anesthesiologists to provide regional anesthesia over the foot and minimize the systemic anesthetic effect in patients with complex medical problems. Successful placement of the block requires recollection of all five of the nerves that must be anesthetized for a successful block.

14.3. **A.** Aspirin may be continued prior to placement of a neuraxial blockade. This is especially true for vascular patients, where the risk of discontinuing the drug is greater than the risk of hematoma formation. The other listed medications should be stopped prior to performing neuraxial anesthesia in order to minimize the risk of spinal (epidural) bleeding and potential neurologic compromise. Each of the anticoagulants has a different set of pharmacokinetics and as such, the time each drug needs to be held varies. The ASRA Consensus Guidelines on regional anesthesia in the anticoagulated patient serves as a ready reference for guiding these decisions.

Clinical Pearls

- Knowledge of lower extremity innervation provides the anesthesiologist with several options to obtain excellent anesthesia for a variety of lower extremity operations.
- Local anesthetic choices are guided by the expected duration of the operation and the degree of expected pain following the procedure.
- Patients who require thienopyridine therapy are not generally candidates for neuraxial anesthesia.

REFERENCES

American Society of Anesthesiologists Committee on Standards and Practice Parameters. Practice alert for the perioperative management of patients with coronary artery stents: A report by the American Society of Anesthesiologists Committee on Standards and Practice Parameters. *Anesthesiology*. 2009;110:22-23.

Horlocker TT, Wedel DJ, Bezon H, et al. Regional anesthesia in the anticoagulated patient: Defining the risks (The Second ASRA Consensus Conference on Neuraxial Anesthesia and Anticoagulation). *Reg Anesth Pain Med.* 2003;28(3):172-197.

Peterson CM, Peterson KP, Jovanovic L. Influence of diabetes on vascular disease and its complications. In: Moore WS, ed. *Vascular Surgery: Comprehensive Review*. 5th ed. Philadelphia, PA: WB Saunders; 1998:146-167.

Case 15

A 36-year-old man has had an increasing numbness of his thumb, his index finger, and the long finger on his right hand for the past 6 months. He was referred by his primary physician to a physiatrist for an electromyography (EMG) study, which showed slowed conduction in the median nerve at the carpal tunnel. He was then referred to a hand surgeon for carpal tunnel release as an outpatient.

The patient's medical history is negative except for diet-controlled diabetes. He has had no previous operations, and thus has no history of previous anesthetics, nor a family history of problems with anesthesia. He has no allergies to medications, does not smoke, and consumes alcohol occasionally at social events. His laboratory results and physical examination by his internist were normal as well. The patient has had nothing to eat or drink since he went to bed last night. He wishes to leave the Surgicenter as quickly as possible after the operation.

On examination, the patient weighs 225 lb and is 5 ft, 8 in tall. His neck appears to be thick and only slightly mobile. His Mallampati classification is a reassuring class I.

- ➤ What type of anesthetic options could be considered for this procedure?
- ➤ What are the indications for i.v. regional anesthesia?
- ➤ What are the risks of i.v. regional anesthesia?

ANSWERS TO CASE 15: Outpatient Anesthesia for Carpal Tunnel Release

Summary: A 36-year-old man with numbness in the distribution of the median nerve presents for carpal tunnel release. His past medical history is remarkable for diet-controlled diabetes mellitus. His laboratory results and physical examination are normal except for morbid obesity and a BMI of 35 kg/m^2.

- **Anesthetic options:** General, intravenous regional, peripheral nerve block, or local with sedation
- **Indications for i.v. regional anesthesia:** Extremity surgery of brief duration (< 90 minutes)
- **Risks of IV regional anesthesia:** Local anesthetic toxicity, injury from tourniquet compression, block failure due to tourniquet pain requiring conversion to general anesthesia

ANALYSIS

Objectives

1. Understand the options for outpatient orthopedic anesthesia.
2. Describe the indications for intravenous regional anesthesia.
3. Recognize the risks of intravenous regional anesthesia.
4. Describe the technical approach to performing intravenous regional anesthesia.

Considerations

This patient is undergoing a minor surgical procedure followed shortly thereafter by discharge from the facility. A carpal tunnel repair can easily be performed using intravenous (i.v.) regional anesthesia, thus allowing the patient to remain fully awake or lightly sedated during the procedure. There is no need for a general anesthetic, so his cognitive functions will remain intact, and he will experience little or no nausea or vomiting.

In addition to the i.v. inserted routinely for the surgery, a small, distal i.v. catheter is inserted into the extremity undergoing surgery. Next the operative extremity is exsanguinated with an Esmarch bandage as the arm is elevated, and a proximal tourniquet is applied. A large dose of local anesthesia (typically 50 mL of 0.5% lidocaine) is then injected through the catheter, quickly rendering the limb insensitive to pain and unable to move. Once the operation is complete, the tourniquet is deflated, the remaining local anesthetic passes into the systemic circulation, and the limb's functions promptly return.

In a comparison of 126 patients undergoing hand surgery (excluding carpal tunnel release and ganglion excision) only 51% of the patients who received intravenous regional required postoperative analgesics compared to 85% of those who received general anesthesia.

APPROACH TO Outpatient Anesthesia for Carpal Tunnel Release

Many orthopedic cases, ranging from minor procedures such as a carpal tunnel repair to more complex cases such as arthroscopic rotator cuff repair are typically performed on an ambulatory basis. Since the patient is to be discharged on the same day as the surgical procedure, the primary goals of the anesthetic necessitate a rapid recovery to normal mentation, minimal side effects, and adequate pain control for discharge. Modern general anesthetics provide these conditions quite effectively.

Yet when compared to peripheral nerve blockade, general anesthetics are associated with higher postoperative nausea and pain scores and a greater need for post-anesthesia care unit time. However, the difference in overall time to discharge has not been reliably reproduced. (It was, however, noted that the discharge process may be sufficiently long as to mask any difference between these two procedures.).

CLINICAL APPROACH

Indications for Intravenous Regional Anesthesia

Intravenous regional anesthesia was first introduced by German surgeon August Gustav Bier in 1908, and is often known as the "Bier block." Dr. Bier had an interest in the use of exsanguinating bandages to provide a bloodless surgical field. He found that by introducing procaine into a cut down peripheral vein distal to a tourniquet, anesthesia would quickly occur in the extremity, and that once the tourniquet was released, anesthesia would rapidly resolve. However, peripheral nerve blockade did not gain significant popularity until the 1960s, when a series of 30 patients receiving intravenous regional anesthesia appeared in *The Lancet*.

Today, i.v. regional anesthesia remains a popular choice for upper extremity surgery including foreign body removal, arthroscopies, carpal tunnel release, de Quervain disease, amputations, plastic surgeries, and synovectomies. In addition to providing anesthesia for surgery, this technique has also for the treatment of palmar hyperhydrosis involving the injection of botulinum toxin, as well as for the treatment of complex regional pain syndrome.

Anesthesia from the i.v. regional technique results from the exposure of small nerve endings and, to some extent, larger peripheral nerves, to local anesthetics thus blocking nerve transmission. Ischemia of the extremity also contributes to the slowing nerve conduction. Unfortunately, the intercostal brachial nerve is not anesthetized because of its origin relative to the tourniquet. This nerve, as well as unmyelinated C-fibers under the tourniquet, are also responsible for the pain related to prolonged tourniquet inflation.

Contraindications

Few absolute contraindications exist for i.v. regional anesthesia. Sickle cell disease is contraindicated, since the use of a tourniquet could potentially trigger a sickle crisis. An allergy to local anesthetics, or presence of infection or the inability to place an intravenous catheter at the site of placement also precludes the use of this technique. Or, patients may simply refuse. Relative contraindications include untreated seizure disorders (since a lidocaine bolus may rapidly enter the systemic circulation), high-grade heart block, bleeding disorders, and hepatic failure.

Risks of Intravenous Regional Anesthesia

Intravenous regional anesthesia has been lauded for its extremely high-safety profile. Early authors proposed that this technique could be used readily by non-anesthesiologists, including in the emergency department for the management of a variety of injuries. However, given the amount of local anesthetic involved, any practitioner utilizing this technique must be familiar with all aspects of local anesthetic toxicity and amply prepared for its management.

Local anesthetic toxicity often initially presents with symptoms period of nervous system excitability culminating in grand mal profound seizure. Cardiovascular toxicity can follow, with significant arrhythmias and the potential for cardiovascular collapse. The tourniquet should have functioning alarms to alert the anesthesiologist of a sudden loss in tourniquet pressure, which could lead to the sudden systemic distribution of a large dose of local anesthetic. After a period of time, usually around 20 minutes, the local anesthetic molecules become fixed to the tissues of the extremity. At this point, deflation of the tourniquet no longer results in a large quantity of the anesthetic being released into the systemic circulation.

Other risks emanate from injury to structures compressed by the tourniquet. The tourniquet for upper extremity surgery tends to be placed well above the antecubital region, but compression of peripheral nerves against bony prominences can lead to prolonged nerve ischemia and subsequent injury. Inattention to the placement of padding around the tourniquet can also contribute to skin injury. Lastly, if the duration of the operation exceeds expectations, the patient may begin to develop an almost uncontrollable tourniquet pain that is not very responsive to analgesics, and which may require deepening the sedation, or even the induction of general anesthesia.

The choice of local anesthetic is relatively straightforward. The duration of action of the local anesthetic in this anesthetic approach is primarily determined by duration of the tourniquet. Therefore, the use of short-acting local anesthetics has been advocated due to the lower risks of serious, persistent cardiovascular complications in the setting of a tourniquet failure. Procaine and lidocaine are the most common choices.

Technique for Intravenous Regional Anesthesia

The patient is prepared for anesthesia as all patients are prepared and according to the guidelines of the ASA. A preoperative evaluation must be performed; patients should have fasted in the usual fashion; appropriate monitors including the standard ASA monitors (pulse oximetry, noninvasive blood pressure, ECG) should all be applied. Standard emergency medications as well as a functioning bag-mask system or anesthesia machine should be available.

Intravenous catheters are placed in both extremities. In the operative extremity, the catheter should be placed as distal as possible and not in the operative field if at all possible. Small doses of premedication may be given for anxiolysis. Some authors promote routine use of benzodiazepines to raise the seizure threshold in the event of systemic vascular uptake of local anesthetic, though excessive premedication may contribute to a prolonged recovery room stay. Infiltration of the intercostal brachial nerve may be performed at this time with 3 to 5 mL of local anesthetic.

Next, a double tourniquet should be placed above the antecubital fossa on the operative extremity. The tourniquet should be padded and carefully inspected to verify absence of any pressure points. Wider tourniquets may be better tolerated, due to the greater surface area of tissue bearing the impact of the tourniquet. The electronic monitoring of the tourniquets must have passed their initial self-check and appear to function appropriately. Most authors recommend an extremity pressure of 250 mm Hg, or at least 100 mm Hg above systemic pressure. The extremity should then be raised above the heart for a few minutes, and an Esmarch bandage applied to exsanguinate the extremity. Once the exsanguination is complete, the proximal tourniquet should be raised.

Once satisfactory inflation of the tourniquet has been achieved, the injection of local anesthetic into the operative extremities intravenous catheter is undertaken. A typical volume of 50 mL of 0.5% lidocaine, or approximately 3 mg/kg, is injected slowly to prevent an excessive intravenous pressure which can overcome the tourniquet's pressure. *During the injection, the patient is questioned for signs of local anesthetic toxicity such as numbness around the mouth, ringing in the ears, headache, or a general sense of feeling bad.* The injection should take approximately 90 seconds to complete. The limb will remain almost white in color, and become rapidly insensitive to pain and lose the ability to move. If the limb's color becomes either dark red or blue, the tourniquet is leaking and local anesthetic could be rapidly absorbed into the circulation if the injection is continued.

After approximately 25 to 45 minutes of anesthesia, the patient may begin to complain of tourniquet pain. At this time, the distal cuff (which is over an area anesthetized by the lidocaine) may be inflated and the proximal cuff deflated. Prior to performing this maneuver, it is useful to pause to reconsider the procedure. This reflation-deflation technique may allow for an additional 15 to 20 minutes of operative time.

At the completion of the operation, the surgeon should be encouraged to infiltrate the wound with local anesthetic to minimize the need for postoperative analgesics in the recovery room. The cuff may then be released briefly (5-10 seconds) and then reinflated for 30 seconds for several iterations (3-6). This may allow for a lower maximum dose of local anesthetic released as a single bolus. If the patient complains of symptoms consistent with local anesthetic toxicity, it may be reasonable to prolong the reinflation period.

Local Anesthetic Toxicity

Signs: Light headedness, tinnitus, headache, circumoral numbness or tingling, metallic taste in the mouth

Symptoms: Muscle twitching, loss of consciousness, grand mal seizure, vascular collapse

Treatment: ("Airway, breathing, circulation"). Oxygen, support ventilation if necessary (local anesthetic toxicity is exacerbated by hypercarbia), anticonvulsants such as a benzodiazepine or thiopental, support the circulation. Intubation may be necessary to protect the airway. Bretylium or cardioversion is given for ventricular arrhythmias, intralipid for bupivacaine toxicity.

Comprehension Questions

15.1. A 24-year-old African American woman presents for revision distal digit amputation of her left hand. She has a history of sickle cell disease, and has had a number of hospitalizations for sickle cell crises. She is treated chronically with large amounts of narcotics for pain management. The patient has had nothing to eat or drink for 8 hours. Which of the following anesthetics are contraindicated for her surgery?

A. General endotracheal anesthesia
B. Axillary nerve block with sedation
C. Intravenous regional anesthesia (Bier block)
D. Sedation with a digital block performed by the surgeon

15.2. A 62-year-old man presents for excision of a ganglion cyst on the wrist under i.v. regional anesthesia. Which of the following local anesthetics would be the best choice?
A. Lidocaine
B. Ropivacaine
C. Bupivacaine
D. Tetracaine

15.3. The ganglion mentioned in the preceding question is quickly excised, and the tourniquet is deflated after 10 minutes of inflation time. The patient becomes agitated and states that he hears a ringing in his ears. He is receiving oxygen through a nasal cannula. What should you do immediately?
A. Administer succinylcholine and intubate the patient.
B. Reinflate the tourniquet.
C. Administer midazolam.
D. Call for help.

15.4. Which of the following is the most common cause of failure of intravenous regional anesthesia?
A. Surgeon use of electrocautery
B. Lack of opioid in the local anesthetic mixture
C. Use of expired local anesthetics
D. Prolonged tourniquet time

ANSWERS

15.1. **C.** Intravenous regional anesthesia is usually an excellent choice for most patients undergoing distal upper extremity surgery. But in this patient, underlying sickle cell disease is a contraindication to the technique because of the induced ischemia of the limb, which may subsequently lead to a sickle cell crisis. Other contraindications to an intravenous regional technique include patient refusal and allergy to local anesthetics.

15.2. **A.** Lidocaine is the best choice for this procedure as it has the greatest safety profile in the event of inadvertent systemic uptake. The duration of the anesthetic is determined by the tourniquet time. The patient should be monitored vigilantly at all times with ASA monitors and functioning tourniquet alarms.

15.3. **C.** Administer midazolam, for the patient's early signs of local anesthetic toxicity. In fact, midazolam, a benzodiazepine, is commonly administered even before the local anesthetic to prophylactically raise the seizure threshold. Reinflating the tourniquet is unlikely to be helpful because the local anesthetic has already entered the blood stream. If the patient's symptoms progress to the point that he cannot protect his own airway or sustain ventilation, it may become appropriate to administer succinylcholine and intubate his trachea.

15.4. **D.** Prolonged tourniquet time is associated with the greatest number of i.v. regional anesthesia failures. Ischemia of the tissues underlying the tourniquet causes pain, transmitted by unmyelinated C-fibers, and resulting in significant discomfort by 30 to 45 minutes. The inflation of second, more distal, tourniquet followed by release of the proximal first tourniquet may allow for an additional 20 to 30 minutes of operative time.

Clinical Pearls

- Tourniquet discomfort defines the duration for which an i.v. regional technique is effective.
- Local anesthetic toxicity is a significant risk in the setting of tourniquet failure. Standard monitors should always be applied and the anesthesiologist must remain vigilant during this anesthetic.
- Benzodiazepines such as midazolam are used to treat local anesthetic toxicity.

REFERENCES

Chan VWS, Peng PWH, Kaszas Z, et al. A comparative study of general anesthesia, intravenous regional anesthesia, and axillary block for outpatient hand surgery: Clinical outcome and cost analysis. *Anesth Analg.* 2001;93:1181-1184.

Crystal CC, McArthur TJ, Harrison B. Anesthetic and procedural sedation for wound management. *Emerg Med Clin North Am.* 2007;25(1):41-71.

Holmes CM. Intravenous regional analgesia. A useful method of producing analgesia of the limbs. *Lancet.* 1963;1:245-247.

Liu SS, Strodtbeck WM, Richman JM, Wu CL. A comparison of regional versus general anesthesia for ambulatory anesthesia: A meta-analysis of randomized controlled trials. *Anesth Analg.* 2005;101:1634-1642.

Van Zundert, Helmstadter A, Goerig M, Mortier E. Centennial of Intravenous Regional Anesthesia. Bier's Block (1908-2008). *Reg Anesth Pain Med.* 2008; 33(5):483-489.

Part 2. Anesthesia for the Subspecialties

Cardiac Diseases

Case 16

A 54-year-old man presents with new-onset "frequent indigestion and diarrhea" over the past 3 months, which his primary care physician ascribes to cholelithiasis. He is scheduled for a laparoscopic cholecystectomy. The surgeon has requested general anesthesia, and an evaluation in the Anesthesia Outpatient Screening Clinic. He has not ordered any laboratory or other tests, but has written on the preoperative tests/orders sheet as "per anesthesia." A postoperative admission to the hospital is planned.

The patient's medical history is remarkable for a hospital admission for 3 days 2 years previously, to rule out a possible myocardial infarction (MI). He was discharged with a diagnosis of "possible non–Q-wave MI." His history is also notable for hypertension, treated with lisinopril hydrochlorothiazide and beta blockers. He has a sedentary lifestyle, but can easily walk up two flights of stairs.

The patient has no history of complications with previous anesthetics or a family history of problems with anesthesia. He has no allergies to medications and does not consume alcohol. He smoked 2 packs of cigarettes per day since age 18, but had quit smoking 2 years ago.

The patient's yearly chest x-ray and ECGs have been "normal" or "unchanged." He missed his yearly ECG and dobutamine stress test 6 months ago, but the two previous studies were normal. The hematological, liver, and kidney function tests were normal as well.

On examination, the patient weighs 89 kg and is 5 ft, 11 in tall. His vital signs are: BP 150/90, HR 90 and regular, respiratory rate 20, and a temperature of 37°C. His neck appears normal and is mobile, he opens his mouth without difficulty, and with his head extended and tongue protruding, his uvula is completely visible. His pulmonary and cardiac examinations are normal.

Laboratory tests ordered by your partner include: Hct 41, WBC 9600, platelets 320,000, Na^+ 138, K^+ 3.4, HCO_3 28, BUN 18, creatinine 1.4, and blood glucose 142. His chest x-ray (CXR) showed "no airspace disease with borderline cardiomegaly," and his ECG, "NSR, rate 86, occasional PACs, borderline LVH, non-specific ST-T changes, unchanged from prior studies."

- What is the appropriate preoperative management of this patient?
- Is any further testing needed, and if so, what?

ANSWER TO CASE 16:

Preoperative Assessment of the Patient with Heart Disease

Summary: A 54-year-old male patient with cholelithiasis is scheduled for an elective cholecystectomy. He has a history of hypertension, tobacco use, and current indigestion with normal exercise capacity and a history of MI 2 years ago.

➤ **Appropriate preoperative management:** Continue the lisenopril on the morning of surgery.

➤ **Further testing:** This is an elective case, in a patient with good functional capacity, without evidence of myocardium at risk, and who is undergoing a low-risk surgical procedure. No further testing is indicated.

ANALYSIS

Objectives

1. Understand the rationale for the 2007 revision of the guidelines for cardiac evaluation before non-cardiac surgery by the American College of Cardiology/American Heart Association (ACC/AHA).
2. Become familiar with the relationship between the level of complexity of the surgical procedure and the level of preoperative testing in the patient with heart disease.
3. Understand the method for and advantages of preoperative cardiac risk stratification for patients undergoing non-cardiac surgical procedures.

Considerations

This is an elective case, so the patient's clinical predictors, such as exercise capacity, and the level of surgical risk guide further diagnostic and therapeutic interventions. His MI was more than 7 days ago, and although he missed the most recently-scheduled stress test, one had been performed following his MI which did not indicate any myocardium at risk, and the patient's functional capacity is good. Inguinal herniorrhaphy is a low-risk procedure. Since this patient is at low risk for a cardiac event and is undergoing a low-risk surgical procedure, he can proceed to surgery without further testing. He is counseled to continue his lisinopril, and to take it as usual on the morning of surgery.

APPROACH TO Preoperative Assessment of the Patient with Possible CAD

CLINICAL APPROACH

Morbidity and mortality from cardiac complications are the most common significant adverse events in the perioperative period. Up to 1% of the 100 million adults having non-cardiac surgery each year will be affected, and of those affected, one in four will die. The goal of any preoperative examination is to lower the risk in the preoperative period by identifying patients with modifiable conditions, and optimizing these conditions prior to surgery. A natural part of this process includes identifying patients with a high risk for perioperative cardiac events.

The 2007 revision of the guidelines for cardiac evaluation before non-cardiac surgery by the American College of Cardiology/American Heart Association (ACC/AHA) reduced the recommendations for preoperative noninvasive stress testing and revascularization. This altered approach was driven by the recognition that unpredictable coronary plaque rupture, of even minor lesions and thrombi cause up to 50% of fatal MIs perioperatively. Revascularization, typically recommended for the more critical stenosis, does not prevent plaque rupture.

The ACC/AHA guidelines are organized in a stepwise approach. Management is determined by the first recommendation that applies to a particular patient. There is no need to progress through the entire algorithm.

Step 1 considers the urgency of the surgery. If emergency surgery precludes further cardiac assessment, the focus of patient management shifts to perioperative surveillance (eg, serial ECGs, enzymes, monitoring), and the reduction of risk (eg, beta blockers with strict control of heart rate, statins, pain management). Clinical predictors, exercise capacity, and the level of surgical risk guide further diagnostic and therapeutic interventions.

Step 2 considers an active cardiac condition. An acute MI, unstable or severe angina, decompensated heart failure, severe valvular disease (eg, severe aortic stenosis), or significant arrhythmias (eg, ventricular tachycardia or atrial fibrillation with a rapid rate) warrant the postponement for all except life-saving emergency surgery. More recent evidence suggests that an acute MI, occurring within the past 7 days, warrants postponing elective surgeries. An MI within the past 8 to 30 days, and with evidence of myocardium at risk (indicated by persistent symptoms or the results of stress testing) represents a high-risk condition. If the recent MI is not accompanied by myocardium at risk, the patient's risk is simply equivalent to that of coronary artery disease any other time.

Step 3 considers the risk of the surgical procedure. Low-risk surgical procedures include endoscopic procedures, superficial procedures, cataract surgery, breast surgery, and most ambulatory surgical procedures. These procedures carry such low risk of an adverse cardiac-event risk (generally < 1%) that even patients at high cardiac risk, provided that they do not have any active cardiac conditions, should proceed directly to surgery without further testing.

Intermediate-risk surgery (1%-5% risk of cardiac complications) includes orthopedic, most intra-abdominal, and intrathoracic procedures. Patients who need vascular surgery are most likely to benefit from further testing.

Step 4 assesses the patient's functional capacity. Asymptomatic patients with heart disease, who have an average exercise capacity (can walk up two flights of stairs or four blocks) can proceed to surgery.

Step 5 considers patients with poor or indeterminate functional capacity scheduled for vascular, intermediate-, or high-risk procedures. This is the last and most complex step. Clinical predictors for cardiac risk were derived from the revised cardiac risk index, identifying ischemic heart disease, heart failure, cerebrovascular disease, diabetes, and renal insufficiency as important patient comorbidities. The number of these clinical predictors alters the recommendations for and likely benefit from cardiac testing. Patients without these clinical predictors may proceed to surgery without further testing.

The ACC/AHA guidelines recommend further testing only "if it will change management." Patients with three or more clinical risk factors, and who need vascular surgery are most likely to benefit from further testing. Patients with one to two clinical predictor(s), and who need intermediate-risk surgery (1%-5% risk of cardiac complications, including procedures such as orthopedic, intra-abdominal and intrathoracic procedures) or vascular surgery can proceed to surgery with heart rate control. Or, they should be scheduled to undergo noninvasive testing if it will change management. The guidelines specifically state, "there are insufficient data to determine the best strategy." Factors to consider are the urgency of the non-cardiac surgery (eg, patients with cancer), the life-expectancy of the individual, and the potential long-term benefits of medical management versus revascularization.

Lastly, the general risk factors for CAD (eg, smoking, family history, hypercholesterolemia, age, and hypertension) have not been shown to predict perioperative cardiac morbidity.

Comprehension Questions

16.1. During the preoperative cardiac assessment for elective surgical procedures, which pieces of information are essential to determine if further testing is warranted?
A. An ECG
B. A dobutamine stress test
C. Information regarding the patient's functional (exercise) capacity
D. A chest x-ray

16.2. Which of the following warrants additional preoperative noninvasive stress testing and possible revascularization prior to non-cardiac surgery?
A. A 45-year-old man with a history of diabetes and poor exercise tolerance, who is scheduled for a colon resection for a mass.
B. A 74-year-old man with chronic, stable angina scheduled for a total knee replacement.
C. A 65-year-old woman with a history of hypertension, chronic atrial fibrillation with a ventricular heart rate of 75 beats per minute scheduled for a carpal tunnel repair.
D. A 58-year-old man with a history of hypertension and a left bundle-branch block undergoing a total knee replacement.

16.3. Which all of the following comorbidities would warrant postponement of an elective operation?
A. Acute MI within the last 30 days
B. Renal failure
C. Heart failure
D. Unstable arrhythmias

ANSWERS

16.1. **C.** According to the AHA/ACC guidelines, information regarding the patient's functional (exercise) capacity, understanding whether the patient has any evidence (or absence) of an unstable cardiac condition, and knowledge of the magnitude of the type of surgery planned for the patient. An ECG is not indicated in patients under 50 years of age (60 in some settings), and a dobutamine stress test is indicated if there is a suspicion of myocardium at risk. Although a chest x-ray can be useful to determine a patient's heart size, it is not otherwise helpful in determining whether further cardiac testing is warranted.

16.2. **A.** This patient is undergoing an intermediate-risk procedure, and has one clinical predictor (diabetes). Since further testing may elucidate a cause for his poor exercise tolerance, additional testing is indicated. The patients in answer B has one clinical predictor (ischemic heart disease), and is scheduled for an intermediate-risk procedure. His condition is stable, and he has good functional capacity. No further testing is indicated. The patient in answer C has no clinical predictors and is scheduled for a low-risk procedure. She does not need further testing. The patient in answer D has no risk factors and is undergoing an intermediate-risk procedure. So no further testing is warranted.

16.3. **D.** D, an unstable arrhythmia, is an active cardiac condition and warrants postponement of all except life-saving surgeries. A, an MI within the past 8 to 30 days, and with the evidence of myocardium at risk (indicated by persistent symptoms or the results of stress testing) represents a high-risk condition, but does not necessarily warrant postponement of surgery. If the recent MI is not accompanied by myocardium at risk, the patient's risk is simply equivalent to that of any other patient with coronary artery disease any other time. Answers B and C, renal failure and heart failure, are clinical predictors of cardiac risk but do not warrant postponing elective surgery. Other clinical predictors include ischemic heart disease.

Clinical Pearls

- Cardiac complications are the leading cause of perioperative morbidity and mortality in the perioperative setting.
- Major clinical risk factors include acute coronary syndromes, decompensated heart failure, clinically significant arrhythmias, and severe valvular disease.
- Intermediate-risk predictors include ischemic heart disease, compensated or prior heart failure, cerebrovascular disease, diabetes mellitus that requires insulin therapy, and renal insufficiency (serum creatinine level > 2 mg/dL).
- Exercise capacity remains an important determinant of perioperative risk.
- Elective major vascular surgery remains the type of surgery with the highest associated risk.

REFERENCES

Fleisher LA, Beckman JA, Brown KA, et al. ACC/AHA 2007 Guidelines on Perioperative Cardiovascular Evaluation and Care for Non-cardiac Surgery. *J Am Coll Cardiol.* 2007;50:e159-241.

Lee TH, Marcantonio ER, Mangione CM, et al. Derivation and prospective validation of a simple index for prediction of cardiac risk of major non-cardiac surgery. *Circulation.* 1999;100:1043-1049.

Case 17

A 72-year-old woman presents with a long history of left shoulder pain recently increasing in intensity, and with a decreased range of motion over the past year. Her orthopedic surgeon has diagnosed a rotator cuff tear, and has scheduled her for an arthroscopic rotator cuff repair. The surgeon plans to perform this procedure in the "beach chair" position. The patient's medical history is significant for severe aortic stenosis and moderate pulmonary hypertension. She experiences dyspnea after walking up one flight of stairs, which has been stable over a significant period of time. She can easily lay flat in bed at night, does not report paroxysmal nocturnal dyspnea, and has not had any recent episodes of syncope. The patient also has hypertension, well-controlled with metoprolol. She has no allergies to medications, and neither smokes nor consumes alcohol. Her review of symptoms is otherwise unremarkable.

The patient is 64 in tall and weights 65 kg. Her physical examination demonstrates a grade III/VI late-peaking systolic murmur, and lungs clear to auscultation. She has mild edema of her bilateral lower extremities. Her laboratory results are significant for a hematocrit of 32%, and are otherwise normal.

➤ What are the most important aspects of the evaluation prior to formation of the anesthetic plan for this patient?

➤ What are the goals for intraoperative hemodynamic management in patients with aortic stenosis?

ANSWERS TO CASE 17:

Severe Aortic Stenosis in Non-Cardiac Surgery

Summary: A 72-year-old woman with severe aortic stenosis and pulmonary hypertension is scheduled for an arthroscopic rotator cuff repair to be performed in the beach chair position.

➤ **Preoperative evaluation:** In patients with aortic stenosis, it is important to carefully probe for signs and symptoms of acute congestive heart failure, a history of syncope or near syncope, and functional exercise capacity prior to the development of an anesthetic plan. An ECG is useful to determine the presence or absence of sinus rhythm, and an echocardiogram unless the patient is currently followed and evaluated by a cardiologist.

➤ **Goals for intraoperative hemodynamic management:** Patients with aortic stenosis include the avoidance of hypotension and tachycardia, and maintenance of a normal sinus rhythm and adequate preload.

ANALYSIS

Objectives

1. Understand the etiology and pathophysiology of aortic stenosis.
2. Become familiar with the signs and symptoms of aortic stenosis, and recognize the importance of decompensated congestive heart failure and syncope in these patients.
3. List the intraoperative hemodynamic goals in patients with aortic stenosis, and the optimal ways of achieving them.
4. Be able to formulate an anesthetic plan for the patient with aortic stenosis presenting for non-cardiac surgery.

Considerations

Since this patient is not symptomatic for her aortic stenosis, is in sinus rhythm and is closely followed by her cardiologist, she can safely proceed with the administration of anesthesia. Rotator cuffs are typically repaired under general anesthesia, with endotracheal intubation. The positioning of the patient in the "beach chair" position predisposes to venous pooling in the extremities resulting in hypotension, which is detrimental in the setting of aortic stenosis. Because of the significant possibility of hypotension following the induction of anesthesia and positioning in this 72-year-old patient, an arterial line for monitoring blood pressure is indicated. Since she is scheduled as the first case of the morning, insensible losses from her NPO status will be minimal, and since blood loss and fluid shifts are minimal for this type of surgery, no central line is indicated.

The optimal induction agent for this patient is etomidate, which causes less vasodilation and myocardial depression than the other anesthetic agents. Fentanyl is an opiate which reduces postoperative pain, and reduces heart rate, a desirable characteristic in patients with aortic stenosis. She will be paralyzed with vecuronium, and the relaxation reversed with neostigmine, and glycopyrrolate carefully titrated to minimize any changes in heart rate or blood pressure.

APPROACH TO Severe Aortic Stenosis for Non-cardiac Surgery

As the average age of the American population increases, an ever-growing number of patients with heart disease will present for non-cardiac surgeries. Patients with aortic stenosis have significantly increased perioperative morbidity and mortality during non-cardiac surgery. An appropriate preoperative evaluation and risk-stratification, accompanied by a thorough understanding of hemodynamic variables is of paramount importance when anesthetizing these patients.

CLINICAL APPROACH

Etiology

Aortic stenosis is the most common valvular lesion in the United States. It is either congenital, or acquired. Congenital aortic stenosis usually results from an incomplete development of the valve commissures, resulting in a unicuspid or bicuspid valve. A bicuspid aortic valve is the most common congenital valvular lesion, and is present in 1% to 2% of the population. This abnormal valve may present cause symptoms at birth, but more commonly, patients present with a murmur on examination in the fifth decade of life. The abnormal valve leaflets are more susceptible to hemodynamic stress which ultimately leads to valve thickening, calcification, and stenosis of the aortic orifice.

Acquired aortic stenosis is due to either calcific disease or rheumatic fever. Since the incidence of rheumatic valvular has declined dramatically over the past 50 years, aortic stenosis resulting from rheumatic fever is a rare occurrence. Calcific disease of a tri-leaflet valve accounts for the vast majority of aortic valve disease, and most likely reflects an inflammatory process with similarities to atherosclerosis. Calcific aortic stenosis occurs more often in males than in females, and symptoms are typically manifest in the seventh decade of life. Regardless of the etiology, the natural course of aortic stenosis is a long, asymptomatic latent period followed by the onset and rapid progression of symptoms.

Pathophysiology

Aortic stenosis is defined as a restriction in the opening of the aortic valve's leaflets leading to an obstruction to flow during systole. This fixed obstruction produces a pressure gradient across the left ventricular outflow tract and aortic root, requiring the ventricle to generate an increased systolic pressure in order to produce flow across the valve. The normal aortic valve area is 2.5 to 3.5 cm^2. Hemodynamic changes due to obstruction are generally not observed until the valve area is less than 1.0 cm^2. Aortic stenosis is considered severe if the peak gradient across the valve is > 50 mm Hg, or if the valve area is < 0.8 cm^2. The definition of the varying degrees of aortic stenosis is detailed in Table 17–1.

Over time, the increased pressures generated by the left ventricle lead to increases in ventricular wall tension in accordance with the law of Laplace:

$$\text{Wall tension} = [\text{Pressure} \quad \text{Radius}]/[\text{Wall thickness} \quad 2]$$

Concentric left ventricular hypertrophy also develops as a compensatory mechanism, to reduce wall tension while allowing the pressure overloaded ventricle to maintain stroke volume. As the walls of the left ventricle become thickened, they become less compliant. Thus filling during diastole is impaired (also known as diastolic dysfunction). Ventricular filling increasingly depends upon an adequate diastolic time, and upon the atrial contraction or "kick" during diastole. Thus, the maintenance of normal sinus rhythm in these patients is very important and tachycardia of any type is poorly tolerated. The maintenance of an adequate preload is also important for the optimal function of a stiff and noncompliant ventricle. However, as atrial pressures increase in response to the increasing left ventricular end diastolic pressures, pulmonary edema and pulmonary hypertension can result.

Signs and Symptoms

Patients with mild to moderate aortic stenosis are generally asymptomatic. Patients with severe aortic stenosis may present with angina, syncope, and/or shortness of breath. Angina can occur in the absence of coronary disease, due to the large, thick ventricle's imbalance between myocardial oxygen supply

Table 17–1 CLASSIFICATION OF THE SEVERITY OF AORTIC STENOSIS

	NORMAL	MILD	MODERATE	SEVERE	CRITICAL
Peak gradient (mm Hg)	0	< 25	25-50	> 50	> 70
Aortic valve area (cm^2)	> 2	1.5-2.0	1.0-1.3	0.7-1.0	< 0.7

and demand. An hypertrophic left ventricle has a greater oxygen demand due to its increased mass, and its generation of higher systolic pressures. The supply of oxygen to the hypertrophic ventricle is reduced by compression of the coronary arteries during systole. Dyspnea and orthopnea may reflect pulmonary edema associated with diastolic congestive heart failure. Syncope results from inadequate cerebral perfusion.

The onset of symptoms in patients with aortic stenosis has significant prognostic implications. Patients with angina have a 50% 5-year survival rate; patients with syncope or dyspnea have survival rates of 50% at 3 and 2 years, respectively. Consequently, the need for surgical intervention is based primarily upon the development of symptoms. Ironically, the aortic valvular area at which symptoms develop is variable.

Preoperative Evaluation

The preoperative evaluation of a patient with aortic stenosis presenting for non-cardiac surgery focuses on identifying patients at high risk. It is imperative that the severity of aortic stenosis be determined prior to any elective surgery. A careful history elicits any symptoms of aortic stenosis including angina, syncope, shortness of breath, and/or signs of heart failure such as peripheral edema, orthopnea, dyspnea on exertion, and paroxysmal nocturnal dyspnea. The patient's general level of activity and exercise tolerance, and the New York Heart Association functional classification of heart disease are also useful tools for estimating the severity of heart disease and estimating prognosis (Table 17–2).

On physical examination a harsh, mid-systolic crescendo-decrescendo murmur heard best over the right sternal border at the second intercostal space is characteristic of aortic stenosis. This murmur may radiate upward toward the carotid arteries. The preoperative physical examination should focus on uncovering signs of heart failure. Thorough auscultation of the chest may reveal rales, wheezing or an S_3 gallop, examination of the neck, jugular venous distension, and examination of the extremities and abdomen, pitting edema or ascites.

Table 17–2 MODIFIED NEW YORK HEART ASSOCIATION FUNCTIONAL CLASSIFICATION OF HEART DISEASE

CLASS	DESCRIPTION
I	Asymptomatic except during severe exertion
II	Symptomatic with moderate activity
III	Symptomatic with minimal activity
IV	Symptomatic at rest

An important tool in evaluating the severity of aortic stenosis is the Doppler and two-dimensional transthoracic echocardiography. If aortic stenosis is symptomatic, elective non-cardiac surgery should be canceled or postponed until after valve replacement surgery. If the patient refuses corrective valve surgery, non-cardiac surgery is accompanied by a mortality risk of approximately 10%. Elective surgery should be postponed or canceled for patients with severe asymptomatic aortic stenosis if the valve has not been evaluated within the past 12 months. Table 17–1 shows the valve areas and peak gradients associated with mild, moderate, and severe aortic stenosis.

Echocardiography will also detail other cardiac valve lesions. A current ECG should also be obtained, and may reveal left ventricular hypertrophy or myocardial ischemia. A chest radiograph may be warranted to rule out pulmonary edema if signs of congestive heart failure are present on examination.

Anesthetic Management

The intraoperative management of patients with aortic stenosis is based upon maintaining a normal sinus rhythm at a rate of 60 to 75 bpm, an adequate preload, and adequate systemic vascular resistance (SVR). In addition to the standard ASA monitors including the measurement of blood pressure and an ECG, invasive monitoring should be considered. Patients with severe aortic stenosis are often intolerant of even brief periods of hypotension. Given the expected hemodynamic perturbations associated with induction of anesthesia, intubation, and varying surgical stimulation, an arterial line is often indicated.

Monitoring of central venous and pulmonary artery pressures may be indicated if the surgical procedure will involve large fluid shifts or the use of vasodilators. As noted in the AHA Guidelines, the substantial risks of PA catheter placement must be weighed against the potential benefit of the data obtained in each individual patient. In this particular patient, the hemodynamic changes associated with reverse Trendelenburg or the "beach chair" position in combination with the severity of her aortic valve disease may warrant placement of a PA catheter.

Alternatively (or in combination with a PA catheter), transesophageal echocardiography may also be used to assess the effect of intraoperative therapeutic interventions. Alterations in cardiac filling and wall motion with therapeutic interventions and patient repositioning are quickly assessed using this relatively low-risk invasive monitor. However, neither the intraoperative use of a pulmonary artery catheter nor transesophageal echocardiography has been shown to change outcomes in patients with aortic stenosis presenting for non-cardiac surgery.

The anesthetic technique employed is of secondary importance as long as the hemodynamic goals of maintaining SVR, a slow heart rate, adequate preload, and normal sinus rhythm are met. Spinal and epidural anesthesia are typically well tolerated in patients with mild to moderate disease. These blocks have been relatively contraindicated in patients with severe disease, but with invasive monitoring and careful titration of agents, spinal and epidural anesthesia have been safely used in patients with severe aortic stenosis.

A balanced general anesthetic technique employing opiates, volatile anesthetics, and muscle relaxants is often employed. Since many agents typically used for the induction and maintenance of general anesthesia cause vasodilation and thus hypotension, careful titration of these agents is of critical importance. Alpha agonists such as phenylephrine treat hypotension, and maintain or increase SVR. Agents that increase inotropy are generally ineffective in patients with aortic stenosis, as the left ventricle is already in a highly contractile state, and the tachycardia often associated with these agents is undesirable. Hemodynamically-significant intraoperative arrhythmias should be promptly treated with synchronized cardioversion. In the event of cardiac arrest, restoring perfusion is important. However, chest compressions are generally ineffective given the extreme hypertrophy that often accompanies significant aortic stenosis. Nonetheless, in the event of an intraoperative arrest, the advanced cardiac life support (ACLS) algorithms should be applied.

Patients with severe aortic stenosis should be monitored closely for at least 24 hours after surgery including minor ambulatory procedures. For major surgeries involving large fluid shifts or patients with significant pulmonary hypertension, postoperative monitoring overnight in the intensive care unit should be strongly considered. In patients with severe aortic stenosis, the risk of cardiac death remains elevated in the immediate postoperative period.

Comprehension Questions

17.1. During your preoperative assessment, a 72-year-old man complains of dyspnea on exertion and intermittent chest pain. Upon auscultation of his heart, you notice a mid-systolic crescendo-decrescendo murmur that radiates to his carotid. This murmur is most characteristic of which valvular lesion?

A. Mitral stenosis
B. Mitral regurgitation
C. Aortic regurgitation
D. Aortic stenosis

17.2. What statement about the pathophysiology of aortic stenosis is most likely true?

A. Patients with aortic stenosis have decreased myocardial oxygen demand as the left ventricular hypertrophy offers a "protective" effect.
B. The increased pressure gradient between the left ventricle and aorta results in eccentric left ventricular hypertrophy.
C. Patients with aortic stenosis can develop impaired left ventricular filling because of diastolic dysfunction.
D. Myocardial ischemia in aortic stenosis is rare in the absence of coronary artery disease.

17.3. You will be taking care of a 72-year-old woman with a history of severe aortic stenosis (valve area 0.7 cm^2) for a laparoscopic cholecystectomy. You are planning a general anesthetic with sevoflurane. What will be the hemodynamic goal for this patient?

A. Low systemic vascular resistance
B. Heart rate between 60 to 75 beats per minute
C. Low preload
D. Increased contractility

17.4. During insufflation of the peritoneum with carbon dioxide, the patient becomes hypotensive (blood pressure 60/48) while the heart rate remains unchanged at 84 beats per minute. You ask the surgeon to decrease the pneumoperitoneum; however, the blood pressure remains low. Which of the following would be the best course of action?

A. Administer an alpha-agonist drug such as phenylephrine.
B. Administer nitroglycerin.
C. Administer a beta agonist, such as dobutamine.
D. Administer an inotropic agent such as epinephrine.

ANSWERS

17.1. **D.** The murmur described is characteristic of aortic stenosis. The murmur of mitral stenosis is a mid-diastolic rumbling murmur, best heard at the apex with the patient in the left lateral position. The murmur of mitral regurgitation is typically a holosystolic murmur that may radiate to the axilla. The murmur associated with aortic regurgitation is a mid-systolic ejection murmur generally heard best at the base of the heart and is transmitted to the jugular notch.

17.2. **C.** The pathophysiology of aortic stenosis involves left ventricular outflow obstruction with the subsequent development of a pressure gradient between the left ventricle and the aorta. This results in concentric left ventricle hypertrophy rather than an eccentric hypertrophy. As a result of left ventricular hypertrophy, myocardial oxygen consumption is increased and patients can develop myocardial ischemia as a result of increased myocardial oxygen consumption and decreased myocardial oxygen supply. Also as a result of left ventricular hypertrophy, ventricular relaxation and filling during diastole is impaired.

17.3. **B.** The hemodynamic goals for patients with aortic stenosis include maintenance of preload, systemic vascular resistance, contractility, and a sinus rhythm, as well as the avoidance of tachycardia. Because of their relatively fixed stroke volume, patients with aortic stenosis are dependent on adequate filling/preload. Tachycardia and rhythms other than sinus rhythm (ie, atrial fibrillation) are poorly tolerated and can be harmful. Patients with aortic stenosis have a fixed resistance at the level of the aortic valve; thus, maintenance of systemic vascular resistance is important to preserve diastolic coronary perfusion gradients. In patients with aortic stenosis, contractility should be preserved.

17.4. **A.** Hypotension is poorly tolerated in patients with severe aortic stenosis. Myocardial ischemia can develop rapidly; hence prompt recognition and treatment of hypotension is critical. In contrast to inotropic agents such as epinephrine or dobutamine, alpha agonists such as phenylephrine are generally regarded as the treatment of choice for hypotension, to restore coronary perfusion pressure. Vasodilators such as nitroglycerin can be harmful because of the potential for hypotension from decreased preload and afterload.

Clinical Pearls

- The hemodynamic goals for managing patients with aortic stenosis include maintaining sinus rhythm, a normal to high preload, normal to high SVR, and slow heart rate. As long as these goals are met, anesthesia can be maintained with many different techniques.
- Alpha agonists such as phenylephrine are the treatment of choice for hypotension.
- With severe aortic stenosis, ventricular relaxation and compliance are altered necessitating higher left ventricular filling pressures. Congestive failure and pulmonary edema may result.
- Arrhythmias are poorly tolerated in patients with severe aortic stenosis, and should be immediately treated with cardioversion.
- Elective (non-cardiac) surgery should be postponed or canceled for patients with symptomatic aortic stenosis, or for those with severe asymptomatic aortic stenosis if the valve has not been evaluated within the past 12 months.
- Cardiopulmonary resuscitation (CPR) is often unsuccessful in this setting.

REFERENCES

ACC/AHA 2007 Guidelines on Perioperative Cardiovascular Evaluation and Care for Noncardiac Surgery: Executive Summary. *Circulation*. 2007;116:1971-1996.

Cook D, Housmans P, Rehfeldt K. Valvular heart disease. In: *Kaplan's Cardiac Anesthesia*. 5th ed. Saunders Elsevier; 2006: 645-690.

Mends LA, Loscalzo J. Acquired Valvular heart disease. In: Andreoli, ed. *Cecil Essentials of Medicine*. 5th ed. Philadelphia, PA: W.B. Saunders Co; 2001: 69-70.

Mittnacht Alexander JC, Fanshawe M, Konstadt S. Anesthetic considerations in the patient with valvular heart disease undergoing non-cardiac surgery. *Semin Cardiothorac Vasc Anesth*. 2008;12(33): 33-59.

Case 18

An 85-year-old gentleman presents to the preoperative testing clinic with the diagnosis of an 8-cm abdominal aortic aneurysm (AAA) requiring repair discovered by his primary care physician during a routine physical examination. The patient's past medical history includes well-controlled hypertension, hypercholesterolemia, benign prostatic hyperplasia, diabetes mellitus, and an 80-pack-year history of smoking. He has no known drug allergies. His medication list includes metoprolol, lisinopril, and lovastatin. He lives on a farm, and often exerts himself physically doing chores or walking long distances.

The patient is 5 ft 10 in tall and weighs 90 kg. His neck is supple, his mouth opening is more than three fingers breadths, and his airway is classed as a Mallampati 1. His lungs are clear with the exception of occasional sonorous rhonchi, and his heart rhythm is slow but without murmurs.

Given the age of the patient and the anatomy of the aneurysm, the surgeon has made the decision to schedule the placement of an endovascular aorto-bifemoral stent. An open repair of the patient's abdominal aortic aneurysm will be performed if the endovascular repair cannot be performed successfully.

➤ What are the preoperative concerns for this patient?

➤ How can tests be used to assess his perioperative risks?

➤ What are the most important factors to remember intraoperatively?

ANSWERS TO CASE 18: Anesthetic Management of Abdominal Aortic Aneurysm

Summary: This is an 85-year-old man with diabetes and a long history of smoking who is undergoing repair of an abdominal aortic aneurysm using an intravascular stent.

- **Preoperative concerns:** The preoperative concerns center on an optimization of his coexisting medical problems such as hypertension, diabetes mellitus, and optimization of his cardiac function.
- **Tests to assess perioperative risks:** In addition to the usual tests obtained before a surgical procedure (hemoglobin, hematocrit, platelet count, chemistry panel, and ECG), preoperative tests are important to assess cardiac function, since the optimization of reversible cardiac disease alters postoperative morbidity and mortality. Appropriate testing includes a history of the patient's functional capacity at the very least, and noninvasive testing such as a stress test or dobutamine stress ECHO may be required if the assessment of functional capacity is complicated by coexisting diseases such as arthritis or a sedentary lifestyle. Similarly, because of his chronic hypertension and diabetes mellitus, an assessment of renal function is also important. The preoperative assessment of hemoglobin and/ or hematocrit aids in preparing for the potential of sudden large blood losses during the procedure.
- **Important factors for intraoperative care:** Important considerations in the intraoperative care of patients undergoing repair of an AAA are the maintenance of a mean arterial pressure sufficient to provide adequate coronary and cerebral perfusion, and the avoidance of hypertensive episodes which could hasten the aneurysm's rupture.

ANALYSIS

Objectives

1. Become acquainted with preoperative workup required for the patient undergoing AAA repair.
2. Be able to compare and contrast an AAA repair by open versus endovascular repair.
3. Identify issues basic to anesthetic choice and management for the patient undergoing AAA repair.
4. Obtain a better understanding of the options for pain management following major vascular surgery.

Considerations

This patient's AAA albeit large was asymptomatic and discovered on a routine physical examination. Though the risk of rupture is a real possibility, the advantages of scheduling his case as an elective procedure following an expeditious preoperative evaluation and preparation outweigh the risks of not proceeding directly to surgery. Optimizing the patient's medical problems minimizes the postoperative complications, and stratifying his perioperative risk provides valuable information which, in turn, affects his intraoperative and postoperative management.

The risks of this procedure emanate from the surgery itself, as well as this patient's pre-existing medical condition. Even when repaired using an endovascular technique, an AAA repair is still major vascular surgery, and carries the risk of a major blood loss. The anatomic location of the aneurysm with respect to ease of repair and the location of the renal arteries, and the duration of the aorta's cross clamp time, also influences the operative risk. All in all, his condition is good compared to many patients who undergo this procedure. He has hypertension, peripheral vascular disease (which also carries the risk of coronary artery disease), long-standing diabetes with the risk of end-organ damage, and a long history of smoking, which suggests the possibility of compromised lung function as well. Nevertheless, his functional capacity is good, exceeding 6 to 8 METs. Thus his ASA Physical Status classification is ASA 3. Combining the risks of this operating with the risks emanating from his medical condition, his attendant risk for this procedure is moderate or high.

This patient prefers general anesthesia, although he understands that regional anesthesia such as an epidural catheter for neuraxial blockade is a viable and safe option as well. He will be monitored using the standard intraoperative monitoring paradigm (ECG, blood pressure cuff, pulse oximetry, capnography, and body temperature). Since he is undergoing an AAA repair, an arterial line will be placed to allow continuous monitoring of arterial pressure and frequent blood gas analysis, and a large bore intravenous (16 gauge or larger) will be placed. The use of central venous pressure (CVP) monitors, pulmonary artery catheters, and/or transesophageal echocardiography (TEE) is optional and should be tailored to specific situations. Given his good functional capacity and lack of significant heart disease, the placement of a CVP line is most likely to be adequate for the monitoring of volume status, in addition to providing additional intravenous access. Urine output should be measured via and recorded at frequent time intervals to assist in the assessment of the adequacy of tissue perfusion.

The most important goal of this patient's intraoperative management is the maintenance of a mean arterial pressure sufficient to provide adequate coronary and cerebral perfusion. This is accomplished by using small doses of anesthetics with minimal side effects in combination, ensuring adequate volume resuscitation, and using vasopressors as necessary. Blood and blood products should be readily available in the event of aneurysm rupture or conversion to open repair.

APPROACH TO

Anesthetic Management of Abdominal Aortic Aneurysm

DEFINITIONS

ABDOMINAL AORTIC ANEURYSM: A focal dilatation of the aorta greater than 50% of its normal arterial diameter. It is often described in relation to the renal arteries as either a suprarenal or an infrarenal abdominal aortic aneurysm.

OPEN REPAIR: Open repair of an AAA involves a midline abdominal incision with excision, the placement of a cross clamp across the width of the aorta above the proximal end of the aneurysm to stop exsanguinations, and replacement by a synthetic graft.

ENDOVASCULAR REPAIR: An endovascular repair is less invasive than an open repair. It is thus associated with less surgical morbidity, enabling it to be considered as a viable therapy for patients considered too ill to be candidates for the traditional open repair. An endovascular repair involves accessing the aorta via bilateral femoral arteries, and then inserting a bifurcated graft across the length of the aneurysm under fluoroscopic guidance.

METABOLIC EQUIVALENT (MET): The metabolic rate consuming 3.5 mL of oxygen per kilogram of body weight per minute or a metabolic rate consuming 1 kcal per kilogram of body weight per hour. (For examples of the energy requirements for common daily activities, please see Table 18–1.)

CLINICAL APPROACH

An AAA is observed at autopsy in 0.5% to 3.2% of the population, and is the primary cause of death in 1.3% of men between 65 and 85 years of age in developed countries. AAAs are more common in men than in women, with a 2:1 preponderance in people under the age of 80, though the frequency of its occurrence approaches 1:1 in older individuals. It is more common in white males than African American males.

Generally, aneurysms that are asymptomatic are followed clinically until they reach 6 cm in diameter, since 6 cm is the maximal size which can be determined by imaging studies alone. Estimating the size or following the progression in size of an aneurysm over 6 cm in diameter requires an invasive intervention.

Abdominal aneurysms requiring treatment are treated surgically by open repair or by endovascular stent placement. Many factors go into the decision-making process which determines the type of repair. The size of the aneurysm, its proximity to the renal arteries, the patient's comorbidities, and operator preference are some of the factors determining the operative approach.

Table 18–1 DAILY ACTIVITIES AND ENERGY REQUIREMENTS

DAILY ACTIVITY	METABOLIC EQUIVALENTS (METS)
Lifting and carrying objects (9-20 kg)	4-5
Lifting and carrying objects > 20 kg	> 6
Walking 1 mile (level) in 20 minutes	3-4
Running/walking on an incline	> 6
Golf	4-5
Gardening (digging)	3-5
Do-it-yourself, wallpapering	4-5
Light housework (ironing, polishing)	2-4
Heavy housework (making beds, scrubbing floors, cleaning windows)	3-6
Competitive sports, swimming, aerobics	> 6
Heavy shoveling, digging ditches	> 6

Abdominal aortic aneurysm repairs, whether open or endovascular, are major vascular procedures with an intermediate risk for perioperative cardiac events. A complete preoperative workup prior to either open or endovascular repair should include a comprehensive history and physical examination. A detailed assessment of the patient's exercise tolerance is of paramount importance, and is typically documented in the record in terms of METs. For patients undergoing procedures with an inherent risk at the intermediate level, who are asymptomatic and able to perform at 4 METs or greater, the American College of Cardiology and the American Heart Association (ACC/AHA) recommends further cardiac testing only if the test will change the course of cardiac management (coronary artery stenting or bypass, or myocardial valve replacement, etc.) prior to the operative procedure.

One of the most important goals of the intraoperative management of AAA repair is the maintenance of a mean arterial pressure sufficient to provide adequate coronary and cerebral perfusion. This may be more important in the patient with an AAA. For example, long-standing hypertension, a common finding in patients undergoing AAA repair, is associated with a shift in the autoregulation curve for cerebral perfusion pressure to the right. This means that the blood pressure over which autoregulation preserves cerebral blood flow is higher in hypertensive patients than in the population as a whole

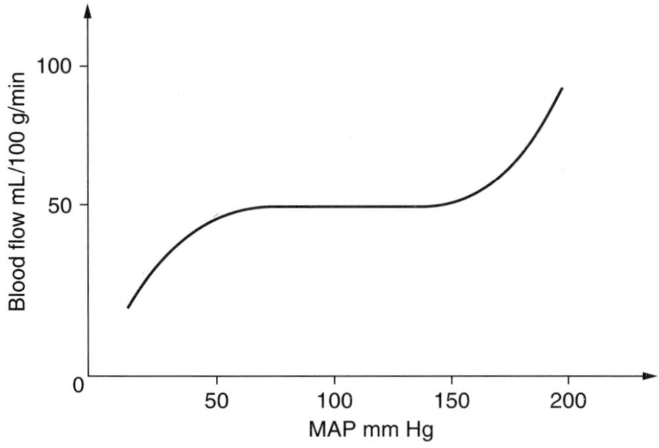

Figure 18–1. Cerebral blood flow is dependent on mean arterial pressure (MAP).

(Figure 18–1). In addition, hypertensive patients may also have left ventricular hypertrophy accompanied by diastolic dysfunction (Figure 18–2). The thickened, hypertrophied ventricle requires more perfusion to meet its oxygen demands. Moreover, coronary perfusion, which happens largely during diastole, may be compromised by diastolic dysfunction.

Monitoring during surgery includes the standard monitors according to guidelines from the American Society of Anesthesiologists (ASA, noninvasive blood pressure monitoring, two-lead electrocardiogram, and end-tidal carbon dioxide concentration, pulse oximetry, and temperature). In addition, for AAA repair, blood pressure is measured by an intra-arterial cannula, and volume status, by central venous pressure monitoring. Urine output is measured periodically to indicate the adequacy of tissue perfusion.

Keeping in mind the hemodynamic goals for this patient, the induction of anesthesia is performed by using agents with minimal cardiovascular effects in combination to minimize the dose of each, in attempt to reduce any undesirable side effects. Prior to induction, an opiate such as fentanyl is administered to reduce the patient's cardiovascular response to endotracheal intubation. Induction is typically accomplished using a combination of midazolam, more fentanyl, and etomidate. Propofol may be added for blood pressure control if indicated; however, given propofol's propensity to cause more peripheral vasodilatation and hypotension, etomidate is probably a better choice as the initial induction agent. The maintenance of anesthesia is achieved by a combination of inhalational agent such as isoflurane or desflurane supplemented by boluses of narcotic agents such as fentanyl.

An endovascular AAA repair may be performed under spinal anesthesia if the aneurysm is infrarenal. Indeed, in patients with severe COPD, spinal may be preferable over general anesthesia, though no demonstrable improvement

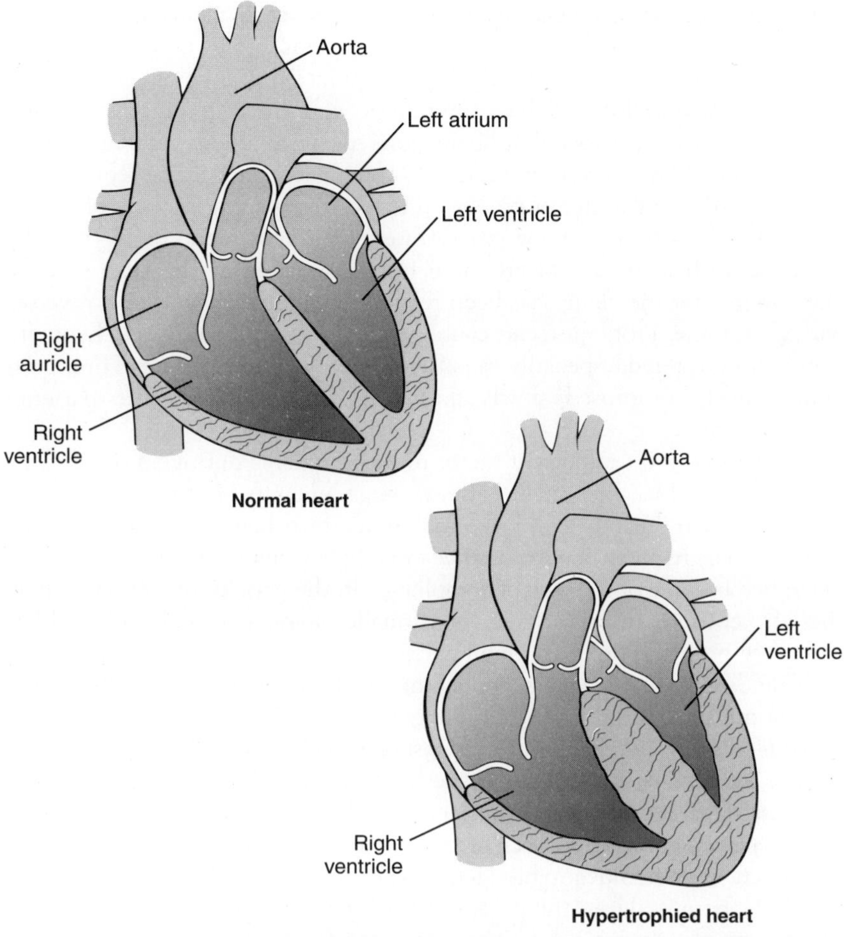

Figure 18–2. Effects of uncontrolled hypertension—left ventricular hypertrophy.

in outcomes has been observed. The main advantage of a spinal is the avoidance of the need for endotracheal intubation which may predispose to the need for postoperative ventilatory support. However, spinal also has two major disadvantages. First, spinal causes a sympathectomy, which can result in hypotension and complicate the assessment of the patient's fluid status. Second, if the operation requires an emergent conversion to an open repair, general anesthesia will be required within an emergent time frame, instead of the typical slow induction while carefully titrating the anesthetic agents to the patient's needs.

The open repair of an AAA requires the placement of both proximal and distal clamps across the width of the aorta to allow the graft to be sutured in place in a bloodless field. Prior to placement of the clamp, the patient is anticoagulated with a heparin. With the aorta cross clamped, the major source of perfusion and oxygenation of the patient's limbs is absent. A local acidemia results, accompanied by the accumulation of inflammatory mediators. The sudden release of these substances when the clamp is removed may cause hypotension, myocardial depression, severe morbidity, and/or death if not recognized and treated promptly. Assuring adequate volume replacement and the ready availability of pressors prior to the opening of the clamp is of paramount importance. Some practitioners also recommend prophylaxis for acidemia with a sodium bicarbonate infusion started at the time of cross clamping. After the clamp has been released, the anticoagulation is reversed with protamine. Protamine can cause profound vasodilatation and hypotension is administered, especially in patients who are hypovolemic. Thus, protamine must be infused slowly and carefully titrated to the patient's hemodynamics.

The second most important factor to be considered during an open AAA repair is blood loss. In normal patients, large amounts of blood loss (greater than 15% of estimated blood volume) result in a hemodynamic instability manifested by hypotension and tachycardia. In "vasculopaths," this response is magnified because of the lack of compliance in the patient's vessels and often, the left ventricle. In this setting, even smaller amounts of sudden blood loss can cause profound drops in blood pressure. Blood loss is treated aggressively with fluids or blood products, depending on the patient's hemoglobin at the time of infusion. If the hemoglobin is greater than 7 g/dL, most practitioners are comfortable with the infusion of a crystalloid such as normal saline or a colloid such as albumin or hetastarch. If the hemoglobin is less than 7 g/dL, blood transfusions should be utilized to support the bleeding and hemodynamics.

The placement of endovascular stent grafts across the AAA is usually not associated with significant blood loss when compared to open procedures, although there is always the potential for aneurysmal rupture or perforation. Stent grafts also do not require the placement of an aortic cross clamp, hence the degree of incurred acidemia is less. Indeed, acidosis, if present, is perhaps more reflective of an inadequate fluid resuscitation than of limb ischemia.

Stents grafts are usually placed with fluoroscopy support, exposing the patient to contrast dye. If stent placement is difficult, the amount of dye used may be significant enough to cause a contrast-induced nephropathy. Data from the cardiac catheterization laboratory (where all interventions are done under fluoroscopy) suggest that prophylactic use of *N*-acetyl cysteine and sodium bicarbonate infusions play an adjunctive role in decreasing the incidence of this syndrome.

If the case has an uncomplicated intraoperative course with, for example, no requirement for inotropes or pressors to support vital signs, a minimal need for transfusion, and normal respiratory patterns and effort, the endotracheal tube may be removed at the end of the procedure. Since patients undergoing AAA repair are at moderate to high risk for perioperative myocardial events, testing for a possible myocardial infarction using serial cardiac enzymes and an ECG are routine. Because of the propensity for a major blood loss and dye load, either of which may adversely affect renal function, renal function is also followed postoperatively.

Pain control is an important part of postoperative management, since pain causes hypertension and tachycardia which may be harmful in the presence of coronary disease, to say nothing of the lack of patient comfort. Pain control enables deep breathing, which is vital to prevent postoperative atelectasis. Atelectasis is problematic because it serves as a nidus for pneumonia, which can necessitate a re-intubation of the trachea as well as the need for mechanical ventilation. In the presence of significant incisional pain, patients splint, and minimize movements that worsen the pain—such as deep breathing and ambulation. Ambulation is key in preventing deep vein thrombosis, improving gut motility and optimizing lung mechanics.

Several options are available for postoperative pain control. Prior to the induction of anesthesia, an epidural or intrathecal catheter may be placed in the operating room. Contraindications to these techniques include localized infection at the site of procedure, thrombocytopenia, and medications that alter coagulation such as preoperative use of antiplatelet agents or anticoagulants such as heparin or warfarin. Epidural or intrathecal techniques reduce the postoperative requirements for parenteral narcotics, and therefore improve patient interaction, decrease somnolence, and provide superior pain control. On the other hand, neuraxial techniques, particularly when an opiate is administered, require close monitoring at a level that is not always available within an institution. Neuraxial techniques also carry the same risks of any regional anesthetic with regards to catheter placement, nerve impairment, or an exacerbation of back pain.

Comprehension Questions

18.1. A 54-year-old man presents with a 5.5 cm AAA for repair. He has a past medical history of well-controlled hypertension and diet-controlled diabetes, and is otherwise in excellent physical condition. Which one of the following tests is most appropriate to perform prior to the scheduled AAA repair?

A. Chemical stress test
B. Exercise stress test
C. Coronary angiography
D. An ECG

18.2. In the face of active bleeding and hypotension, fluid resuscitation is performed with which of the following?
A. Colloid such as hetastarch or albumin
B. Crystalloids
C. Blood and blood products
D. As indicated by the hemoglobin and hematocrit

18.3. What actions are indicated prior to the opening of an aortic cross clamp?
A. Be sure that the patient is euvolemic.
B. Obtain additional i.v. access.
C. Ensure an adequate depth of anesthesia.
D. Administer protamine to antagonize the heparin-induced anticoagulation.

ANSWERS

18.1. **D.** An ECG. This gentleman is in excellent physical condition. On further questioning he states he plays tennis for an hour everyday, is compliant with his medications, doesn't smoke and has a very healthy diet. In this setting, additional cardiac testing does not give any additional information. While an AAA repair is considered a moderate- to high-risk procedure for cardiac events, testing should only be performed in the setting of positive symptoms and in the event that results from the test would alter management strategy. In this patient with stable and active exercise tolerance, cardiac testing over and above an ECG will be of low yield.

18.2. **D.** Management of bleeding in the operating room is somewhat of an art. Sudden torrential bleeding which depletes greater than 15% of the patient's blood volume is usually an emergency and needs to be promptly resuscitated with blood transfusion and cell salvage techniques. If the patient is hemodynamically stable and demonstrates mild hypotension and tachycardia (all signs that point to less than 15% blood volume loss), resuscitation with crystalloids or colloids may be appropriate.

18.3. **A.** "Be sure that the patient is euvolemic." Removing the cross clamp in an hypovolemic patient can be life threatening, due to the sudden reduction in systemic vascular resistance and myocardial suppression that accompanies the release of acidotic mediators with the clamp's removal. Ensuring an adequate blood volume is an important part of the anesthetic plan, especially at this critical point in the procedure.

Any required i.v. access should already be in place, and the depth of anesthesia should be stable. Protamine is administered to antagonize the heparin-induced anticoagulation when the anticoagulation is no longer needed, that is, after the graft has been placed and the clamp has been removed.

Clinical Pearls

- Because of its lower morbidity, an endovascular (as opposed to open) approach to aortic aneurysm repair has expanded the population of patients with AAA who are candidates for surgical treatment.
- Patients that present for AAA, whether by open technique or by stent, often have other comorbidities such as hypertension, diabetes, and cardiac disease which significantly impact anesthetic management.
- Invasive monitoring such as arterial blood pressure and central venous pressure provide valuable information such as the "beat-to-beat" arterial pressure, volume status, and cardiac functionality both in the operating room and intensive care unit. In the setting of AAA repair, the benefits of invasive monitoring far outweigh the attendant risks.
- AAA repair is a moderate- to high-risk procedure that carries the possibilities of complications such as myocardial infarction and stroke in the perioperative period.

REFERENCES

Baril DT, Kahn RA, et al. Endovascular abdominal aneurysm repair: Emerging developments and anesthetic considerations. *J Cardiothorac Vasc Anesth*. 2007;21:730-742.

Norris EJ. Abdominal aortic reconstruction. In: Miller RD, ed. *Miller's Anesthesia*. 6th ed. Philadelphia, PA: Churchill Livingstone; 2005.

Case 19

A 59-year-old man with a left indirect inguinal hernia was admitted for left-sided herniorrhaphy. He had undergone a coronary artery bypass surgery (CABG) 6 months ago, and an automatic implantable cardioverter defibrillator (AICD) was implanted 4 months ago because of recurrent episodes of ventricular tachycardia (VT) unresponsive to amiodarone therapy.

The patient's medical history is remarkable for one episode of an irregular cardiac rhythm 2 months ago that responded to activation of the AICD. He denies any other episodes since that event. He also notes a history of hypertension, which is treated with lisinopril. He denies symptoms of angina, dyspnea on exertion, or paroxysmal nocturnal dyspnea. He has no history of complications with previous anesthetics or a family history of problems with anesthesia. He has no allergies to medications, does not smoke or consume alcohol.

Echocardiography revealed a left ventricular ejection fraction (LVEF) of 25% with trace mitral regurgitation. The chest x-ray showed an AICD in situ and an enlarged heart size. The hematological, liver, and kidney function tests were normal. On examination, the patient weighs 180 lb and is 5 ft, 10 in tall. His neck appears to be normal and mobile. He opens his mouth without difficulty, and with his head extended and tongue protruding, his uvula is completely visible. His lung and cardiac examination is normal.

- How are AICD devices managed in patients undergoing surgery?
- What factors are important to address preoperatively in the patient with an AICD?
- What are the special concerns applicable to patients with an AICD in the operative setting?

ANSWERS TO CASE 19:
Automatic Implantable Cardiovertor Defibrillator

Summary: A 59-year-old man with a left indirect inguinal hernia admitted for a left-sided herniorrhaphy. He has a history of recurrent episodes of ventricular tachycardia (VT), which has been treated with an AICD device.

- **AICD in surgery:** An AICD is disabled before the start of surgery using a noninvasive programming device. It is reprogrammed (reactivated) in post-anesthesia care unit (PACU) postoperatively.
- **Important factors:** Most patients with an AICD have poor left ventricular function, with a low ejection fraction and coexisting systemic disease. Primary management of the patient includes evaluation and optimization of his coexisting disease, and evaluating the defibrillator. Most patients with an AICD carry a wallet-sized card which lists the specific type of device. If not already easily accessible in the patient's medical record, this information should be added. The AICD is also interrogated preoperatively to determine whether it is operating properly, whether it has fired and if so, what conditions triggered the firing. This can provide useful information for the patient's intraoperative management, when the device will be turned off. At this time, arrangements should also be made for the AICD to be turned off prior to the surgery, and back on in the PACU after the procedure.
- **Special concerns:** Ensure the safety of the patient and of the operating room personnel. Electromagnetic interference from the electrocautery or from external defibrillation can affect the AICD. If unintentionally left in the activated mode, sudden movements such as those occurring during positioning, or muscle fasciculations such as with succinylcholine can cause the device to fire inappropriately, potentially posing a hazard to operating room personnel and the patient.

ANALYSIS

Objectives

1. Become familiar with the preoperative care of a patient with an AICD.
2. Understand how AICDs are managed in the perioperative setting.
3. Understand the special intraoperative concerns in patients with an AICD.

Considerations

An inguinal herniorrhaphy is readily amenable to repair under a regional anesthetic approach such as a spinal or a peripheral field block. Because of this patient's left ventricular dysfunction and the type of surgery, an epidural anesthetic was chosen. An epidural has the advantage of administering multiple doses of an anesthetic as opposed to a single dosed spinal, allowing the level of sensory block to be carefully titrated so that it is sufficient, without being too high.

The patient's AICD was turned off prior to the procedure, and an external pulse generator and external pacing were kept ready in the operating room (OR). External counter shock paddles were also checked and brought into the operating room, so they were immediately available. The monitoring during surgery included a continuous two-lead electrocardiogram (lead II and V5), a pulse oximeter, and a noninvasive arterial pressure monitor. An epidural catheter was inserted, and after a test dose, ropivacaine was injected and a T10 sensory block obtained. Oxygen was given via nasal prongs at 4 L/min. The patient did not require any sedation. His AICD was re-activated in the PACU postoperatively.

APPROACH TO Automatic Implantable Cardiovertor Defibrillator

Automatic internal cardiac defibrillation has significantly reduced the risk of sudden cardiac death in patients with known life-threatening ventricular arrhythmias. The ability of an AICD to provide therapy within 5 to 15 seconds of arrhythmia detection allows a defibrillation success rate approaching 100%.

An ICD system consists of a pulse generator and leads for detection and therapy of tachyarrhythmias. It may provide antitachycardia, antibradycardia pacing, synchronized or nonsynchronized shocks, telemetry, and diagnostic storage. Many devices use adaptive rate pacing to modify the pacing rate for changing metabolic needs. The AICD batteries contain up to 20,000 J of energy. Most AICD designs use two capacitors in series to achieve the maximum voltage for defibrillation. High energy discharges of 10 to 40 J, delivered asynchronously are used to treat ventricular fibrillation (VF). Cardioversion with energy exceeding 2 J results in skeletal and diaphragmatic muscle depolarization. This is painful to the conscious patient, although if sleeping or syncopal, the patient may be unaware that the device has fired.

AICDs terminate VF successfully in 98% of cases. Supraventricular tachycardia (SVT) remains the most common etiology of inappropriate shock therapy. According to one report, antitachycardia pacing successfully terminated spontaneous VT in greater than 90% of cases. Approximately 20% of AICD patients require pacing for bradycardia, and 80% of those requiring pacing benefit from dual chamber pacing. ICD devices are placed adjacent to the heart via either a central transvenous route or epicardial location.

For 25 years, the accepted method for ensuring appropriate function of an AICD has included the intentional induction of ventricular fibrillation (VF) to ensure that the ICD will sense, detect, and defibrillate VF. At the time of implantation, this method is used to determine the smallest possible shock that will successfully manage the arrhythmia. Occasionally, these "AICD checks" cause complications, and rarely, death. The risks of implant testing include those related to VF (circulatory arrest, albeit brief), those related to shocks of the myocardium, or the combination of circulatory arrest and shocks. In general, the poorer a patient's myocardial function, the slower he or she will recover from the induced arrest. With better understanding of defibrillation coupled with today's improved technology, and use of AICDs for primary prevention of ventricular tachycardia (VT) or VF, some question the need for either defibrillation testing or any assessment of defibrillation efficacy at ICD implantation. However, the device is to be periodically checked to determine that its leads are functioning appropriately, and the clinical parameters under which it has fired are appropriate.

For a pacemaker-dependent patient undergoing surgery, the AICD should be reprogrammed to an asynchronous mode, the tachycardia sensing and adaptive rate pacing functions turned off, and alternative facilities for pacing should be available. Sudden movements such as fasciculations following succinylcholine, or sudden movements during positioning may otherwise trigger the device to inappropriately fire.

The use of electrocautery in the presence of a functioning AICD is particularly hazardous. If the AICD is inadvertently left on during surgery, electrocautery treatment for hemostasis during surgery may inappropriately signal the AICD that the patient has developed a malignant dysrhythmia. The detection of the "false rhythm abnormality" by the AICD would trigger the delivery of a therapeutic shock. Even worse, electrocautery has been associated with the reprogramming of the AICD to a ventricular rate of 300, with disastrous results.

In patients with an AICD, the cautery grounding tool should be placed as far as possible from the AICD (at least 15 cm), and in such a way that the pulse generator and the leads are not in the current pathway between the device and the electrocautery. Only the lowest possible energies and short bursts of cautery should be used to minimize adverse effects of electromagnetic interference. If electrocautery is to be used within 15 cm of AICD, a compatible programming device and a pulse generator should be accessible in the operating room. In the event that external defibrillation is required, the pads or paddles should be placed 10 cm from the pulse generator and implanted electrodes. The use of sutures instead of cautery, or bipolar instead of unipolar cautery can also be employed to minimize the risk of an AICD malfunction. In all cases, the AICD is reactivated after the electrocautery is no longer required.

A magnet placed over the AICD will inactivate the defibrillator function (not the pacemaker function) appropriately during surgery. When the magnet is removed, normal function returns. However, use of a magnet should not be substituted for inactivating the defibrillator device prior to the procedure, and reprogramming it afterwards.

The perioperative management of patients with a cardiac rhythm management devices is as complicated and constantly evolving as its corresponding field of technology. Understanding of the basic principles as to how these devices function, and how to make use of available resources such as consulting the provider responsible for device follow-up or even the device manufacturer, is strongly encouraged to make anesthesia safer for these high-risk cases.

Comprehension Questions

19.1. A 72-year-old man presents for a left colon resection for cancer. He has an AICD which was placed 2 years prior to this admission. The preoperative visit confirms that the patient's medical condition is optimized, an ECG is performed, and the device is interrogated to determine its activity history. Just prior to surgery, which of the following actions is appropriate?

A. Have a pacemaker/AICD technician available in the operating room to reprogram the device if needed.
B. Deactivate the defibrillator.
C. Place external pacing pads.
D. Put a magnet over the pacemaker/defibrillator.

19.2. Optimal perioperative management of a patient with an AICD includes which of the following?

A. Placing the electrocautery pad ("grounding") on any large surface area of the patient's body is appropriate.
B. Reactivating the AICD following a surgical procedure is required.
C. The immediate availability of external pacing or defibrillation equipment is not necessary.
D. The patient may have his AICD turned off the day prior to surgery at his primary care physician's office.

19.3. Muscle fasciculations following succinylcholine, sudden patient movement such as may occur in positioning, and the use of electrocautery may result in which of the following?

A. Cause a deactivated defibrillator to fire in the operating room.
B. Cause an active defibrillator to fire inappropriately in the operating room.
C. Necessitate the use of a magnet.
D. Interfere with the delivery of a shock if it is needed.

ANSWERS

19.1. **B.** Immediately prior to the procedure, the AICD's defibrillator mode is deactivated, and it is reactivated immediately post-op in the PACU. Alternatively, and if compatible with the type of defibrillator, a magnet may be placed over the defibrillator to temporarily inactivate it. However, some AICD's may be reprogrammed in an uncontrolled fashion by a magnet, leading to rapid ventricular rate and catastrophe. It is not necessary to place external pacing pads, or to have a pacemaker/AICD technician available in the operating room.

19.2. **B.** The patient may have his AICD turned off at the hospital, immediately prior to surgery. External pacing or defibrillation equipment must be immediately available. Placing the electrocautery pad ("grounding") on any large surface area of the patient's body is appropriate, provided the pad is at least 15 cm away from the AICD, and that it is placed in such a way that the pulse generator and the leads are not in the pathway between the device and the electrocautery. Reactivation and evaluation of the AICD following the procedure is required.

19.3. **B.** Muscle fasciculations, sudden patient movement, and electrocautery may trigger an active AICD to fire inappropriately in the operating room. A magnet placed over the AICD inactivates the defibrillator function, or reprograms the defibrillator in an uncontrollable fashion.

Clinical Pearls

- The preoperative evaluation of a patient with an AICD includes an evaluation and optimization of the underlying heart disease and left ventricular function as well as determination that the AICD is functioning well.
- The perioperative monitoring of such a patient is mainly guided by the degree of left ventricular function, and the type of surgery.
- The AICD is deactivated prior to the procedure and reactivated afterward.
- An external cardiac defibrillator should always be available in the operating room, with the external defibrillator pads in place so that an effective cardioversion or defibrillation can be performed without interfering with the surgical field.
- Any electromagnetic force can interfere the functioning of the AICD.
- It is essential to monitor patients with an AICD continuously in the postoperative period until the vital signs are stable.

REFERENCE

Practice Advisory for the perioperative management of patients with cardiac rhythm devices: Pacemakers and implantable cardioverter-defibrillators. *Anesthesiology*. 2005;103:186-198.

Case 20

A 44-year-old woman is scheduled for a vaginal hysterectomy for dysmenorrhea that has failed medical therapy. Although she had been otherwise healthy, over the past year, she has increasingly noticed exertional dyspnea, particularly when shopping in large stores. These symptoms have worsened, to the point that she sometimes felt as though she was about to "pass out." She consulted her primary physician several months ago. After an extensive workup, she was diagnosed with idiopathic pulmonary hypertension, and treated with amlodipine, a calcium channel blocker, and furosemide. The administration of another medication by permanent central indwelling catheter has been discussed, but is not warranted at this time.

The patient's vital signs on presentation include a blood pressure 102/56 mm Hg, heart rate 90 bpm, 94% O_2 saturation. On physical examination, she has clear lungs to auscultation, mild ankle edema, a 2/6 systolic murmur, and an S_4 gallop. The ECG shows right axis deviation and right ventricular hypertrophy. An echocardiogram demonstrates mild right ventricular (RV) enlargement, and a right ventricular systolic pressure (RVSP) of 35 mm Hg. Following the induction of anesthesia, her oxygen saturation decreases to 90%, blood pressure falls to 80/43 mm Hg, and her heart rate increases to 110 bpm.

- ➤ What should the preoperative evaluation include?
- ➤ What is the impact of the anesthesia and surgical procedure on pulmonary hypertension?
- ➤ What are the goals of anesthetic management?

ANSWERS TO CASE 20: Pulmonary Hypertension

Summary: A 44-year-old woman with pulmonary hypertension and right heart failure presents for a vaginal hysterectomy under general anesthesia.

- **Preoperative evaluation:** The evaluation of patients with pulmonary hypertension should focus on identifying the severity of the disease, the patient's baseline cardiac function, and assure that the patient's condition is optimized prior to surgery. It typically includes an arterial blood gas, a chest radiograph, ECG, echocardiography, and right heart catheterization.
- **Effect of anesthetic and surgical techniques on pulmonary hypertension:** Anesthesia and surgery can dramatically affect artery (PA) pressure and right heart function. Acidemia, hypoxia, hypercarbia, and hypotension in the perioperative period can worsen both pulmonary hypertension and right ventricular failure.
- **Goals of anesthetic management:** Goals are directed toward maintaining the stability of pulmonary and systemic arterial pressure, the maintenance of normal sinus rhythm, and the appropriate volume status, oxygenation, and ventilation.

ANALYSIS

Objectives

1. Understand the pathophysiology of pulmonary hypertension.
2. Be able to conduct a preoperative evaluation in a patient with pulmonary hypertension.
3. Understand the implications of anesthesia in the setting of pulmonary hypertension, and develop anesthetic management plan accordingly.
4. Manage the perioperative complications in a patient with pulmonary hypertension.

Considerations

This patient with pulmonary hypertension presents a unique challenge in anesthesia management. A vaginal hysterectomy typically requires general anesthesia, although, general anesthesia can exacerbate pulmonary hypertension and right heart failure. So in addition to the routine monitors as described by the American Society of Anesthesiologists, arterial blood pressure monitoring should be performed to provide beat-to-beat BP measurements, as well as the ability to frequently sample arterial blood gases. Blood gases are useful in the analysis of acid-base status, hemoglobin, and electrolytes. Given the status of her right ventricular dysfunction, it is not unreasonable to monitor her central venous pressure (CVP). If the surgical procedure were more complex or her condition had progressed, then a pulmonary artery catheter might also be indicated.

The major goal of an anesthetic is to avoid situations that might exacerbate her pulmonary hypertension. These include acidemia, hypoxia, hypercarbia, sympathetic stimulation, hypotension, and the use of drugs which exacerbate pulmonary hypertension such as nitrous oxide. Narcotics increase the carbon dioxide threshold, so even patients who are well narcotized require a higher end-tidal carbon dioxide level to initiate spontaneous respiration. Such a well narcotized state may worsen pulmonary hypertension and precipitate RV failure as well.

APPROACH TO Pulmonary Hypertension

DEFINITIONS

PULMONARY HYPERTENSION: A sustained elevation of the pulmonary artery pressure, which can be idiopathic or secondary to diseases of the respiratory or cardiovascular systems.

COR PULMONALE: A right ventricular enlargement and dysfunction secondary to acute or chronic pulmonary hypertension.

CLINICAL APPROACH

Pathology of Pulmonary Hypertension

The pulmonary circulation is a low-pressure circulation. Elevation of the pulmonary vascular pressure can result from cardiac and respiratory disorders such as primary pulmonary hypertension, congenital heart disease, acquired valvular dysfunction, cardiomyopathy, myocardial infarction, acute and chronic thromboembolism, chronic respiratory disease, collagen vascular disorders, and end-stage liver disease. An elevated pulmonary artery pressure leads to increase in the right ventricular afterload, an increase in preload, tachycardia, and impaired contractility. The increased demand for oxygen in the face of a decreased perfusion of the right ventricle further perpetuates impairment of the right ventricular contractility, increases right ventricular pressure, and causes right ventricular failure. In patients with pulmonary hypertension, the perioperative risk for cardiopulmonary complications is related to the severity of the pulmonary hypertension and the degree of right ventricular dysfunction. Hypoxia, hypercarbia, and acidemia during anesthesia contribute to elevation of the pulmonary artery pressure.

The preoperative evaluation of a patient with pulmonary hypertension should focus on the severity of the disease and the presence of cor pulmonale. Clinical signs and symptoms of right ventricular failure and valvular incompetence include jugular venous distention, peripheral edema, liver congestion, heart murmurs, and additional heart sounds. The patient's ECG can demonstrate right axis deviation, right bundle-branch block (RBBB), right atrial enlargement, $S_1Q_3T_3$ pattern, and electrolyte abnormalities. Echocardiography and cardiac catheterization are utilized to assess ventricular function and pressures, as well as pulmonary vascular resistance, and the response to intravenous or inhaled vasodilators. The respiratory system should be comprehensively evaluated and optimized prior to elective surgery.

The treatment for pulmonary hypertension includes continuing any pulmonary vasodilators, diuretics, and inotropes during the perioperative period. The surgical procedure, as well as the anticipated effects on the pulmonary circulation and the heart guides the choice of general or regional anesthetic technique.

Vaginal hysterectomy procedures can sometimes be done under regional anesthesia. Neuraxial regional anesthesia is associated with decrease in venous return and systemic blood pressure and the need for intravenous fluid load, all of which may exacerbate cardiac dysfunction. The maintenance of optimal fluid balance is critical in these cases. The right ventricular function is preload dependent; however, fluid overload can easily precipitate right heart failure. Neuraxial anesthesia such as spinal or epidural carries risks from the need for fluid preload, and the sympathectomy-induced hypotension, and are not be an optimal choice. In addition, the avoidance of hypercarbia and hypoxia due to heavy sedation is important, and the maintenance of hemodynamic stability is critical.

The prevention of endogenous catecholamine release during intubation and emergence can be achieved with opiates, intravenous anesthetics, and local anesthetics. Hypotension as a result of anesthetic induction, intraoperative fluid overload, excessive anesthesia, or blood loss is detrimental to right ventricular perfusion and should be avoided. The selection of an induction agent such as etomidate, administered slowly and at a reduced dose, facilitates the maintenance of a normal blood pressure. An invasive arterial blood pressure monitor aids in careful hemodynamic control, and monitoring adequacy of oxygenation and ventilation. If significant hemodynamic instability and fluid shifts are anticipated, central venous and pulmonary artery pressure monitoring as well as transesophageal echocardiography are indicated to guide fluid, inotrope, or pressor management.

Blood loss can result in hypovolemia, tachycardia, and decrease in oxygen-carrying capacity, all of which can precipitate right ventricular failure and should be corrected promptly. For some procedures, laparoscopic techniques have the benefit of less blood loss, pain, and stress. However, patients with pulmonary hypertension may not tolerate the detrimental effects of the hypercarbia from the CO_2 insufflation, or the reduction in preload while increasing afterload which is associated with pneumoperitoneum.

Comprehension Questions

20.1. A 45-year-old man with pulmonary hypertension presents to the emergency room with shortness of breath, jugular venous distension, peripheral edema, BP 87/46 mm Hg, HR 122 bpm, pulse oximeter oxygen saturation (Spo_2) 91%, and hemoglobin 8.5 g/dL. Match the treatment (left column) with the order in which it would be administered.

A. Transfusion of red blood cells	1. First
B. Fluid bolus of 1 L normal saline	2. Second
C. Oxygen via face mask	3. Third
D. Furosemide dieresis	4. Fourth
E. Norephrine vasopressor infusion	5. Not at all

20.2. A 37-year-old woman with primary pulmonary hypertension, treated with intravenous epoprostenol infusion, is scheduled for emergency appendectomy. Which of the following statements regarding her anesthetic plan is correct?

A. Aggressive premedication with opiates is recommended.
B. Induction with standard dose of propofol will help in the control of hemodynamics.
C. Vasopressor use to treat hypotension is indicated.
D. The epoprostenol infusion should be discontinued to avoid hypotension.
E. Large fluid bolus before induction is indicated to avoid hypotension.

20.3. A 32-year-old woman with pulmonary hypertension secondary to mitral stenosis is undergoing laparoscopic nephrectomy for a renal mass. Half an hour after the start of the surgery, her Spo_2 is 89%, her end-tidal CO_2 is 55, BP 89/47, and HR 120. She has received 1 L of i.v. fluids. Which of the following is the most likely diagnosis for her hemodynamic compromise?

A. Left ventricular myocardial infarction (MI)
B. Ventilatory failure
C. Excessive IV fluid administration
D. Hypovolemia due to blood loss
E. Pulmonary embolism
F. A CO_2 embolus from insufflation

ANSWERS

20.1. **C, 1.** Supplemental oxygen will improve oxygenation. Transfusing blood will increase oxygen carrying capacity and pulmonary artery pressure, but it will take time before the blood is available. Thus, **E, 2,** the vasopressor infusion is started next, to improve RV perfusion and contractility, and **D, 3**, the patient is diuresed to reduce the RV pressure. Answer B, a large fluid bolus, would further increase the RV pressure and worsen RV failure, and should not be done at all.

20.2. **C.** Hypotension should be treated with vasopressors to maintain RV perfusion and contractility. Premedication with high dose of opiates can lead to respiratory depression and hypercarbia and should be avoided. Induction agents should be used carefully and in reduced dose to avoid hypotension. Fluid overload can precipitate RV failure and fluids should be administered gradually and incrementally.

20.3. **B.** Ventilatory failure during laparoscopy with CO_2 insufflation can lead to hypoxemia and hypercarbia, which elevates the pulmonary artery pressure and leads to right ventricular failure. **E** is a possible but less likely diagnosis. Patients with pulmonary hypertension are also at risk for pulmonary embolism in the perioperative period secondary to thromboembolic disease. **C**, excessive intravenous fluid administration, can also precipitate RV failure, although that would not be anticipated after only 1 L of saline. **F**, a CO_2 embolus from insufflation is an unlikely possibility: CO_2 emboli are usually catastrophic and temporally related to insufflation. **D**, hypovolemia secondary to blood loss is a possibility, although the surgeons have not noticed any bleeding. Answer **A** is incorrect. This young patient without risk factors for CAD is unlikely to have an MI of the left ventricle.

Clinical Pearls

- Patients with pulmonary hypertension may have considerable cardiac dysfunction and have increased risk of heart failure with hemodynamic alterations.
- Patients with pulmonary hypertension require a comprehensive preoperative evaluation which identifies the severity of the disease and baseline cardiac function, and assures that the patient's condition is optimized prior to surgery.
- Both anesthetic and surgical techniques can worsen pulmonary hypertension and precipitate heart failure.
- The perioperative management of patients with pulmonary hypertension is critical to the reduction of cardiopulmonary complications and improvement of outcomes.

REFERENCES

Klinger J. Pulmonary arterial hypertension: An overview. *Semin in Cardiothorac Vasc Anesth.* 2007;11:96-103.

MacKnight B, Martinez E, Simon B. Anesthetic management of patients with pulmonary hypertension. *Semin Cardiothorac Vasc Anesth.* 2008;12:91-96.

Ramakrishna G, Sprung J, Ravi B, Chandrasekaran K, McGoon M. Impact of pulmonary hypertension on the outcomes of noncardiac surgery. *J Am Coll Cardiol.* 2005;45:1691-1699.

Subramaniam K, Yared J. Management of pulmonary hypertension in the operating room. *Semin Cardiothorac Vasc Anesth.* 2007;11:119-136.

Case 21

A 28-year-old Haitian woman presents to labor and delivery at 38 weeks' gestation for a repeat elective cesarean section. She has had an uneventful pregnancy with a singleton fetus. The patient's past medical history is significant for mitral stenosis. During her pregnancy, she noticed dyspnea on exertion with walking one flight of stairs, which has remained stable. She is unable to lay flat in bed, and props herself up on two pillows to sleep. She has taken Coumadin in the past, but has taken low-molecular-weight heparin since becoming pregnant. With the consent of her cardiologist, she has not taken any anticoagulant for the past 2 days. Her only other medication is prenatal vitamins. She has no known drug allergies, does not smoke, and has not consumed any alcohol since becoming pregnant. The patient is 5 ft 3 in tall and weighs 75 kg. Auscultation of the chest reveals a III/VI diastolic murmur. Her lungs are clear to auscultation, though she has +2 edema of both lower extremities to the knee. She has very mild jugular venous distension.

- What additional information should be obtained in the preoperative evaluation?
- What are the intraoperative hemodynamic goals?
- What special monitors should be considered because of the mitral stenosis?

ANSWERS TO CASE 21: Mitral Stenosis for Non-Cardiac Surgery

Summary: A 28-year-old woman with mitral stenosis presents for an elective cesarean section.

- **Preoperative evaluation:** The preoperative assessment in the patient with mitral stenosis should include questions to elicit any signs and symptoms of pulmonary edema, pulmonary hypertension, or congestive heart failure. It is important to note the patient's exercise tolerance, as well as medication taken with particular attention to anticoagulant agents. The patient should also have an ECG and transthoracic echocardiogram performed preoperatively.
- **Intraoperative hemodynamic goals:** Maintenance of sinus rhythm if at all possible, the prevention of tachycardia and/or systemic vasodilatation, and the careful maintenance of preload.
- **Special monitoring:** An arterial line and possibly a pulmonary artery catheter. If she has a general anesthetic, a transesophageal echocardiography probe should also be considered. This is in addition to the standard monitors specified by the American Society of Anesthesiologists.

ANALYSIS

Objectives

1. Understand the pathophysiology and etiology of mitral stenosis.
2. Become familiar with the signs and symptoms of mitral stenosis.
3. Know the intraoperative hemodynamic goals of mitral stenosis.
4. Be able to formulate an anesthetic plan for the patient with aortic stenosis presenting for non-cardiac surgery.

Considerations

Besides the need to monitor the cardiovascular status, the patient in this case is happily complicated by an impending birth. So, many medications administered to the mother could affect the fetus as well. Routine caesarean sections are usually performed under spinal and/or epidural anesthesia to minimize the circulating concentrations of anesthetics which might cause fetal depression. However, both spinal and epidural anesthesia cause sympathectomy, which in turn reduces preload and afterload, neither of which are well tolerated in patients with mitral disease. However, for patients with mild or moderate disease, an epidural with its indwelling catheter, can be intermittently dosed to gradually achieve the desired sensory level, while concomitantly administering alpha blockers to control preload and afterload.

The general anesthetic for a typical cesarean section is characterized by the administration of an induction anesthetic agent before the patient is paralyzed and incubated. No additional anesthetic is administered until the baby has been delivered. The period between induction and delivery of the infant is often marked by classic signs of "light" anesthesia such as tachycardia and hypertension, neither of which is well tolerated by a patient with mitral stenosis.

Whatever the choice, monitoring is an important consideration. Simply measuring central venous pressure may not provide sufficient information regarding a possible increase in pulmonary artery pressure, which could lead to pulmonary edema. Although it has not been shown to alter mortality, pulmonary artery pressure monitoring should be considered. If a general anesthetic is used, a transesophageal echocardiogram (TEE) probe can provide superior information. However, the TEE probe cannot remain in place throughout the postoperative period.

APPROACH TO Mitral Stenosis for Non-Cardiac Surgery

The incidence of mitral stenosis has decreased drastically in the United States over the past 50 years; however, it continues to remain a major health problem in developing countries. Patients with mild mitral disease have a minimally increased risk of adverse cardiac outcomes in the setting of non-cardiac surgery. However, patients with severe disease or associated pulmonary hypertension (PHT) have a significantly increased risk of perioperative morbidity. Two-thirds of patients with mitral stenosis are women.

Etiology

Mitral stenosis can be congenital, but the vast majority of cases are acquired, most commonly from rheumatic fever. The most common etiology of acquired mitral stenosis is rheumatic fever. In susceptible individuals, inflammatory changes following a group A *Streptococcus* infection can lead to valvular disease as a delayed complication. After the widespread institution of antibiotic treatment for group A streptococcal infection was initiated in the United States, the incidence of this complication has decreased dramatically. Other less common causes of acquired mitral stenosis include infective endocarditis, connective tissue disorders, rheumatoid arthritis, atrial myxoma, carcinoid disease, sarcoidosis, and iatrogenic stenosis after mitral valve surgery. Congenital mitral stenosis is rare and usually associated with a more complex cardiac malformation such as hypoplastic left heart syndrome.

Pathophysiology

Mitral stenosis occurs when thickening, fibrosis, or calcification of the valve leaflets, or fusion of the leaflet commissures obstruct flow from the left atrium to the left ventricle. The normal mitral valve orifice is 4 to 6 cm^2. Symptoms generally occur when the orifice is narrowed to less than 2.5 cm^2. Patients may initially develop symptoms only during exercise, or other states which increase cardiac output. However, as the disease progresses and the valve narrows to less than 1.5 cm^2, mitral stenosis is considered severe and patients often have symptoms at rest.

A stenotic mitral valve limits diastolic inflow of blood from the left atrium to the left ventricle. As a result, a pressure gradient develops between the two chambers and left atrial pressures increase to maintain flow across the valve. The increase in left atrial pressure decreases pulmonary venous inflow, thereby increasing pulmonary vasculature pressure. Over time, pulmonary hypertension can result and ultimately, right ventricular failure. A second consequence of the increased left atrial pressure is chamber dilation. As the left atrium dilates, atrial fibrillation often develops. An enlarged left atrium is also susceptible to areas of stasis, and thus thrombus formation. Because of the obstruction to inflow, in mitral stenosis the left ventricular end-diastolic volume is low resulting in low stroke volume and cardiac output.

Signs and Symptoms

Patients with mitral valve abnormalities due to rheumatic disease tend to present with symptoms in the third to fourth decades of life: most commonly, dyspnea and orthopnea. Pregnancy, which also occurs during these decades, produces hemodynamic changes that may unmask previously undiagnosed disease. Rarely, patients may have hemoptysis due to rupture of dilated bronchial veins. With severe mitral disease, patients have signs of right ventricle failure such as peripheral edema and jugular venous distension.

Preoperative Evaluation

The preoperative evaluation of a patient with mitral stenosis presenting for non-cardiac surgery focuses on identifying high-risk patients. Parturients with severe PHT can have mortality rates of up to 40% during pregnancy and in the postpartum period. A careful history should be obtained to search for symptoms of dyspnea, orthopnea, paroxysmal nocturnal dyspnea, arrhythmias, or peripheral edema. The patient's functional capacity and exercise tolerance should be determined, since a patient with good exercise tolerance and functional capacity can undergo low-risk surgery without further invasive testing. In parturients,

Table 21–1 MODIFIED NEW YORK HEART ASSOCIATION FUNCTIONAL CLASSIFICATION OF HEART DISEASE

CLASS	DESCRIPTION
I	Asymptomatic except during severe exertion
II	Symptomatic with moderate activity
III	Symptomatic with minimal activity
IV	Symptomatic at rest

the prepregnancy classification using The New York Heart Association functional class (Table 21–1) has been strongly associated with both maternal and fetal complications during childbirth.

On physical examination, a characteristic low-pitched, rumbling diastolic murmur at the left ventricular apex is heard with the patient lying in the left lateral decubitus position. In patients with mild disease, this murmur may only be heard when the heart rate is elevated and the flow across the mitral valve is increased. The preoperative physical examination also focuses on uncovering signs of heart failure. Auscultation of the chest may reveal rales, wheezing, or an S_3 gallop, examination of the neck may reveal jugular venous distension, and examination of the extremities and abdomen may reveal pitting edema or ascites.

The severity of mitral valve stenosis should be determined prior to any elective surgery. Doppler and two-dimensional transthoracic echocardiography are valuable tools to assess the pathology and grade the severity of mitral stenosis. Echocardiography will also detail other cardiac valvular lesions, as well as providing information with regard to right ventricular function and detecting left atrial thrombus formation if present. A current ECG should be obtained and may reveal atrial fibrillation. A chest radiograph may be warranted to rule out pulmonary edema if signs of congestive heart failure are present on examination.

Anesthetic Management

The intraoperative management of patients with mitral stenosis is based upon preventing tachycardia, maintaining afterload, and carefully maintaining of preload. Attention to preload and intravascular volume is most important to minimize exacerbation of pulmonary vascular congestion. In patients with PHT, it is also of critical importance to avoid further increasing pulmonary vascular resistance, by preventing hypercarbia and hypoxemia. In the presence of severe pulmonary hypertension, agents that cause pulmonary vascular vasodilation may also need to be employed.

Premedication for an anxious patient may be indicated to prevent tachycardia. However, over-sedation should be avoided as this can precipitate hypoxemia and hypercarbia thereby worsening PHT. SpO_2 should be monitored continuously, and supplemental oxygen provided. Rate control medications such as beta blockers, calcium channel blockers, and digoxin should be continued until the time of surgery. To promote intraoperative hemostasis, Coumadin should be discontinued preoperatively and a heparin bridge instituted if necessary.

In addition to standard ASA monitors, an arterial line may be indicated. In patients with PHT, the placement of a pulmonary artery catheter should be considered although there are no data that demonstrate an improvement in outcome with the intraoperative use of this device. Transesophageal echocardiography may be useful to monitor ventricular function and preload.

A variety of anesthetic techniques can be employed as long as the hemodynamic goals of avoiding tachycardia or pulmonary vasoconstriction and maintaining adequate preload and systemic vascular resistance are met. Spinal and epidural anesthesia are typically well tolerated in patients with mild to moderate disease, but are relatively contraindicated in patients with severe disease. However, with invasive monitoring and careful titration of agents to prevent hypotension, spinal and epidural anesthesia have been safely used in patients with severe mitral stenosis.

For general anesthesia, a balanced technique employing opiates, volatile anesthetics, and muscle relaxants is most often employed. The judicious, careful titration of the induction agent to prevent hypotension is of critical importance. Alpha agonists such as phenylephrine are the agents of choice to treat hypotension, as they increase SVR and may even cause a reflex bradycardia. Beta-adrenergic agents which cause tachycardia and vasodilation are undesirable in patients with mitral stenosis.

Comprehension Questions

21.1. During your preoperative assessment, a 28-year-old woman complains of dyspnea on exertion. Upon auscultation of her heart, you notice a mid-diastolic rumbling murmur. This murmur is most characteristic of which valvular lesion?

A. Mitral stenosis
B. Mitral regurgitation
C. Aortic regurgitation
D. Aortic stenosis

21.2. Which of the following statements about the pathophysiology of mitral stenosis is accurate?

A. Patients with mitral stenosis generally have an under-loaded left ventricle.

B. The increased pressure gradient between the left atrium and left ventricles results in left ventricular hypertrophy.

C. Patients with mitral stenosis have decreased left atrial pressure.

D. Diastolic filling of the left ventricle is increased in mitral stenosis because of the increased pressure gradient between the left atrium and left ventricle.

21.3. What are the intraoperative hemodynamic goals in the management of a pregnant patient undergoing an urgent caesarean section with mitral stenosis?

A. Tachycardia, low systemic vascular resistance, high pulmonary vascular resistance.

B. Tachycardia, avoid marked decreases in systemic vascular resistance, avoid increases in pulmonary vascular resistance.

C. Avoid tachycardia, avoid marked decreases in systemic vascular resistance, and avoid increases in pulmonary vascular resistance.

D. Avoid tachycardia, avoid marked decreases in pulmonary vascular resistance.

ANSWERS

21.1. **A.** The murmur described is characteristic of mitral stenosis. The murmur of mitral stenosis is a mid-diastolic rumbling murmur, best heard at the apex with the patient in the left lateral position. The murmur of mitral regurgitation is typically a holosystolic murmur that may radiate to the axilla. The murmur associated with aortic regurgitation is a midsystolic ejection murmur generally heard best at the base of the heart and is transmitted to the jugular notch. The murmur associated with aortic stenosis is a mid–systolic crescendo-decrescendo murmur that often radiates to the carotids.

21.2. **A.** The pathophysiology of mitral stenosis involves impaired diastolic filling of the left ventricle because of an obstruction at the level of the mitral valve. This results in a pressure gradient between the left atrium and the left ventricle. Consequently, left atrial pressure rises while the left ventricle is under-filled. As left atrial pressure increases, pulmonary venous return is impaired and pulmonary hypertension with right ventricular failure can occur.

21.3. **C.** The hemodynamic goals of mitral stenosis include the avoidance of tachycardia, as tachycardia will decrease diastolic filling of the left ventricle and can precipitate pulmonary congestion. Factors that can worsen pulmonary hypertension, such as hypercarbia and hypoxemia, should be avoided. Systemic vascular resistance as well as contractility should be maintained. Lastly, preload or volume status should be maintained carefully to promote stroke volume while minimizing the risk of pulmonary congestion.

Clinical Pearls

- Pulmonary hypertension and right ventricular failure are often observed in patients with mitral stenosis and can be precipitated by hypercarbia and hypoxemia. Pharmacological treatment with medications that vasodilate the pulmonary vasculature may be required.
- Patients with mitral stenosis often present in atrial fibrillation; however, it is important to remember that tachycardia is poorly tolerated and should be prevented or treated.
- As left atrial pressure increases with mitral stenosis, so does pulmonary venous pressure. This increase in pulmonary venous pressure can precipitate pulmonary edema.

REFERENCES

Cook D, Housmans P, Rehfeldt K. Valvular heart disease. In: *Kaplan's Cardiac Anesthesia*. 5th ed. Philadelphia, PA: Saunders Elsevier; 2006:645-690.

Mends LA, Loscalzo J. Acquired valvular heart disease. In: Andreoli, ed. *Cecil Essentials of Medicine*. 5th ed. Philadelphia, PA: W.B. Saunders Co; 2001:69-70.

Mittnacht Alexander JC, Fanshawe M, Konstadt S. Anesthetic considerations in the patient with valvular heart disease undergoing non-cardiac surgery. *Semin Cardiothorac Vasc Anesth*. 2008;12(33):33-59.

Case 22

A 75-year-old man with severe coronary artery disease is scheduled for coronary artery bypass surgery under general anesthesia. He experiences a tightness in his chest, and shortness of breath with exercise. These symptoms are increasing in frequency, and relieved by 0.2 mg of nitroglycerine within 2 minutes.

He has diabetes and well-controlled hypertension. His medications include metoprolol, metformin, and nitroglycerine. He has never had surgery, and has no known allergies to any medications. He continues to smoke 1 pack per day, and has done so for almost 40 years. His review of systems is otherwise negative.

The patient's blood chemistries are normal, his hemoglobin is 13, and hematocrit 39. His chest x-ray is normal, but his ECG showed inverted T waves in leads II and III, and aVF. A cardiac catheterization showed multiple occlusions of left main artery, left anterior descending artery (LAD), left circumflex artery (CX), and right coronary artery (RCA), and an ejection fraction of 55%. The echocardiogram showed no valvular disease, and confirmed the ejection fraction.

- ➤ What are the components of a cardiopulmonary bypass (CPB) machine?
- ➤ Why do patients have to go on CPB?
- ➤ What are the most common complications of CPB?

ANSWERS TO CASE 22: Management of a Patient on Cardiopulmonary Bypass Machine

Summary: A 75-year-old male patient with history of diabetes and hypertension with no past surgical history is undergoing coronary artery bypass graft (CABG) surgery. As part of the procedure, he will be placed on cardiopulmonary bypass.

- **Components of coronary bypass machine:** An oxygenator, a heat exchanger for warming and cooling, a venous reservoir, and pumps.
- **Reason for CPB machine:** Because of the likelihood of hemodynamic instability during cardiac surgery without it. CPB also allows the surgeons to access parts of the heart that would not otherwise be accessible.
- **Most common complications of cardiopulmonary bypass:** Acute complications: hypotension, anemia, light anesthesia, lack of suitable neuromuscular blockade. The most common long-term complications are postoperative cognitive dysfunction, renal failure, and disseminated intravascular coagulopathy (DIC).

ANALYSIS

Objectives

1. Understand the basics of the CPB machine.
2. Understand why CPB is necessary in some patients but not in others.
3. Become familiar with the common complications of CPB, and how they may be prevented.

Considerations

The special concerns in the patient preparing for cardiopulmonary bypass are the continuance of his "cardiac" medications, particularly beta blockers, on the morning of surgery. Discontinuance of beta-blocker therapy has been associated with an adverse outcome in some cohorts of patients. As with all elective cases, the patient must be NPO. Blood and blood products must be ready and available in advance, and the CPB readied by the perfusionist.

A large-bore peripheral intravenous line is placed to facilitate transfusion if necessary, and similarly, an arterial catheter is placed for instantaneous blood pressure measurement and for the repeated arterial blood gas sampling. Large-bore central venous access is obtained, but a pulmonary artery catheter may or may not be used for CABG surgery.

After standard monitors are placed, anesthesia was induced using 2 mg of midazolam, 100 mg lidocaine, 20 mg of etomidate, and 100 mg of succinylcholine. The patient was easily intubated using Miller #3 blade with an 8.0 endotracheal tube. Blood pressure is carefully controlled, with either vasopressors for hypotension, or contrarily, a vasodilator anesthetic such as propofol or labetalol for hypertension.

The chest is opened by sternotomy, and the internal mammary artery and saphenous vein are dissected. In preparation for CPB, 3 mg/kg of heparin is administered as per surgeon's request, and the heparin-induced anticoagulation confirmed by the activated clotting time (ACT). After the ACT has reached 480, the patient is placed on the cardiopulmonary bypass machine (CPB, the "pump"). The patient's ventilator is turned off.

APPROACH TO
Management of a Patient on Cardiopulmonary Bypass Machine

The CPB Machine

In its simplest form, the CPB machine consists of pumps, an oxygenator, a heat exchanger which can either heat or cool the blood, a venous reservoir. In preparation for CPB, the entire "pump" system is "primed," or filled with a crystalloid solution. Large cannulae from the pump are also flushed with crystalloid, and then connected to smaller cannulae that have been inserted into the patient's heart and allowed to fill with blood. Thus, one liquid-filled tube is inserted into another liquid-filled tube to minimize air emboli. The venous cannula drains blood from the patient to the CPB machine by gravity. An aortic (arterial) cannula delivers blood pumped from the CPB machine to the patient. The heart is isolated from this aortic cannula, the CPB circuit, and the body by the aortic clamp. While on CPB, the patient's circulatory volume expands by the amount of fluid used to prime the pump and its associated cannulae.

Heparin is administered prior to the institution of CPB to prevent clotting which could occlude the cannula and the CPB machine. The efficacy of the heparin is measured by the activated clotting time (ACT) to confirm anticoagulation prior to the institution of bypass. This large dose of heparin can be associated with hypotension, which should be anticipated and promptly treated with vasopressors if necessary. Tragedies have occurred when the patient was placed on CPB but not anticoagulated: either the heparin was inadvertently omitted, or following a medication error, protamine, a heparin antagonist, was administered accidentally. To prevent the accidental administration of protamine, by convention, protamine is kept in a location that is different from the other anesthetic drugs, and the package or vial remains unopened until it is needed.

CLINICAL APPROACH

Most patients undergoing cardiac surgery will need to be placed on CPB to allow surgery to be performed on a motionless heart under controlled circumstances (Figure 22–1). Without CPB, surgery would be performed on a beating heart, substantially increasing the degree of technical difficulty. Moreover, some cardiac

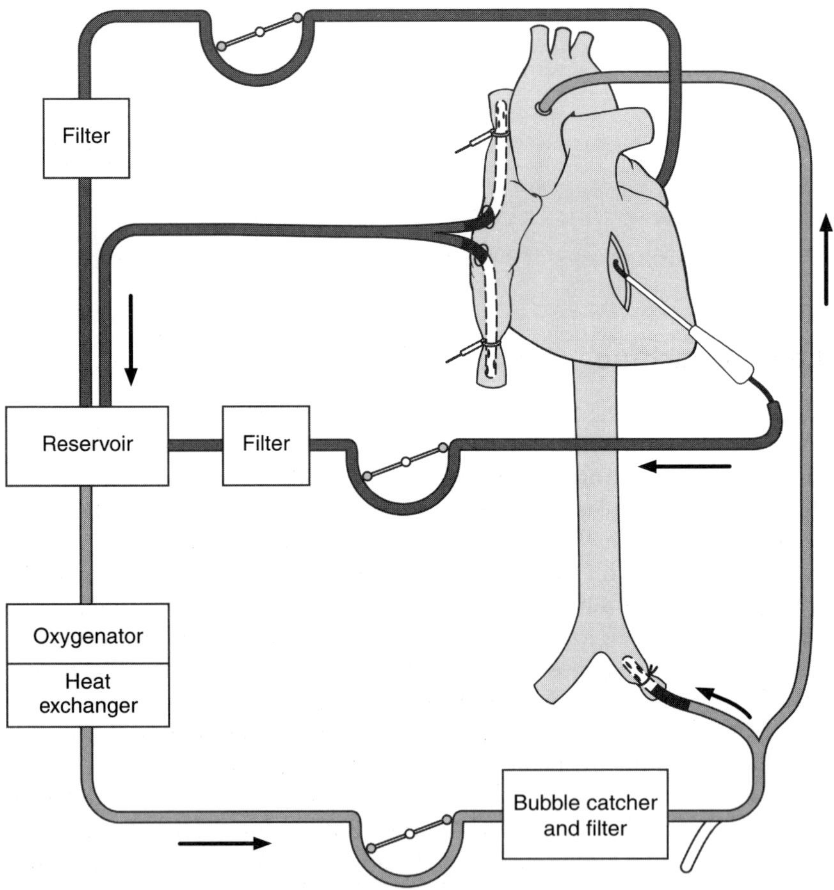

Figure 22–1. Diagram demonstrating how a patient is connected to the cardiopulmonary bypass machine. [dark grey] represents alternate pathways from patient to pump. [light grey] represents alternate pathways from pump to patient. (*Redrawn with permission from Dr. Joseph Reeves-Viets.*)

lesions are anatomically difficult to access in the beating heart, and manipulation of the heart in and of itself can make the patient unstable.

In addition to possible myocardial damage, the most common complication of CPB is short-term memory loss (cognitive defect), which can occur in a significant proportion of patients. The need to reduce the risk of postoperative cognitive dysfunction is probably the most important indication for an "off pump" CABG procedure.

Other complications associated with CPB include:

1. Hypotension
2. Renal failure
3. Light anesthesia and intra-op awareness
4. Coagulopathy and bleeding, including DIC
5. Stroke
6. Death

Hypotension following the institution of CPB generally indicates one of three things. After the patient's blood mixes with the 2 L of crystalloid used to "prime the pump" (usually Plasmalyte), the hematocrit can be seriously reduced, even by as much as 10%. If the hematocrit falls to below 24%, blood transfusions should be given. Hemodilution also reduces blood viscosity and systemic vascular resistance, and thus decreases the blood pressure. Hypotension resulting from hemodilution should be anticipated, and any tendency toward hypotension should be treated early with a vasopressor like phenylephrine or norepinephrine. Hypotension can also result from the dilution of catecholamines by the crystalloid "pump prime," and is also treated with vasopressors such as phenylephrine or norepinephrine. Less common, but equally critical causes of hypotension post institution of CPB include inadequate pump flow, kinked tubing, and aortic dissection following cannula placement.

It is also possible for components of the CPB machine to stimulate an allergic reaction, thus resulting in hypotension. In some patients, when the patient's blood comes in contact with the components of CPB machine, chemical mediators are released causing vasodilation. Currently, there are no diagnostic tests which are immediately available to confirm this scenario. Vasopressors are the appropriate treatment, and may also include a vasopressin infusion. Similarly, simply traversing the CPB machine causes a constant injury to the blood components. In some patients, disseminated intravascular coagulopathy (DIC) may result. DIC also can be a part of systemic inflammatory response syndrome (SIRS). Both syndromes can be triggered by an unusually long CPB run, and both can be associated with stroke, renal failure, diastolic dysfunction of the myocardium, and death.

Hemodilution also increases the volume of distribution of anesthetic agents, potentially leading to light anesthesia and even intra-op awareness. Estimates of the incidence of awareness in cardiac surgical procedures vary, but may approach 10%. Many centers advocate neurophysiologic monitoring for awareness in cardiac surgical patients. Levels of neuromuscular blocking agents and narcotics are also decreased significantly, possibly allowing patient movement as well. To anticipate this situation, just prior to the institution of bypass patients should receive an additional neuromuscular blocking agent, a narcotic, and a benzodiazepine (which may provide amnesia) to ensure therapeutic levels. Once CPB has been initiated, an inhalational anesthetic can be administered using a vaporizer mounted on the CPB machine.

Myocardial injury is unavoidable during CPB, since the heart largely reverts to anaerobic metabolism accompanied by the release of inflammatory mediators, and operative trauma. Myocardial stunning, apoptosis, and myocardial infarction may result. In an attempt to protect the myocardium and minimize such complications, oxygen consumption is reduced by cooling the heart and inducing asystole with potassium containing cardioplegia solution.

Following the surgery, the patient is warmed to a core temperature of 36°C (known as the "rewarming period"). Once this temperature is reached, he or she is "weaned" from bypass by incrementally reducing the venous drainage into the pump and the pump's arterial flow out into the patient. This is an incremental process, as vasodilation from warming increases the circulating volume. Appropriate volume resuscitation is estimated by the pulmonary artery pressure. Arterial pressure is also monitored closely. If too high, stroke or bleeding may result; if too low, organ hypoperfusion with stroke, renal failure, and multiple system organ failure can result.

As the patient is warmed, the cardioplegia stopped, and the aortic clamp separating the heart from the CPB circuit and body is opened, the heart usually begins beating on its own. The anesthesiologist resumes mechanical ventilation, confirms that the core temperature is indeed 36° C or above, that the hematocrit and arterial blood gases are suitable, and that the perfusionist has an adequate remaining volume in the pump's reservoir to maintain circulating volume as bypass is discontinued. (For the anesthesiologist's checklist prior to separating from bypass, please see Table 22–1.) Should ventricular fibrillation occur, the patient is promptly cardioverted to avoid any unnecessary increases in myocardial oxygen consumption.

Table 22–1 ANESTHESIOLOGIST'S CHECKLIST PRIOR TO "COMING OFF" BYPASS

- Confirm that the patient's core temperature is ≥ 36°C.
- Confirm that mechanical ventilation has resumed.
- Confirm that the CPB reservoir contains sufficient volume to maintain MAP, PAP, and CI as bypass is discontinued.
- Ensure that arterial blood gases are conducive to the discontinuance of bypass.
  - pH ≥ 7.30
  - K ≤ 5.5 (K^+ is contained in cardioplegia and packed RBCs, and increased by acidosis)
  - Hct ≥ 24

"Coming off bypass" is often a tumultuous period as the heart, postarrest, progresses toward the resumption of normal function. The post-bypass heart usually requires support in the form of vasopressors and inotropes, in particular, epinephrine, norepinephrine, dobutamine, and milrinone. Cardioplegia often impairs electrical conduction in the heart, so pacing is often required and the need for cardioversion for ventricular fibrillation is not unusual. The delicate balance between the progressive vasodilation that accompanies warming, the possibility of continued surgical bleeding, and a heart that may be prone to failure make separation from bypass one of the most challenging periods in anesthesiology and cardiac surgery.

Rarely but occasionally, there is a malfunction of the CPB machine. This usually reflects a problem of the machine, but can also result from the failure of both the main and auxiliary power sources of the institution. In this event, the CPB can be powered by a hand crank. As might be expected, a malfunction of the CPB machine can also lead to stroke, renal failure, and death. A good understanding of the working of the CPB machine, as well as the physiologic changes it induces is important for the anesthesiologist managing these complicated procedures.

Comprehension Questions

22.1. Which of the following cardiac surgery may be done without using CPB?
   A. Mitral valve repair
   B. Coronary artery bypass surgery
   C. Tricuspid valve surgery
   D. Replacement of the ascending aorta

22.2. Why do patients who are going to be on CPB need a higher dose of heparin (at least 3 mg/kg) when compared to a vascular case which does not need CPB machine?
   A. Use of oxygenators on CPB
   B. Tubing in the CPB machine
   C. Heat exchanger in CPB machine
   D. Using kinetic pump on CPB machine

22.3. What is the most common complication of CPB machine?
   A. Renal failure
   B. Myocardial infarction
   C. DIC
   D. Short-term memory loss

22.4. Shortly after the institution of CPB, the patient became severely hypotensive (mean blood pressure of 30 mm Hg or less) and started moving on the OR table. Which is the most likely cause of this scenario?

A. Myocardial infarction resulting from sudden exposure to the cold solution.

B. Hemodilution from mixing the 2 L of crystalloid "pump prime."

C. Hemodilution has significantly reduced the hematocrit and increased the SVR.

D. Hemodilution has caused a myocardial infarction.

ANSWERS

22.1. **B.** Even though majority of the CABG surgeries are done on CPB machine, some of them can be done without CPB machine ("off pump"), depending on the patient's anatomy. Good candidates for "off pump" procedures include patients with one vessel disease like a single LAD occlusion not involved with hemodynamic instability, or in a patient who is at a high risk for stroke (calcified aorta etc).

22.2. **A.** The oxygenator is the most thrombogenic component of the CPB machine. Heparin dose of 1 mg/kg, which is normally used in vascular cases, is not enough to prevent clots with certainty in the CPB machine. On the other hand, a heparin dose of 1 mg/kg is sufficient to prevent clots in the other components of CPB.

22.3. **D.** Short-term memory loss (cognitive defect) is the most common complication of CPB, though DIC and renal failure are very common complications as well. The need to reduce the risk of postoperative cognitive dysfunction is the most important indication for an off pump CABG procedure.

22.4. **B.** On the CPB machine, the additional saline in the pump prime is associated hemodilution. Concentrations of the medications decrease, leaving the patient lightly anesthetized and not paralyzed, possibly resulting in movement. This could be prevented by giving additional doses of neuromuscular blocking agents and narcotics just prior to the institution of bypass, and adding an inhalation anesthetic from the CPB machine. Hemodilution can also reduce hematocrit sufficiently to reduce SVR, resulting in hypotension. Hypotension should be promptly treated with vasopressors. Should the hematocrit fall below 24%, blood should be transfused.

Clinical Pearls

- Familiarity with the CPB machine and its functions are vital for the anesthesiologist.
- Recognizing and promptly treating (or even pretreating in anticipation of the complications that occur while on CPB can avoid disastrous consequences. Vasopressors should be used immediately, the hematocrit checked, and other less likely scenarios considered if appropriate.
- Instituting cardiopulmonary bypass in a patient who is not anticoagulated can have disastrous consequences.

REFERENCES

Stoelting RK. Anticoagulants. In: Stoelting RK, ed. *Pharmacology and Physiology in Anesthetic Practice*. 2nd ed. Philadelphia, PA: J.B.Lippincott Company; 1991:466-476.

Yao FS, Scubas N. Ischemic heart disease and coronary artery bypass grafting. In: Yao FS, ed. *Anesthesiology*. 6th ed. Philadelphia, PA: Lippincott Williams & Wilkins; 2007:131-197.

Case 23

A 65-year-old man with severe claudication secondary to peripheral vascular disease is scheduled for a right femoral-popliteal artery bypass. He has type II diabetes treated with NPH insulin, and hypertension treated with metoprolol. He also has coronary artery disease treated by coronary artery bypass surgery several years ago, and has been asymptomatic from his heart disease since that time. The patient's past surgical history includes a femoral popliteal bypass on the other side, and a vasectomy, without problems with anesthesia. He is allergic to iodine and seafood. The patient's pertinent labs include a hematocrit of 35, a potassium of 3.8, and an ECG which showed an old inferior myocardial infarction. By echocardiogram, his ejection fraction is 25%.

Mindful of his coronary artery disease, anesthesia is induced with etomidate, and the patient is paralyzed with succinylcholine and intubated easily. The anesthetic is maintained with desflurane, fentanyl is added for analgesia. His vital signs remain stable throughout. As the arterial anastomosis is begun, the surgeons request that the patient be given 7,000 units of heparin. The heparin is administered, and the anastomosis is completed expeditiously and with minimal blood loss. At the end of the surgery, they request that protamine be administered to reverse the heparin.

Suddenly, the patient became severely hypotensive with blood pressure of 60/30 mm Hg, and a heart rate of 130 bpm. He is cold and clammy in appearance.

- ➤ What most likely triggered the events?
- ➤ How should this patient be treated?
- ➤ Are special monitors indicated?

ANSWERS TO CASE 23:
Protamine Reaction in a Patient Undergoing Vascular Surgery

Summary: A 65-year-old man with a history of multiple vascular procedures, coronary artery bypass surgery, and vasectomy, undergoing femoral-popliteal artery bypass surgery, suddenly became severely hypotensive after protamine is administered.

- **Triggering events:** The temporal correlation is highly suggestive of a protamine reaction.
- **Treatment:** Volume, either crystalloid or colloids, should be infused, and vasopressors such as phenylephrine or norepinephrine should be administered. Inotropes such as epinephrine and/or milrinone should be added if needed.
- **Special monitors:** If patient is not responding to the above interventions, a pulmonary artery catheter and/or transesophageal echocardiography probe may be placed.

ANALYSIS

Objectives

1. Learn to recognize the protamine reaction.
2. Understand the risk factors for protamine reaction.
3. Become familiar with the different types of protamine reactions, and treatment of each.

Considerations

The fact that the patient is severely hypotensive shortly following the administration of protamine strongly suggests a protamine reaction. Since the pressure measured by an arterial line can be artifactual, it is confirmed by another method such as a blood pressure cuff. However, the patient's cold, clammy appearance is consistent with the hypotensive measurement being correct. Next, other potential causes of severe hypotension must be excluded. The differential diagnosis includes bleeding from the surgical site resulting in hypovolemia, excessive anesthetic agent, ongoing myocardial ischemia, pulmonary embolism, etc.

Protamine reactions are not uncommon, especially in patients who were exposed to protamine in the past such as during previous vascular surgeries and a coronary artery bypass surgery. This patient also has additional risk factors for a protamine reaction including an allergy to iodine and seafood, treatment with NPH insulin, and (although controversial) a history of vasectomy.

This patient's pressure is 60/30. He is treated by stopping the protamine, calling for help, and notifying the surgeons so that they can assess the surgical site for bleeding and help in the resuscitation if needed. Vasopressors including phenylephrine and a fluid bolus are administered. If patient does not respond, epinephrine, and then milrinone are added. To aid in treatment decisions such as whether vasoconstriction, volume, or inotropy are needed, an invasive arterial pressure monitor and pulmonary catheter are inserted.

APPROACH TO Protamine Reaction in a Patient Undergoing Vascular Surgery

DEFINITION

PROTAMINE REACTION: An hemodynamic response to protamine, ranging from mild hypotension to cardiorespiratory arrest.

CLINICAL APPROACH

Heparin is a direct inhibitor of thrombin, and a potent anticoagulant used frequently in cardiovascular surgical procedures. For example, if a patient was cannulated and placed on cardiopulmonary bypass without heparin, the cannulae would clot and the patient would die. However, such potent anticoagulation also predisposes to significant surgical bleeding, so it is typically reversed at the end of the case. Protamine is the only drug currently approved by the FDA to reverse heparin. It is a strong base, which combines with heparin, a strong acid, to form a stable salt which does not have any anticoagulant effect.

Protamine can produce different hemodynamic reactions which can range from mild hypotension to severe hemodynamic instability including cardiorespiratory arrest. The mechanisms for these reactions can be quite different. Depending on the cause, the mechanisms of protamine reactions can be divided into four types:

TYPE 1: Systemic hypotension from rapid injection: A predictable side effect of the drug, prevented by diluting and injecting the protamine slowly. This most common protamine reaction, can be accompanied by severe hypotension from massive peripheral vasodilatation. The best way to prevent this kind of reaction is to anticipate the resultant hypotension, particularly in patients who are hypovolemic and vasoconstricted at the time protamine is administered. This type of protamine reaction is treated by stopping or slowing the protamine, while infusing fluids. Treatment with intravenous fluids, vasopressors like phenylephrine or norepinephrine may be necessary to help restore the blood pressure. Insertion of another large-bore i.v. may be warranted.

TYPE 2: Protamine reaction secondary to histamine release: Protamine can cause histamine release and thus produce hypotension. Histamine-induced hypotension is suggested by tachycardia, and flushing. Treatment is combination of H_1 blocker like diphenhydramine and H_2 blocker like ranitidine. The patient also might require additional fluids and vasopressors. Since it may be difficult to determine the signs of histamine release, it is recommended to administer diphenhydramine and ranitidine intravenously anyway.

TYPE 3: Anaphylactic or anaphylactoid reaction: The patient experiences severe hypotension, tachycardia, and possibly bronchospasm. The response may be immediate or delayed. It is most commonly an anaphylactic reaction associated with an IgE-mediated antibody response, although an anaphylactoid response without antibody involvement is also possible.

This reaction is more common in patients who have had multiple exposures to protamine, or diabetic patients who are on NPH insulin for prolonged period of time. Additional risk factors include allergies to seafood and iodine, and though controversial, having had a vasectomy.

Anaphylactic reactions usually present with severe hemodynamic instability including cardiovascular collapse, and possible bronchospasm. Like any other anaphylactic reaction, treatment of choice is epinephrine and volume resuscitation. Vasopressors may also be needed along with volume resuscitation. Steroids such as hydrocortisone may also be given for anaphylaxis, even though benefit of this drug is controversial.

TYPE 4: Protamine reaction with severe pulmonary vasoconstriction and right ventricular failure: Probably the most severe reaction, it is fortunately very rare. This reaction may be difficult to distinguish from type 3 unless patient has pulmonary artery catheter or TEE probe in place. It is mediated by complement C5b. It is optimally treated with an inodilator like milrinone, which causes pulmonary vasodilatation and inotropy. In the event that it is uncertain whether a reaction is type 3 or type 4, therapy can be begun with epinephrine, and milrinone added if required.

The most important way to reduce the morbidity and mortality from a protamine reaction is to prevent and/or attenuate the reaction with anticipation and vigilance. In patients at high risk, such as those with a history of previous multiple exposures to protamine, NPH insulin, an allergy to seafood and iodine, and perhaps those who have had a vasectomy, the intensity of the reaction can be decreased significantly by the prophylactic administration of H_1- and H_2-receptor antagonists and steroids.

One of the most deadly medication errors involves the mistaken administration of protamine—either instead of heparin, in combination with heparin, or in place of another intended drug. Indeed, to prevent even the possibility of this complication, standard practice is not to even draw the protamine up into a syringe until it is to be used. Protamine in and of itself produces a DIC-like coagulopathy, due to the inactivation of factor 2 and platelets. Patients appear "oozy," and bleed almost as though heparinized. However, in reality, this clinical picture is quite different from heparinization. Heparin and protamine-induced bleeding can be distinguished by the activated clotting time, which is elevated by heparin. The ACT is unaffected by protamine, since protamine is not a direct thrombin inhibitor.

Comprehension Questions

23.1. Which of the following statements is most accurate regarding the treatment of protamine reactions?

A. To reduce bleeding, continue the protamine until the heparin is satisfactorily reversed.
B. Administer diuretics to reduce "third spacing."
C. Steroids are contraindicated in this situation.
D. If inotropy is required in addition to vasoconstriction, then milrinone may be indicated in addition to the epinephrine.

23.2. A 72-year-old female patient is undergoing aortic valve surgery on cardiopulmonary bypass machine. After separation from bypass machine, surgeons asked the anesthesiologist for protamine. What is the best site for the injection of protamine?

A. Central line in the right internal jugular vein
B. Peripheral i.v.
C. Left atrial injection by surgeons
D. Pulmonary artery port of the pulmonary artery catheter

23.3. A 56-year-old man with history of unstable angina and diagnosed coronary artery disease comes to the operating room for coronary artery bypass surgery. The surgeons just finished triple vessel bypass on cardiopulmonary bypass, and just "came off pump." The patient is allergic to protamine, and has a history of severe hypotension followed by cardiac arrest with protamine infusion during the previous vascular surgery. What should be used for reversal of heparin now to prevent bleeding from heparin-induced anticoagulation?

A. Try protamine again.
B. Hexadimethrine.
C. Transfuse blood products until ACT (activated clotting time) is normal and close the chest.
D. Bivalirudin as anticoagulant in the place of heparin.

ANSWERS

23.1. **D.** The treatment for a protamine reaction is also the treatment for an allergic drug reaction. First, the administration of the drug is stopped. Epinephrine, vasopressors, fluids, and steroids are administered, although the later is controversial. If additional inotropy is required in addition to vasoconstriction, then milrinone may be indicated in addition to the epinephrine.

23.2. **C.** Injecting a high dose of protamine into the central line or the PA port of Swan-Ganz catheter can produce severe pulmonary hypertension and right ventricular failure due to the activation of the C5b complement pathway. Most commonly, protamine is administered slowly through the peripheral IV, giving ample time for dilution before it reaches pulmonary vasculature. Protamine can still elicit pulmonary hypertension and right ventricular failure if given rapidly and in large quantity through the peripheral IV, since despite dilution, the pulmonary vasculature can be exposed to a large quantity of the drug. For these reasons, protamine should ideally be administered distal to the pulmonary vasculature, which means through the left atrium. Occasionally the surgeons administer protamine from the operative (sterile) field in this manner.

23.3. **C.** No suitable alternative is currently available for protamine. When faced with this situation, the best course is to transfuse blood products like fresh frozen plasma and platelets, and ask the surgeons to observe for bleeding until activated clotting time returns to normal and bleeding has stopped. As this patient had a severe reaction from protamine during his previous surgery, the protamine should not be repeated.

Hexadimethrine is a variant of protamine currently under investigation but not approved by FDA, perhaps because it produces nephrotoxicity and pulmonary hypertension. There is no role for the heparin alternative, bivalirudin, in this case since the patient does not have heparin-induced thrombocytopenia and thrombosis.

Clinical Pearls

- A high degree of suspicion, vigilance, and anticipation helps to prevent and/or attenuate protamine reactions.
- It is important to recognize the risk factors for protamine reactions including: previous multiple exposures to protamine, an allergy to seafood and iodine, treatment with NPH insulin, and a history of vasectomy. Patients at high risk should be pretreated with H_1 and H_2 antagonists to prevent or at least decrease the intensity of the reaction.
- Understanding the different types of protamine reactions is important, since the type of reaction carries different implications for treatment. Distinguishing between types 3 and 4 may require the insertion of a pulmonary artery catheter or TEE probe.

REFERENCES

Stoelting RK. Anticoagulants. In: Stoelting RK, ed. *Pharmacology and Physiology in Anesthetic Practice*. 2nd ed. Philadelphia, PA: J.B. Lippincott Company; 1991:466-476.

Yao FS, Skubas N. Ischemic heart disease and coronary artery bypass grafting. In: Yao FS, ed. *Anesthesiology*. 6th ed. Philadelphia, PA: Lippincott Williams & Wilkins; 2007:131-197.

Pulmonary Diseases

Case 24

A 22-year-old college student presents for outpatient surgery. He is scheduled for an arthroscopic repair of the anterior cruciate ligament of his left knee, which he injured during a basketball game a month ago. He reports that his only chronic medical problem is asthma. He has been diagnosed with mild, intermittent asthma and he takes fluticasone/salmeterol inhalational powder 250/50 daily. He reports not having an asthma attack in a year, but is feeling, "a little tight today because it's cold outside." As he is young, healthy, and to undergo a low-risk surgical procedure, no further preoperative testing is performed.

- ➤ What are the key pieces of information relevant in the preoperative evaluation of a patient with asthma?
- ➤ What are some considerations for an asthmatic having general anesthesia?
- ➤ What therapies can be used perioperatively to minimize the risk of an asthmatic attack?

ANSWERS TO CASE 24:
Anesthesia in a Patient with Reactive Airways

Summary: A 22-year-old patient with mild, intermittent asthma with new sports-induced injury for outpatient knee surgery.

- **Preoperative evaluation of asthma:** It is important to know what triggers the attacks, their frequency and severity, and medications which the patient is taking and has taken on the day of surgery.
- **Major considerations for an asthmatic patient having anesthesia:** Include whether or not the patient's condition is optimized prior to the procedure, the type of airway device required (if any), and the avoidance of drugs which release histamine.
- **Perioperative medications:** Beta-2 agonists administered via aerosolized treatment, or the patient simply using his or her own inhaler can be used to minimize the risk of an attack in the perioperative period.

ANALYSIS

Objectives

1. Understand the preoperative evaluation of patients with symptomatic reactive airway diseases.
2. Compare general anesthesia versus other modes of anesthesia, and delineate their benefits and drawbacks for the asthmatic patient.
3. Discuss various preoperative and intraoperative treatments for bronchospasm.

Considerations

This patient has mild, persistent asthma, and is experiencing mild symptoms preoperatively. During a more detailed history, he states that cold weather is a trigger for asthma, and that he takes an inhaler as a preventative medication daily, and uses an albuterol inhaler as a "rescue" medication for bronchospasm less than twice a month. This suggests that his asthma is relatively mild and well controlled. He also reports a more severe episode last winter, requiring outpatient treatment with a course of steroids. On the morning of the operation, he did take his daily inhaler, but has not taken any inhalational albuterol. It would be prudent to have the patient use an albuterol inhaler to decrease the likelihood of bronchoconstriction intraoperatively.

The anesthesia options for this patient, given that he is having a knee surgery, include general or regional anesthesia. Regional anesthesia with or without sedation is preferable for this patient in order to avoid instrumentation of the airway and thereby minimize risks of airway irritation and hyperreactivity. If for some reason a general anesthesia is necessary, then using a laryngeal mask airway is preferable to an endotracheal tube, since the latter acts as a foreign body in the patient's trachea and can thus cause bronchospasm.

APPROACH TO
Anesthesia in a Patient with Reactive Airways

DEFINITION

SUPRAGLOTTIC AIRWAY DEVICES: Airway adjuncts such as a laryngeal mask airway (LMA) which are positioned in the pharynx or hypopharynx above the vocal cords.

CLINICAL APPROACH

Preoperative Evaluation

Preoperative evaluation of a patient with asthma includes a detailed asthma history, and a focused physical examination. The history should include the following: recent upper respiratory infection, allergies, possible bronchospasm "triggers" (such as smoke, pets, dust, cold, or seasonal changes), medications used for symptom prevention and treatment, and occurrence of dyspnea at night or early morning. It is also useful to know the frequency and severity of the attacks. For example, is his asthma sufficiently severe to warrant steroids, if so, when did he last need and/or take steroids? Is he dependent on steroids to control his asthma? Have any of the attacks warranted hospitalization? If so, when, and how frequently? How is he feeling today? For an elective procedure, is the patient's condition optimized on the day of surgery?

Along with a detailed history, it is important to perform a focused preoperative physical examination. This examination should include observation for respiratory distress and accessory respiratory muscle usage, pursed lips during exhalation, signs of hypoxemia and breathlessness during speaking, and auscultation of the lung fields. Any wheezing, rhonchi, or deceased air movement should be noted.

Spirometry is a simple and acceptable means of assessing airway obstruction preoperatively. A decrease of 15% or more in FEV_1 is considered clinically significant. Similarly, and particularly in the older patient with COPD, the magnitude of any response to bronchodilators (if present) is helpful to determine the preoperative course. A chest x-ray is not necessary, as it will not provide diagnostic information. If a patient is having significant respiratory distress and signs of hypoxemia, the procedure should be delayed, and an arterial blood gas analysis and pulmonologist consult should be ordered.

Preoperative management may include beta-2 adrenergic agonists and/or corticosteroids. Both have been shown to improve preoperative lung function and to decrease wheezing. For patients receiving general anesthesia, preoperative medications decrease the rate and severity of bronchospasm during intubation and other airway manipulations in both symptomatic and asymptomatic asthmatics. Studies have found that the preoperative administration of methyl prednisolone and salbutamol minimizes bronchoconstriction resulting from intubation. Bronchoconstriction occurs most often with general anesthesia, and especially with intubation and at emergence. The choice of a neuraxial or peripheral nerve block instead of general anesthesia could avoid many of the anesthesia-associated triggers of asthma.

Intraoperative Course

It is unlikely that regional or monitored anesthesia care (MAC) will cause an exacerbation of bronchospasm intraoperatively. However, if the patient declines regional anesthesia, or if the regional anesthetic is inadequate or inappropriate for the surgical procedure, then general anesthesia may be necessary. Bronchospasm generally occurs at the induction of general anesthesia and manipulation of the airway. The choice of induction drugs and airway device can impact airway reactivity. Propofol is an excellent choice for induction, in that it blunts the airway reflexes and relaxes airway musculature. Ketamine is also an option, because it causes bronchodilation. However, ketamine increases airway secretions and causes tachycardia, which can make it less favorable. If ketamine is used, excessive secretions can be blocked with an antisialagogue, such as glycopyrrolate, prior to induction.

Most opioids are desirable adjuvants to induction. Indeed, pretreatment with a large dose of opioids can blunt the foreign body response to intubation. Similarly spraying lidocaine into the trachea also blunts the foreign body response, as does intravenous lidocaine in a dose of 2 mg/kg.

Drugs which cause histamine release may also exacerbate bronchoconstriction. Morphine is a well-known member of this category, so opioids that do not cause histamine release, such as fentanyl, are preferred. Similarly, the selection of a neuromuscular relaxant that does not cause histamine release is necessary for asthmatic patients. Succinylcholine can cause histamine release, but given that it provides the most rapid neuromuscular relaxation, there are times its benefits outweigh its risks, such as for a patient with mild asthma and a full stomach, or an anticipated difficult airway.

The type of devices used to secure the patient's airway can significantly affect airway hyperreactivity. Endotracheal intubation causes more severe bronchospasm than placement of supraglottic devices such as a laryngeal mask airway (LMA) that do not enter the trachea, and thus do not exert a foreign body response. Use of an LMA or mask ventilation is desirable if appropriate for the surgical procedure, since these techniques cause less airway irritation than intubation.

All volatile anesthetics cause bronchodilation. However, they are also pungent, and can irritate the airway. Sevoflurane and halothane are the least pungent volatile anesthetics, and therefore the best choices for maintenance of anesthesia in patients with reactive airway disease. Desflurane is the most irritating, and can cause coughing and airway irritation, especially at high doses in a patient who is not deeply anesthetized prior to its inhalation.

Even after meticulous selection of induction drugs, airway management, and maintenance anesthesia, bronchospasm can still occur intraoperatively. Severe, refractive bronchospasm is one of the most frightening scenarios that an anesthesiologist faces. Prompt recognition and an immediate treatment for bronchospasm is imperative when caring for an asthmatic patient. If an intubated patient experiences bronchospasm, ventilation becomes more difficult. Higher peak inspiratory pressures are needed to deliver the same tidal volume. The end-tidal capnograph may show a tracing with a steep slope (see Figure 24–1), reflecting the obstruction, and prolongation of exhalation during bronchospasm. If bronchospasm is so severe that adequate tidal volumes for gas exchange cannot be delivered, the patient will become hypoxemic. Auscultation of the patient's lung fields may yield wheezing and/or decreased air movement.

Prior to administering medications to treat bronchospasm, the anesthesiologist needs to search for a definable trigger for the bronchospasm, and if a trigger is identified, eliminate it immediately. However, in the case of intubation-triggered bronchospasm, it may or not be appropriate for the endotracheal tube to be removed. The second issue is whether depth of anesthesia is appropriate. Bronchospasm can reflect an inadequate depth of anesthesia. If this is the case, then additional anesthetics should be administered immediately. Both intravenous and inhalation agents can be utilized to rapidly deepen the level of anesthesia in order to halt the bronchospasm.

The use of beta-2 agonists, such as albuterol, to increase bronchodilation is appropriate. However, when using an inhaled beta-2 agonist intraoperatively,

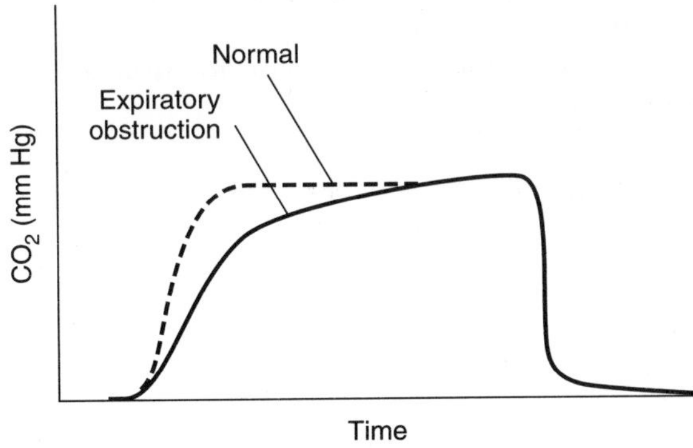

Figure 24–1. Effect of airway obstruction on the capnograph. *(Reprinted from: Morgan GE Jr, Mikhail MS, Murray MJ, eds. Clinical Anesthesiology, 4th ed. New York, NY: McGraw-Hill, 2006:575.)*

very little actually reaches the airways during positive pressure ventilation, so more than the usual dosage will be needed. Beta-2 agonist delivery can be improved if the drug is administered into the inspiratory limb of the breathing circuit near the endotracheal tube. In addition, the action of the beta-2 agonists may be greater if the ventilator's inspiratory to expiratory time (I:E) ratio is altered to lengthen the expiratory time. If inhalational beta-2 agonists do not attenuate the bronchospasm, then epinephrine should be considered. An intravenous bolus of 25 to 50 μg of epinephrine will reduce or eliminate bronchospasm in most patients. If bronchospasm persists despite increased depth of anesthesia and appropriate treatment, the patient may be suffering from status asthmaticus. Status asthmaticus necessitates even more aggressive intervention, cessation of the most operations, and treatment in the intensive care unit. While corticosteroids can be effective in preventing intraoperative bronchospasm if given prior to the operation, they are not effective in treating acute bronchospasm.

Postoperative Care

The symptoms of asthma can still occur after extubation and prior to discharge from the post-anesthesia care unit (PACU). While it is less likely to happen at this time than intraoperatively, the patient should still be observed for dyspnea, wheezing, and oxygen desaturations in the postoperative period. Should symptoms occur, the treatment involves the elimination of triggers and administration of beta-2 agonists via aerosolized respiratory treatment, such as nebulized albuterol and ipratropium. Once this is completed and the patient has recovered from anesthesia, his risk of bronchospasm returns to baseline.

Comprehension Questions

24.1. Which of the following is an aspect of a comprehensive perioperative evaluation of the asthmatic patient?

A. History of wheezing and treatments for asthma
B. Chest x-ray
C. An ECG
D. Computerized tomography of the lungs

24.2. At which of the following times during a general anesthetic is bronchospasm most likely?

A. Induction
B. Intubation
C. LMA insertion
D. Extubation

24.3. Which of the following is the first treatment for an anesthetized patient experiencing bronchospasm?
A. Administer inhalational beta-2 agonists
B. Administer additional anesthetic(s)
C. Administer neuromuscular blocking agent
D. Administer intravenous epinephrine

ANSWERS

24.1. **A.** A focused history and physical examination are absolutely necessary. Should the history and physical examination yield information that would require further evaluation, bedside spirometry and/or arterial blood gas analysis can also give important information as to the state of the patient's asthma. Answer **B**, a chest x-ray, will not give information regarding the asthmatic state of a patient nor will it show bronchospasm. Chest tomography is unlikely to be helpful in the preoperative evaluation of the asthmatic patient.

24.2. **B.** Although bronchospasm can occur at all the times posed in this question, initial manipulation or instrumentation of the airway is the most likely time for bronchospasm to occur. During general anesthesia, intubation is more likely to cause bronchospasm than other methods of airway management, such as the laryngeal mask airway.

24.3. **B.** Administer additional anesthetic(s) to deepen the level of anesthesia, is the first treatment for bronchospasm because it is quick to administer. Inhalational beta-2 agonists, volatile anesthetics, and intravenous drugs with beta-adrenergic activity (epinephrine) can all attenuate bronchospasm. **C**, neuromuscular blocking agents, have no effect on bronchospasm. In fact, some neuromuscular blocking agents can precipitate a bronchospasm if they cause histamine release.

Clinical Pearls

- Information obtained during the preoperative examination, pretreatment with beta-2 agonists, and/or steroids can help predict the risk and prevent or reduce the incidence of bronchospasm during the perioperative period.
- Airway manipulation, especially endotracheal intubation, is the most likely time that bronchospasm will occur.
- The treatment of intraoperative bronchospasm includes eliminating any triggers, increasing depth of anesthesia, and administering drugs with beta-2-adrenergic activity.

REFERENCES

Barash PG, Cullen BF, and Stoelting RK (eds). *Clinical Anesthesia*. 5th ed. Philadelphia, PA: Lippincott, Williams and Wilkins; 2006.

Burburan, SM, Xisto, DG, Rocco, PR. Anaesthetic management in asthma. *Minerva Anestesiol*. 2007;73:357-365.

Case 25

A 53-year-old woman with long-standing chronic obstructive pulmonary disease (COPD) presents for a laparoscopic cholecystectomy. Her past medical history includes hypertension well-controlled with lisinopril, a 40-pack-year history of smoking, and resultant COPD.

The patient states that she can do her own grocery shopping, but that she often has to stop and rest when she gets short of breath. She states that she had the flu 6 to 7 months ago, which aggravated her COPD resulting in hospitalization. She currently uses an Advair inhaler (a long-acting beta agonist) and Spiriva (a long-acting anticholinergic agent). Approximately once a week she also uses a Ventolin inhaler for breakthrough therapy. The patient was recently referred to a pulmonologist, who added oral steroids to her regimen. Since the adjustment of her medical regimen, she has had more energy to devote to activities.

Her vital signs are BP of 140/80 mm Hg, a heart rate of 85 bpm, and her respiratory rate is of 24 breaths per minute. She does not use accessory muscles of respiration, and can speak in complete sentences. Her laboratory blood tests are normal.

- What are your concerns during preoperative evaluation for this patient?
- What are the ventilator strategies for this patient?
- What are the likely postoperative concerns for this patient?

ANSWERS TO CASE 25:
Chronic Obstructive Pulmonary Disease

Summary: This 53-year-old woman is a controlled COPD patient presenting for a laparoscopic cholecystectomy under general anesthesia.

- **Preoperative evaluation:** In patients with COPD should include the history regarding the adequacy of long-acting inhaler therapy, the frequency of pneumonia and bronchitis, and duration of oral steroid therapy including when it was last administered. Several bouts of pneumonia per year as well as frequent requirements for short-acting agents signify inadequate outpatient therapy, and significantly increase the patient's risk of surgery.
- **Ventilator strategies:** COPD results in loss of elastic recoil of the alveoli in the lungs. As a result, the alveoli need a longer time to exhale. Thus the inspiratory/expiratory ratio needs to be adjusted on the ventilator. Since the patient has been on an indefinite number of days of steroid therapy, adrenal insufficiency needs to be considered in the differential diagnosis of refractory hypotension should it occur.
- **Likely postoperative concerns:** In the post-anesthetic period this patient is at the highest risk for pulmonary complications including but not limited to hypoxia, bronchospasm, and pneumonia.

ANALYSIS

Objectives

1. Understand the issues involved in the preoperative evaluation and assessment of suitability for surgery in a patient with COPD undergoing elective surgery.
2. Understand the intraoperative management of ventilation under general anesthesia in a patient with COPD.
3. Understand postoperative complications in a patient with severe COPD.

Considerations

This is a 53-year-old obese woman who presents for a laparoscopic cholecystectomy under general anesthesia. She has moderately severe COPD, which seems to be under reasonable control. However, she is currently treated with long-acting beta-2 agonists, which have been shown to actually increase the mortality in patients with asthma. She has required steroids in the past 6 months, which suggests that her COPD is moderately severe. In addition, the exposure to steroids also predisposes the patient to the possibility of adrenal insufficiency.

The standard monitors recommended by the American Society of Anesthesiologists (ASA) are sufficient, and there is no real indication for invasive monitoring in this case. During induction and maintenance, agents such as thiopental and desflurane should be avoided since the former can cause bronchoconstriction, and the later is the most irritating general anesthetic to the airway. Following the induction of general anesthesia, the ventilator's inspiratory/expiratory ratio is adjusted to accommodate the patient's prolonged expiratory phase, and a small amount of PEEP is added to decrease work of breathing. Both of these maneuvers result in optimal peak and plateau pressures.

The patient's pulmonary function tests indicate that she has small airways and an element of broncho-reactivity. This renders her susceptible to bronchospasm, and also responsive to bronchodilator agents. The patient should be asked to use her inhalers prior to surgery.

Laparoscopic cholecystectomy is typically associated with little blood loss, so the fluid management should be judicious given the higher likelihood for pulmonary edema in this patient. Indeed, a common saying is "keep the lungs dry," and it applies to many if not most pulmonary surgical procedures. The presence of COPD exacerbates the possibility of atelectasis, pneumonia, and hypoxemia in the postoperative period. Pain control is an important consideration in the postoperative period. The use of narcotics may potentiate respiratory depression and failure in the setting of atelectasis, while inadequate pain control may result in splinting and inadequate respiratory effort, which will exacerbate atelectasis as well.

APPROACH TO Chronic Obstructive Pulmonary Disease

DEFINITIONS

COPD: Chronic obstructive pulmonary disease (COPD) is a slowly progressive lung disease that results in progressive shortness of breath and a declining activity level. It includes a spectrum of illnesses such as emphysema and chronic bronchitis.

LAPAROSCOPIC CHOLECYSTECTOMY: Surgical procedure of removal of the gall bladder via small incisions on the abdomen. The entire abdominal cavity is visualized by means of a laparoscope inserted after creation of a pneumoperitoneum.

CLINICAL APPROACH

Preoperative Evaluation

The preoperative evaluation for any patient prior to surgery includes assessment of exercise tolerance. In the setting of COPD, focused questioning may reveal a subtle decline in exercise over a period of years (eg, using a push lawn mower to a power lawn mower to paying someone to mow the lawn). Primary care physicians often have a low threshold for cardiac stress testing, to ferret out presence of concomitant cardiac disease.

In a patient with proven COPD, the next assessment should be the adequacy of therapy. A stable inhaler regimen with minimal use of breakthrough inhalers, no requirement for oral steroids, and an absence of frequent bronchitis/pneumonia represent "stable" COPD. A subset of patients with COPD has alveolar thickening and loss of lung area, resulting in a decrement in diffusion capacity for carbon monoxide (DLCO). A low DLCO implies an impaired oxygen uptake by the alveolus, and may necessitate implementation of home oxygen therapy. Other causes of low DLCO are cardiac insufficiency, anemia, and pulmonary hypertension.

Pulmonary function tests may identify a response to bronchodilator therapy, if it is present. Oddly, broncho-reactivity is most common in the moderate stage of COPD. Resting arterial blood gas testing helps identify the level of baseline ventilation as evidenced by degree of arterial carbon dioxide (CO_2) retention, as does the bicarbonate (HCO_3) level. In the presence of an elevated $Paco_2$, there is typically a conservation of HCO_3 by the kidney. Thus, elevated CO_2 in patients with COPD is often accompanied by a concomitant increase in HCO_3. It is important to have baseline CO_2 and HCO_3 levels, as they determine the intraoperative ventilation strategies. Hyperventilation in these patients, in attempt to normalize CO_2, leads to renal bicarbonate wasting and metabolic acidosis.

Intraoperative Management

In patients with a significant bronchospastic component to their COPD, patients should be asked to use their inhalers prior to the induction of general anesthesia. Routine monitoring is appropriate. Thiopental and histamine-releasing drugs such as morphine and succinylcholine should be avoided if possible. Laryngoscopy and intubation should only be attempted after ensuring an adequate depth of anesthesia, or bronchospasm may result. One option involves spraying the trachea with 4% lidocaine prior to intubation. While the lidocaine does anesthetize the trachea and reduce the foreign body response to intubation, the spray occasionally also provokes a foreign body response. Use of this maneuver varies widely by practitioner.

The anesthetic maintenance regimen typically includes a combination of inhaled agents and narcotics. Respiratory management should take into account the pathophysiology of COPD, which involves the loss of alveolar elasticity and impaired ventilation/perfusion mismatch (V/Q). The extent of V/Q mismatch in COPD reflects the extent of lung tissue destroyed. During exacerbations of COPD, V/Q mismatch worsens. Ventilator management includes a long exhalation time to counter the loss of alveolar elasticity. The judicious use of PEEP can improve oxygenation in the setting of hyperinflation. PEEP also increases the intrathoracic pressure somewhat, and if excessive, can impair venous return. The optimal level of PEEP does not decrease cardiac output (blood pressure can be used as a surrogate for cardiac output).

The emergence from general anesthesia is a critical time for patients with COPD. Rapid shallow breaths of low tidal volume are consistent with respiratory failure. This breathing pattern can be followed by progressive hypercapnia, respiratory muscle fatigue, and respiratory failure. Noninvasive positive pressure ventilation (NPPV) increases patient comfort while decreasing the work of breathing, and over the long term decreases mortality. NPPV is commonly administered in the form of bi-level positive airway pressure (BiPAP) by means of a specialized BiPAP mask. This form of ventilation decreases atelectasis, improves oxygenation, and also decreases work of breathing. However, it does require concerted patient cooperation.

Fluid management in patients with COPD is targeted toward euvolemia. In the presence of significant lung dysfunction, even a minor fluid overload can precipitate pulmonary edema and delay tracheal extubation. Neuraxial blockade is the preferred anesthetic in a patient with severe COPD if the procedure is amenable, as there is a decreased incidence of respiratory depression and failure.

In addition to bronchospasm, other complications should be considered when caring for a patient with COPD. Sudden cardiovascular collapse could represent a ruptured emphysematous bleb, particularly if mechanical (positive pressure) ventilation is used. And if the patient is on steroids, the presence of sustained hypotension after anesthetic causes have been eliminated, the possibility of adrenal insufficiency secondary to prolonged steroid use should be considered. It is common practice to administer supplemental "stress-dose" of steroids; typically, hydrocortisone is administered every 6 hours for the first 24-hour period. However, this practice and steroid regimen are entirely empirical, and has not been shown to influence outcomes.

Postoperative Management

Postoperative pain relief is vital in the presence of COPD. Pain increases patient splinting and predisposes them to atelectasis and pneumonia. However, narcotics are also associated with respiratory depression and the requirement for re-intubation. BiPAP is an option as a treatment for hypoxemia. Weaning from BiPAP is dictated by patient comfort (no use of accessory muscles, adequate oxygenation, and ventilation) as well as pulse oximetry.

Comprehension Questions

25.1. A 50-year-old man with stable severe COPD has just undergone a radical prostatectomy. His intraoperative course was uncomplicated. Currently he is in the post-anesthesia care unit (PACU) with a respiratory rate of 28, SpO_2 94% on 6 L oxygen by a simple facemask. When breathing, he uses his alae nasi and intercostal muscles. Pain is controlled with a patient controlled analgesic regimen. The nurse calls you to assess this patient, as he doesn't "look right." What is your first step?

A. Intubate the trachea
B. Institute BiPAP after getting an arterial blood gas
C. Administer naloxone
D. Administer diuretic

25.2. What is the role of PEEP?

A. Improves oxygenation
B. Decreases atelectasis
C. Decreases cardiac output
D. Decreases the risk of pneumothorax

25. 3. In the preoperative clinic, a 50-year-old woman presents for a laparoscopic adrenalectomy for a benign adenoma. She has a history of progressive shortness of breath over the past couple of years, and a slight but steady decrease in her functional capacity. She needs oxygen at night to help her breathe. Her past medical history includes well-controlled hypertension (with one drug, onset of disease 3 years ago). She is not obese but does appear to use accessory muscles of respiration. What would your differential diagnosis include?

A. Cardiac failure
B. COPD exacerbation
C. Asthma
D. Being in poor physical shape

ANSWERS

25.1. **B.** General anesthesia with intubation and positive pressure ventilation most often causes a small degree of atelectasis, which is usually clinically insignificant. In patients with COPD, any loss of lung function can precipitate respiratory distress and failure. This patient demonstrates increased work of breathing by use of accessory muscles and is mildly hypoxemic. Both of these symptoms can be alleviated by use of BiPAP, which will both open up atelectatic alveoli as well as decrease work of breathing. If NPPV fails as evidenced by rising

CO_2 and no change in work of breathing, it is appropriate to intubate the trachea and institute controlled ventilation. There is no evidence of pulmonary edema to warrant use of a diuretic prior to NPPV. Overuse of narcotics commonly results in a low respiratory rate with large tidal volumes progressing to apnea. Serial arterial blood gas analysis will assess adequacy of both oxygenation and ventilation and thereby guide success of therapy.

25.2. **D.** PEEP prevents total collapse of alveoli at end exhalation. The stinting open of the alveoli prior to the next breath helps increase the amount of lung mass participating in gas exchange. PEEP decreases V/Q mismatch by decreasing atelectasis and thereby improves both oxygenation and ventilation. PEEP increases intrathoracic pressure, which can be impedance to venous return and cardiac output. PEEP increases, not decreases, the risk of pneumothorax.

25.3. **B.** COPD presents as slowly progressive shortness of breath and fatigue. Exacerbations are marked by hypoxemia, and an increase in respiratory work secondary to bronchitis or inadequate control. Her hypertension is not long standing and has been controlled with a single agent. While cardiac or coronary artery disease is in the differential diagnosis, the likelihood of this being a primary event is unlikely. A stress test should be performed if inhalers do not alleviate her symptoms. New-onset asthma presents with a more acute picture and is lower on list of probable diagnosis. In this patient, being physically out of shape is an unlikely explanation for shortness of breath requiring oxygen at night.

Clinical Pearls

- Frequency of COPD exacerbations indicates medical control of this disease process.
- Loss of alveolar elasticity favors auto-PEEP development in the presence of incorrect ventilator management.
- Fluid management needs to be precise to avoid alveolar flooding and hypoxia while maintaining euvolemia.
- Postoperative respiratory complications tend to increase length of stay and worsen patient satisfaction. They can range from hypoxia and bronchospasm to ventilator dependence and respiratory failure.

REFERENCES

Licker M, Schweizer A et al. Perioperative medical management of patients with COPD. *Int Chron Obstruct Pulmon Dis*. 2007;2:493-515.

Miller RD. Anesthetic management of concomitant diseases: Chronic obstructive pulmonary disease. In: *Miller's Anesthesia*. 6th ed. Philadelphia, PA: Elsevier; 2005: Chapter 27.

Case 26

A 65-year-old Caucasian man presents to the anesthesia preoperative clinic for an evaluation in anticipation of a video-assisted thoracoscopic (VATS) resection of a right lower lobe squamous-cell carcinoma. His symptoms include shortness of breath after climbing two flights of stairs, and a chronic morning cough with yellow productive sputum.

His past medical history includes a smoking history of 1 pack per day for 40 years and chronic obstructive lung disease (COPD). He also has hypertension and a review of his medical record shows multiple blood pressure readings which were elevated. His only medication is amlodipine.

The patient is 70 in tall and weighs 70 kg. His vital signs include BP = 170/90 mm Hg, heart rate = 90 bpm, respiratory rate (RR) = 20 breaths per minute, and Temp = 97.2°F. His airway examination demonstrates a supple neck with full range of motion, a hyomental distance of 6 cm, and an airway classification of Mallampati 2. Scattered expiratory wheezes are audible on auscultation of his chest. The rest of his physical examination was unremarkable.

Preoperative tests include a complete blood count (CBC), chemistry-7, coagulation profile, chest x-ray, and ECG. Pertinent findings on preoperative tests include hemoglobin = 12 (an Hct of 35). The rest of his preoperative tests are unremarkable.

- What pulmonary function tests may help to assess this patient's surgical risk and why?
- What are the most important intraoperative concerns in a patient undergoing lung resection?
- Why is postoperative analgesia important in these patients?

ANSWERS TO CASE 26: Thoracoscopic Lung Resection

Summary: This is a 65-year-old man with a 40-pack-year smoking history and a past medical history of hypertension and COPD being scheduled for a thoracoscopic resection of right middle lobe squamous cell carcinoma. Additional concerns found during anesthesia preoperative evaluation include poorly-controlled hypertension and mild anemia.

➤ **Pulmonary function tests:** Since a vital capacity of at least three times the tidal volume is needed to produce an effective cough, pulmonary function tests (PFTs) can predict increase risk of postoperative pulmonary morbidity. PFTs are also useful to determine the degree of severity of his lung disease and to evaluate the degree of reversibility with bronchodilator treatment prior to proceeding with surgery. Predictors of perioperative morbidity include:

1. $FEV_1 < 2$ L
2. $FEV_1/FVC < 0.5$
3. Vital capacity (VC) <15 cc/kg
4. Arterial blood gas with hypoxemia and/or hypercarbia

If the FEV_1/FVC value is low on the PFT, then this supports the diagnosis of COPD in this patient. Unlike patients with restrictive lung disease who will have a normal FEV_1/FVC value, patients with obstructive lung disease will have a low FEV_1/FVC due to a markedly low FEV_1.

➤ **The three most important intraoperative concerns:** (1) Maintaining hemodynamic stability, (2) maximizing oxygenation and maintaining adequate ventilation during one lung ventilation, and (3) avoiding overhydration of fluid replacements.

➤ **Importance of adequate analgesia:** This allows patients to effectively perform incentive spirometry and enables the pulmonary toilet functions to clear airway secretions, both of which reduce atelectasis and thereby improve ventilatory function. Conversely, it is also important to avoid oversedating these patients, for essentially the same reasons.

ANALYSIS

Objectives

1. Identify preoperative anesthesia concerns as it pertains to patient undergoing surgery for lung resection.
2. Become acquainted with use of a double lumen tube, and some of the factors to consider when choosing a right-versus left-sided tube.

3. Understand the intricacies of intraoperative anesthetic management of patients undergoing lung resection.
4. Identify postoperative concerns for patients post lung resection.

Considerations

This patient is an ASA-3, with poorly controlled hypertension, tobacco use, chronic obstructive lung disease (COPD), squamous-cell lung carcinoma, and anemia. The fact that he can climb two flights of stairs before developing shortness of breath indicates that he has a MET of > 6, indicating that he has an adequate cardiopulmonary reserve to undergo an intermediate risk procedure.

He has not had pulmonary function tests, and is currently not receiving bronchodilator therapy. A pulmonary function test (PFT) should be requested to determine severity of COPD and to determine if patient responds to bronchodilator treatment. If PFTs indicates good bronchodilator response, he should be referred to his primary care physician (PCP) to initiate bronchodilator treatment.

Since his surgery date is 2 weeks following the preoperative evaluation, he will also benefit from referral to his PCP for optimization of his blood pressure prior to surgery. Patients with long-standing uncontrolled or poorly controlled hypertension will have a right shift of the cerebral autoregulatory curve, and as a result, require a higher blood pressure tó maintain adequate cerebral perfusion. Hemodynamic liability, especially acute hypotension, may occur with general anesthesia and predisposes these patients to a higher risk of ischemic strokes during surgery.

It is important to ensure that cross-matched blood is available during surgery since patient has mild anemia and is undergoing a procedure with potential for large blood loss. He should give consent for general anesthesia with invasive (arterial and CVP) monitoring, possible thoracic epidural catheter placement, and blood transfusion therapy.

APPROACH TO Thoracoscopic Lung Resection

DEFINITIONS

VATS (VIDEO-ASSISTED THORACOSCOPIC SURGERY): A procedure involving the use of advanced video technology, computers, and high-tech electronics to perform surgeries within the chest.

DOUBLE LUMEN TUBE: A specialized endotracheal with two separate ventilation lumens .

UNIVENT: A single lumen endotracheal tube with a build-in endobronchial blocker .

WEDGE RESECTION: A surgical procedure to remove a triangle-shaped slice of tissue.

LOBECTOMY: A surgical procedure to remove an entire lobe of an organ.

PNEUMONECTOMY: An entire resection of a lung.

LEFT LATERAL DECUBITUS POSITION: Lateral position during surgery in which the patient's body will be lying on the left side.

CLINICAL APPROACH

In 2009, the National Cancer Institute reports 219,440 new cases of lung cancer and 159,390 deaths from lung cancer in the United States. These numbers include small-cell- and non–small cell-lung carcinomas. The cancer mortality rate is usually expressed as the number of deaths due to cancer per 100,000 population. That is,

Mortality Rate = (Cancer Deaths/Population) 100,000

The overall outcome of patients with lung cancer depends on early detection and treatment. The benefits of preoperative optimization must be weighed against the risks of delaying the early surgical treatment of his lung cancer. COPD is common in this population, and preoperative optimization reduces the incidence of pulmonary complications after surgery. Similarly, preoperative blood pressure control can decrease the incidence of hemodynamic lability and incidence of stroke during the perioperative period.

The preparation for pulmonary resection includes cross-matched blood, which is immediately available because of the potential of large blood loss during surgery. This is particularly true in the cancer patient, who may be anemic. It is preferable to place a large-bore (preferably 16 gauge or larger) peripheral intravenous (PIV) in the arm on the operative side. Since patients are placed in the lateral decubitus position (nonoperative side down) during surgery, there is a potential for vascular compression of the upper extremity on the nonoperative side (the "down" arm). Should vascular compression of the "down" arm occur due to a position related problem, then an i.v. placed in the "down" arm would be rendered useless during surgery. This is the reason why the PIV is recommended to be placed in the upper extremity on the operative ("up") side.

After the i.v. is placed, the placement of an arterial catheter will allow a room air blood gas to be sent prior to induction of anesthesia. Additional monitors for this patient include: (1) arterial line and (2) central venous pressure (CVP) monitoring. The strongest clinical indication for an arterial line placement in this case is to provide serial sampling of arterial blood gas in order to monitor arterial oxygen and carbon dioxide levels during surgery. Room air blood gas is also useful in determining the degree of severity of lung disease, and will be invaluable later in the case as one lung ventilation is established. A right thoracoscopic surgical approach requires that this patient be placed in a left lateral decubitus position (left side down and right side up). Placing the arterial line in the "anatomically down" arm will allow early detection of axillary artery and brachial plexus compression during surgery. A central line is usually placed in order to provide rapid access for fluid resuscitation and to provide close monitoring of central venous filling pressures in order to avoid overhydration during surgery. Besides standard monitors and equipments, additional equipment should include a fiberoptic bronchoscope, a CPAP device, a vascular clamp to facilitate one lung ventilation, a double lumen tube, and in case of difficulty intubation, a standard endotracheal tube with a stylette.

With the possible exception of endoscopic procedures, surgical procedures on the lung require general endotracheal anesthesia. If the likelihood of an open thoracotomy is high, then patients will benefit from the preoperative placement of a thoracic epidural for postoperative pain control. The epidural may also be used during the intraoperative period to decrease intravenous use of narcotics, and therefore, facilitate early endotracheal extubation of patients at termination of surgery. If a thoracic epidural catheter is considered and there are no contraindications, then it is preferred to place the thoracic epidural catheter between levels of T_4 and T_7 prior to the induction of general anesthesia. Patient cooperation during thoracic epidural catheter placement is essential. Therefore, at a maximum, light sedation can be provided to facilitate this procedure.

Once the proper surgery protocol including patient identification and surgical marking is completed, the patient is transported into the operating room. Following the application of standard monitors (ECG, noninvasive blood pressure [NIBP], pulse oximetry) and connection of arterial line for continuous blood pressure monitoring, 100% oxygen is administered prior to the induction of general anesthesia.

Unlike routine general anesthesia cases, one lung ventilation is needed to maximize the surgical exposure when using a thoracoscopic approach. One lung ventilation can be achieved by using a double-lumen endotracheal tube (Figure 26–1) or a single-lumen endotracheal tube with a built-in endobronchial

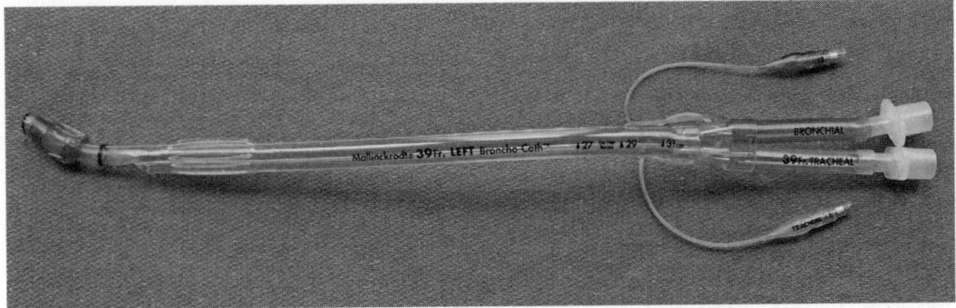

Figure 26–1. Double-lumen endotracheal tube. The most distal tip of the double-lumen tube is always the bronchial lumen. A left pneumonectomy will require a right-sided double-lumen tube for one lung ventilation. Otherwise, a left-sided double-lumen tube is preferred by most since it is easier to position than a right-sided double-lumen tube.

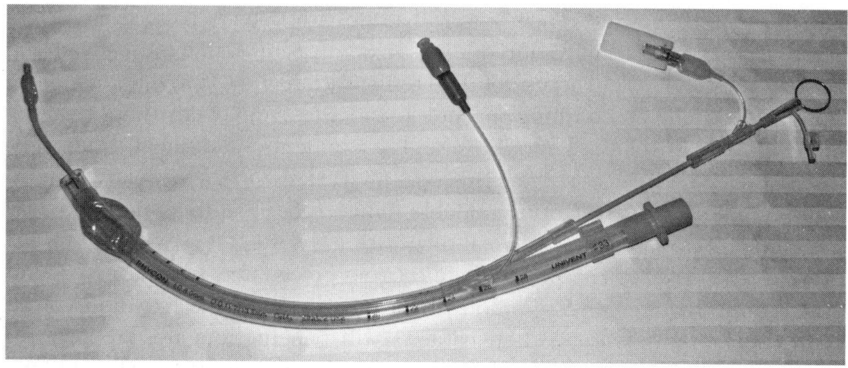

Figure 26–2. Univent endotracheal tube. This is a single-lumen endotracheal tube with a built-in endobronchial blocker. Using fiberoptic bronchoscopy, the endobronchial blocker can be positioned into the desired bronchus to achieve one lung ventilation. The advantage of the Univent tube is that it is easier to place than the double lumen tube. The disadvantages are that suctioning of the nonventilated lung cannot be achieved and continuous positive airway pressure (CPAP) cannot be applied during one lung ventilation.

blocker such as the Univent tube (Figure 26–2). The advantages of a double-lumen endotracheal tube include better lung isolation, the ability to provide continuous positive airway pressure (CPAP), and better access for endotracheal suctioning of airway secretions. For patients with a difficult airway and need one lung ventilation, a Univent tube may offer the advantage of easier endotracheal insertion than a double-lumen endotracheal tube.

Double-lumen endotracheal tubes are available in both left-sided and right-sided versions and in 28F, 35F, 37F, 39F, and 41F. Most male adult tracheas accommodate a 39F or 41F DLT, while most female adult tracheas accommodate a 35F or 37F. Though it is actually easier to intubate the right mainstem bronchus due to its larger size and less acute angle with the trachea, it is very difficult to align the small orifice made for the right upper lobe with the right upper lobe bronchus, often leading to right upper lobe atelectasis. Although counterintuitive, a left-sided double lumen tube is actually easier to position for one lung ventilation than a right-sided double lumen tube, and obviously does not carry the risk of right upper lobe collapse. A left-sided double lumen tube is preferred by most anesthesiologists, unless the patient is undergoing a left pneumonectomy (which includes bronchial resection), and therefore requires a right-sided double lumen tube.

If the patient does not appear to have a difficult airway, general anesthesia is induced, and laryngoscopy performed to visualize the vocal cord for direct placement of the double-lumen tube. Once the trachea is intubated, ventilation is confirmed by listening for presence of bilateral breath sounds and by detecting the presence of end-tidal carbon dioxide using capnography. In addition to auscultation, the proper placement of the double-lumen tube is confirmed by fiberoptic bronchoscopy through the tracheal lumen of the double-lumen tube. The trachea and carina are used as a marker to identify the carina, which in turn identifies the right and left mainstem bronchi. Once the carina is identified, it is interesting to identify the anterior and posterior parts of the trachea. The posterior trachea does not have tracheal rings: rather, it consists of soft tissue with a smooth surface. Looking straight at the carina, if tracheal rings are noted on the anterior part of the bronchoscope screen, then the right main bronchus will be located on the right side of the screen. If the bronchial lumen of the double-lumen tube has already advanced into the left main bronchus (a desirable outcome if one is using a left double-lumen tube), the left mainstem bronchus may not be visualized. A left endobronchial intubation is also verified by advancing the fiberoptic bronchoscope through the tube's tracheal lumen, into the right mainstem bronchus. From the carina, the visualization of three bronchial lumens distal to the main bronchus correctly identifies the right main bronchus. The correct placement of the double-lumen tube in the left main bronchus is confirmed by visualization of bronchial lumen placed in the left main bronchus, and visualization of a slight herniation of the bronchial cuff into the trachea after it is inflated with 3 cc of air.

Once the double-lumen tube is secured, the patient's neck is prepped for central line placement. Unless otherwise contraindicated, it is recommended to place the central line on the same side of the surgical procedure. An iatrogenic pneumothorax is always possible following central line placement. So if it occurs, it's preferable that the pneumothorax be on the operative side where the chest is open anyway, and where a chest tube will be placed.

The next step is to position the patient into the lateral decubitus position. During position, it is important to keep the neck in a neutral position, and to ensure that the eyes and ears are free from being compressed. A chest roll is placed under the arm distal to the left axilla, making sure brachial plexus and axillary vasculature are not being compressed. The right arm is placed on a specialized arm board (sometimes called the "airplane") to allow adequate surgical exposure of the right chest. It is important to make sure that all pressure points are well padded during patient positioning. After the patient is well positioned, the position of the double-lumen tube is confirmed one more time. This can be achieved by listening over the lung fields during one lung ventilation, and by using the fiberoptic bronchoscope.

During surgery, both lung fields are ventilated until the surgeon requests one lung ventilation. Take note of the tidal volume and peak airway pressure during normal ventilation. One goal of one lung ventilation is to provide nearly the same tidal volume and peak airway pressure as with double lung ventilation, in order to maintain adequate oxygenation and ventilation and avoid barotrauma. When one lung ventilation is requested, a clamp is applied to the tracheal lumen of the DLT. This will cease ventilation to the right lung, produce a quiet surgical field, and allow better surgical exposure. Ventilation and oxygenation to the left lung is maintained through the left bronchial lumen of the double-lumen tube. It is important to note (and document) the tidal volume, peak airway pressure, end-tidal carbon dioxide tension, and pulse oximetry, both prior to clamping the tracheal lumen, as well as after. Adjustments to ventilator settings maintain oxygenation and ventilation, and avoid the barotrauma caused by high-peak airway pressures during one lung ventilation. Whether to use a high FiO_2 (1.0) or a lower FiO_2 remains controversial. Clearly, maintenance of an acceptable $PaCO_2$, One concern of using a high FiO_2 during surgery, especially with one lung ventilation, is that it causes absorption atelectasis, potentially increasing the degree of shunting caused by the collapsed alveoli. The concept of high FiO_2 causing oxygen toxicity is a theoretical concern, unless the patient has been previously exposed to chemotherapeutic agents such as bleomycin or busulfan.

Approximately 10 to 15 minutes after initiation of one lung ventilation, an arterial blood gas is sampled to monitor arterial oxygen and carbon dioxide tensions. One major goal during OLV is to keep the PaO_2 between 150 to 200 mm Hg. If PaO_2 falls below 150 mm Hg, continuous airway pressure (CPAP) can be applied to the nondependent (nonventilated) lung and positive end-expiratory pressure (PEEP) can be added to the dependent (ventilated) lung to improve oxygenation.

After the right middle lobectomy is completed, the surgeon will request to return to two lung ventilation. After 10 to 15 minutes on two lung ventilation, another arterial blood gas is obtained to determine if oxygenation and ventilation is significantly affected after lobectomy. Optimization of oxygenation and ventilation during this time is important if patient is to be considered for extubation at termination of surgery. Maneuvers such as endotracheal suctioning to remove airway secretions and nebulization with bronchodilator agents may help to improve oxygenation prior to extubation. If extubation cannot be achieved at the end of surgery, once the patient is moved to a supine position, the double-lumen tube is replaced by a single-lumen endotracheal tube.

If a thoracic epidural catheter is placed for this patient, this epidural can be used to supplement anesthesia and analgesia and decrease intravenous narcotic administration during surgery. This allows the patient to be comfortable and yet awake enough to respond to coaching deep breathing exercises. Hypotension is a concern with intraoperative use of thoracic epidural catheters, since infusions or boluses of these catheters using dense concentration local anesthetic may result in hypotension. A dilute epidural regimen using 0.0625% to 0.125% of bupivacaine and 2 to 5 μg/cc of fentanyl infusing at 5 to 10 cc/h started just prior to surgical incision may be considered as an alternative. Providing adequate analgesia so that patient can be comfortable to perform deep incentive spirometry and to produce an effective cough to clear airway secretions is essential during the postoperative period. These maneuvers will help reexpand the lungs, decrease atelectasis, and improve lung function after surgery.

Another concern during lung resection surgery is avoiding excessive fluid resuscitation. Central venous pressure monitoring can help guide fluid management during this case, although the absolute number provided by the CVP is not necessarily accurate in either the lateral position, or in the presence of an open chest. Excessive fluid resuscitation during lung resection surgery, especially lobectomy and pneumonectomy, predisposes patients to an increase risk of right heart failure and cardiac dysrhythmias, especially atrial fibrillation, during the postoperative period. Indeed, during lung surgery, even normal amounts of fluid are often considered to be "excessive."

Comprehension Questions

26.1. What is the smoking history of a patient who smokes 2 packs per day for 50 years?
A. 40 pack years
B. 50 pack years
C. 80 pack years
D. 90 pack years
E. 100 pack years

26.2. A vital capacity of at least how many times the vital capacity is needed to produce an effective cough?
A. One
B. Two
C. Three
D. Four
E. Five

26.3. Which of the following values on the pulmonary lung test is useful in differentiating between restrictive and obstructive pulmonary disease?
A. FVC
B. FEV_1
C. FEV_1/FVC
D. RV/TLC
E. MVV

26.4. Which of the following values will predict an increase risk of postoperative pulmonary complications?
A. $PaO_2 > 80$ (room air arterial blood gas)
B. $PCO_2 > 50$
C. $FEV_1 > 2$ L
D. $FEV_1/FVC > 0.5$
E. VC > 15 cc/kg

26.5. Which of the following maneuvers can help improve oxygenation during one lung ventilation?

A. Increasing the concentration of an inhaled anesthetic to aid bronchodilation
B. Adding mild suction to the nondependent (nonventilated) lung
C. Adding PEEP to nondependent (nonventilated) lung
D. Adding PEEP to the dependent (ventilated) lung

26.6. Which of the following tests would be useful in determining the surgical risk for a patient with COPD, complaining of severe shortness of breath after one flight of stairs, and who has a new left bundle-branch block on the preoperative ECG?

A. Exercise stress test
B. Pulmonary function test
C. Chemical stress test
D. Echocardiography

ANSWERS

26.1. **E.** Total pack years of smoking is calculated by multiplying the number of packs the patient smokes a day with the total number of years smoked (2 packs/day 50 years = 100 pack years).

26.2. **C.** A vital capacity of at least three times the tidal volume is needed to produce an effective cough.

26.3. **C.** A low FEV_1 is indicative of airway obstruction. However, the ratio of FEV_1/FVC is more useful in differentiating between restrictive and obstructive pulmonary disease. This ratio is normal in restrictive lung disease and low in obstructive lung disease. Both FEV_1 and FVC decrease with restrictive lung disease. As a result, the FEV_1/FVC ratio will be normal. FEV_1 is markedly decreased with obstructive lung disease. As a result, the FEV_1/FVC ratio will be low.

26.4. **B.** The presence of hypercarbia on an arterial blood gas (ABG) is predictive of increased postoperative pulmonary complications. Other predictors of postoperative pulmonary complications include: (1) an FEV_1 lower than 2 L, (2) the ratio of FEV_1/FVC of less than 0.5, (3) the VC of less than 15 cc/kg, and (4) the presence of hypoxemia on the arterial blood gas.

26.5. **D.** Adjusting the minute ventilation, respiratory rate, and tidal volume help improve oxygenation during one lung ventilation. In addition, PEEP can be applied to the dependent (ventilated) lung and CPAP can be applied to the nondependent (nonventilated) lung to improve oxygenation during one lung ventilation. With respect to answer **C**, positive end-expiratory pressure (PEEP) cannot be added to the nondependent lung because the nondependent (operative) lung is not ventilated, and PEEP can only be added to a ventilated circuit. Increasing the concentration of an inhaled anesthetic to aid bronchodilation is only helpful if the patient is wheezing. Adding mild suction to the nondependent (nonventilated) lung will not affect oxygenation.

26.6. **D.** The presence of a new left bundle-branch block (LBBB) on the preoperative ECG may indicate cardiac disease. Since this patient has low functional capacity due to shortness of breath with exertion, it is important to determine if his dyspnea is due to COPD and lung cancer or cardiac disease caused by myocardial ischemia. A chemical stress test (myocardial perfusion scan and dobutamine stress echo) will help to determine if dyspnea is due to cardiac or pulmonary pathophysiology. Shortness of breath with exercise can indicate a severely depressed systolic myocardial function, and stress-induced ischemia.

Clinical Pearls

- It is important to thoroughly evaluate the patient undergoing lung surgery to determine the risk for anesthesia and surgery.
- Early detection and treatment of lung cancer offers better outcome. If time permits, then patient's medical problems need to be optimized prior to surgery.
- For patients scheduled for lung resection surgery, especially with lobectomy and pneumonectomy, it is important to determine whether or not the patient has enough pulmonary reserve to undergo the surgical procedure. Pulmonary function tests, room air arterial blood gas, split lung function test, and pulmonary artery balloon-occlusion test can help predict patient's postoperative outcome after lung resection surgery, and are especially important prior to a pneumonectomy.

REFERENCES

Barash PG, Cullen BF, Stoelting RK. *Clinical Anesthesia*. 5th ed. Philadelphia, PA: Lippincott Williams & Wilkins; 2006.

National Cancer Institute. www.cancer.gov. 2009.

Stoelting RK, Miller RD. *Basics of Anesthesia*. 4th ed. New York, NY: Churchill Livingston; 2000.

Case 27

A 29-year-old man presented to the hospital with a 5-week history of fatigue, nonproductive cough, increasing dyspnea, and pleuritic chest pain. He had no history of hemoptysis, night sweats, or fevers, and his medical history was otherwise unremarkable. On physical examination, the patient was noted to be tachypneic and dyspneic at rest, with seemingly prolonged expiration and accessory muscle use. His blood pressure was 116/71 mm Hg, the pulse 74 bpm, the respiratory rate 18 breaths per minute, the temperature 36.3°C, and the oxygen saturation 88% while the patient was breathing room air. On auscultation of the chest, breath sounds were normal. Blood chemistry and hematology values were all normal, except for hypoxemia and a mild respiratory alkalosis (partial pressure of oxygen [Po_2] = 53 mm Hg, arterial oxygen saturation [Sao_2] = 86%, partial pressure of carbon dioxide [Pco_2] = 30 mm Hg, and pH = 7.48; fraction of inspired oxygen [Fio_2] = 1). A chest radiograph showed a small left pleural effusion with a large mass in the anterior and middle mediastinum abutting the heart and hilar structures. Subsequent computed tomographic examination showed a mass in the anterior mediastinum measuring 12.3 5.6 11 cm. It compressed the tracheobronchial tree posteriorly.

- What are the most serious outcomes in patients with a mediastinal mass?
- How can the risk of these complications be reduced?
- What is the optimal anesthetic plan?

ANSWERS TO CASE 27: Anterior Mediastinal Mass

Summary: A 29-year-old man with a symptomatic anterior mediastinal mass undergoing diagnostic mediastinoscopy.

- ➤ **Most serious outcome:** Airway obstruction and hemodynamic instability including cardiac arrest, especially with the administration of general anesthesia in patients with anterior mediastinal masses. Although the possibility for a disastrous outcome still exists, improvements in the intraoperative management of these cases have rendered severe intraoperative respiratory or cardiovascular collapse less likely. Major life-threatening complications now occur more frequently postoperatively.
- ➤ **Minimizing risks:** The primary goal during general anesthesia is the maintenance of spontaneous ventilation if at all possible. Positioning the patient either sitting and leaning forward at a 45 degree angle, or moving from supine to lateral or prone may help prevent cardiovascular or respiratory collapse. Cardiopulmonary bypass may also be indicated.
- ➤ **Anesthesia plan:** Preoperative studies (CT, transthoracic echocardiography) determine the structural abnormalities and facilitate coordinated planning between the anesthesia and surgical teams. Local anesthesia with sedation, regional anesthesia, or general anesthesia with the maintenance of spontaneous ventilation represent appropriate anesthetic options. Of course, it is imperative to monitor gas exchange and hemodynamics while maintaining spontaneous ventilation until either the airway is definitively secured or the procedure is completed.

ANALYSIS

Objectives

1. Understand the complications, including respiratory and cardiovascular collapse, including the inability to resuscitate, that can ensue on induction of general anesthesia.
2. Become acquainted with the technique for extubating a patient with a mediastinal mass.
3. Examine what have been identified as suitable methods to care for this group of patients.

Considerations

In this patient with a mediastinal mass, monitoring during surgery includes a continuous two-lead electrocardiogram (lead II and V5), oxygen saturation, and direct arterial pressure catheter. Anesthesia is induced with an inhalational agent such as sevoflurane, with the patient sitting at a 45 degree angle and breathing spontaneously. In contrast, an induction with intravenous agents could well be associated with apnea. Respiration can be assisted if necessary, but tracheal intubation is achieved without the use of neuromuscular blockade.

Consistent with the CT scan, fiberoptic bronchoscopy will likely reveal a severe (> 70%) compression of the lumen of the lower third of the trachea. If possible, the end tracheal tube is advanced distal to the tracheal compression under fiberoptic guidance. This will allow ventilation of both lungs, and subsequent bronchoscopic examination. An uncomplicated left anterior mediastinoscopy revealed a high-grade Hodgkin lymphoma at biopsy. The conclusion of the procedure, the patient was successfully extubated awake, while again, sitting at a 45 degree angle.

APPROACH TO Anterior Mediastinal Mass

Anesthesia in patients with anterior mediastinal masses has been associated with airway obstruction and hemodynamic instability, including cardiac arrest. However, due to the increased awareness by the medical community of the significance of this syndrome, there has been a significant decline in intraoperative fatalities during general anesthesia. Major airway complications in these patients are now more likely to occur in the PACU, instead of the operating room.

Since an anterior mediastinal masses vary in anatomy, pathology, and the proposed surgical procedure, there is the need to individualize management for each patient. Masses may be benign or malignant tumors, cysts, or aneurysms, and may originate from the lung, pleura, or any of the components of the anterior mediastinum. Etiologies include (in order of frequency): lymphoma (Hodgkin or non-Hodgkin), thymoma, germ cell tumor, granuloma, bronchogenic carcinoma, thyroid tumors, bronchogenic cyst, and cystic hygroma. Possible diagnostic or therapeutic surgical procedures include sternotomy, thoracotomy, cervical mediastinoscopy, anterior parasternal mediastinoscopy, or video-assisted thoracoscopic biopsy.

Patients typically present with signs or symptoms that include chest pain, dyspnea, cough, sweats, superior vena cava obstruction, hoarseness, syncope, or dysphagia. Patients may also be asymptomatic, and have a mass diagnosed on screening chest radiograph or computed tomography (CT) scan. Signs and symptoms which should alert the anesthesiologist to the possibility of an increased risk of airway complications are increased dyspnea, orthopnea, or cough when supine. An increased risk of cardiovascular collapse is suggested by syncopal symptoms or pericardial effusion. Patients with severe symptoms cannot voluntarily lie supine even for a short duration. Similarly, placing them in the supine position following the induction of anesthesia can have disastrous consequences.

The preoperative preparation of the patient with an anterior mediastinal mass includes a chest radiograph and a CT scan prior to any surgical procedure. In addition, the anesthesiologist must personally examine the imaging studies to plan the airway management. The CT scan will show the site, severity, and extent of the airway compromise. In patients who are unable to tolerate the supine position due to the compressive effects of the mass, the scan can be performed in either prone or lateral position. Patients with cardiovascular symptoms should also have transthoracic echocardiography to assess for cardiovascular compromise. Flow-volume loop studies have not been shown to be of benefit in the perioperative assessment or management of these patients.

The intraoperative administration of anesthesia for patients requires careful planning and execution to maintain airway patency and patient safety. It is imperative to monitor gas exchange and hemodynamics while maintaining spontaneous ventilation until either the airway is definitively secured or the procedure is completed. Induction is best achieved with a volatile agent such as sevoflurane by a slow, intravenous titration of propofol to ensure that apnea does not ensue, and possibly with the addition of ketamine. Alternatively, dexmedetomidine may also be a useful adjunct. Intubation of the conscious patient prior to induction is also a practical approach in some patients. If muscle relaxants are required, assisted ventilation should first be gradually taken over manually to assure that positive-pressure ventilation is tolerated and only then can a short-acting muscle relaxant be administered.

The development of airway or vascular compression requires that the patient be awakened as rapidly as possible and other options for surgery implemented. If intraoperative airway compression occurs, possible remedies include changing the patient's position from supine to lateral or prone, or by passing a rigid bronchoscope distal to the obstruction. Lastly, in severely compromised patients who cannot tolerate general anesthesia, cannulation of the groin for the use in cardiopulmonary bypass should be performed preemptively. In some cases, it may also be appropriate to begin cardiopulmonary bypass electively, and not just to be ready in a standby mode.

Comprehension Questions

27.1. Patients with positional dyspnea exacerbated by laying supine warrant which of the following preoperative assessments before a surgical procedure?

A. A CT of the chest
B. An ENT consult
C. Pulmonary function studies—flow volume loops
D. Pulmonary function studies—response to bronchodilators

27.2. Safe anesthetic care for a patient with a symptomatic anterior mediastinal mass includes which of the following?

A. Induction with propofol and succinylcholine followed by laryngoscopy and endotracheal intubation.
B. Positioning the patient supine.
C. Maintaining controlled ventilation and PEEP at all times.
D. Preoperative discussion with the surgeon about the radiologic imaging studies, perioperative plan, and contingency options which may include cardiopulmonary bypass.

ANSWERS

27.1. **A.** Patients with positional dyspnea exacerbated by lying supine warrant a physical examination of their head and lungs, a CT scan of the chest, and a chest radiograph before a surgical procedure. Pulmonary function studies including flow-volume loops or the response to bronchodilators are not helpful in predicting possible compression of the airway. If these tests are normal, then an ENT consult to examine possible pharyngeal or tracheal pathology would be indicated.

27.2. **D.** Safe anesthetic care for a patient with a symptomatic anterior mediastinal mass includes maintaining spontaneous ventilation and airway patency at all times, positioning the patient in a sitting or upright position, and preoperative discussion with the surgeon about the radiologic imaging studies, formulation of a perioperative plan, and contingency options which may include cardiopulmonary bypass. Answer **A**, bolus intravenous propofol and succinylcholine followed by laryngoscopy and endotracheal intubation is contraindicated in patients with a mediastinal mass unless cardiopulmonary bypass has been instituted.

Clinical Pearls

- Anesthesia in patients with anterior mediastinal masses has been associated with airway obstruction and hemodynamic instability including cardiac arrest.
- Maintenance of spontaneous ventilation is the anesthetic goal whenever possible.
- Major life-threatening complications now occur more frequently postoperatively.

REFERENCE

Current Opinion in Anesthesiology. 2007;20:1-3.

Neurological/Neurosurgical Disorders

Case 28

A 51-year-old man with a tempero-parietal metastatic melanoma presents for left craniotomy and tumor excision. Over the past few days, he has experienced new-onset right upper extremity weakness and grand mal seizures. The patient's past medical history is significant for mild systemic hypertension, and melanoma on the right side of his neck. His past surgical history is significant for wide local excision and lymph node dissection of right side of his neck. His current medications include atenolol 25 mg once a day, prednisone 20 mg tid, and dilantin 100 mg tid. The patient's lab test results are normal. His hemoglobin is 14 g%, platelet count is 140,000, and his INR is 1.0. Serum electrolytes are within normal limits. His ECG is normal with sinus rhythm of 66 bpm. CT scan shows a 3 4 cm lesion in the left tempero-parietal cortex with edema around the tumor, and a 2-mm midline shift.

- ➤ What preoperative information is especially useful for the anesthesiologist regarding patients undergoing a craniotomy?
- ➤ How can intracranial pressure (ICP) be reduced?
- ➤ Why are patients observed in an ICU setting postoperatively, and what are the implications of a new abnormal finding?

ANSWERS TO CASE 28:
Craniotomy for Brain Mass Excision

Summary: A 51-year-old man presents with metastatic melanoma, a 2-mm midline shift, and the new onset of a motor deficit.

- **Preoperative information:** In addition to the usual pre-anesthetic assessment, the preoperative assessment for a patient with a space occupying lesion (SOL) includes knowledge of the size and site of lesion and its vascularity, and whether the patient has any neurological deficits, and if so, whether they are stable or worsening in intensity. Any symptoms of an elevated ICP and/or impending herniation warrant special attention.
- **Ways to reduce intracranial pressure:** The anesthetic is designed to actively reduce and avoid any further increases in ICP, and to maintain cerebral perfusion. The elevation of ICP can worsen the cerebral edema, the midline shift, and ultimately, the neurological deficit. Increases in ICP are minimized by ensuring an adequate depth of anesthesia for painful parts of the case such as the application of head pins. ICP can be reduced by moderate hyperventilation, mannitol, and/or furosemide.
- **Reason for observation in ICU postoperatively:** Postoperatively, the strict control of blood pressure and periodic assessment of mental status and motor function are essential. Any acute deterioration in mental status or a new deficit suggests worsening cerebral edema or an intracranial bleed and requires an immediate intervention such as a CT scan or MRI.

ANALYSIS

Objectives

1. Learn the elements of a preoperative evaluation specific for patients with a SOL.
2. Become familiar with the relationship between arterial pressure, intracranial pressure, and cerebral perfusion pressure.
3. Understand the factors that influence intracranial pressure (ICP), and the methods to control ICP.
4. Understand the effects of anesthetic agents on ICP and cerebral metabolic rate for oxygen ($CMRO_2$).
5. Be able to describe an anesthetic plan for craniotomy.

Considerations

This patient has a SOL with a midline shift and new onset of a neurological deficit. He is receiving medical management for the cerebral edema and elevated

ICP. The preoperative assessment of this patient includes knowledge of the size and site of lesion and its vascularity. This information can be obtained by physical examination and evaluating the radiological images and medical record.

The goal of the anesthetic is to avoid any further increase in ICP. Further increases in ICP can worsen the cerebral edema and midline shift, and contribute to worsening of the neurologic deficit. Invasive blood pressure monitoring is required. However, in this case, the elevation of ICP is not severe enough to require intraoperative ICP monitoring.

General anesthesia is induced with thiopental or propofol, and muscle relaxation can be achieved with vecuronium. After endotracheal intubation, anesthesia is maintained with nitrous oxide/oxygen and low concentrations of an inhalational agent. A nicardipine infusion is used to treat hypertension, and fentanyl is administered for pain control.

The anesthetic technique is also designed to actively reduce ICP and maintain cerebral perfusion. The careful control of blood pressure, moderate hyperventilation, and use of diuretics such as furosemide and mannitol help to reduce the ICP. To minimize bleeding at the surgical site, the patient is extubated with minimal coughing and bucking, and strict control of blood pressure is maintained during emergence.

This patient will be monitored postoperatively in an intensive care setting to ensure the strict control of blood pressure and periodic assessment of mental status and motor function. Any acute deterioration in mental status or a new onset neurodeficit suggests a worsening of the cerebral edema or an intracranial bleed and must be addressed immediately.

APPROACH TO Craniotomy for Brain Mass Excision

DEFINITIONS

ICP: Normal ICP is 5 to 15 mm Hg and reflects the relationship between the rigid cranial vault and its contents; that is, the brain, blood, and the CSF. Sustained ICP of 15 to 20 mm Hg is considered elevated ICP.

CEREBRAL COMPLIANCE: When intracranial volume increases such as with a SOL, one of the other components (eg, CSF) is initially displaced, and ICP remains relatively normal. But as these "buffering mechanisms" are exhausted and intracranial volume continues to increase, intracranial pressure then increases as well potentially resulting in brainstem herniation (Figure 28–1).

CEREBRAL AUTOREGULATION: Autoregulation maintains a constant level of cerebral blood flow (CBF) over a wide range of mean arterial pressures. Autoregulation is impaired by cerebral edema, brain injury, and inhaled

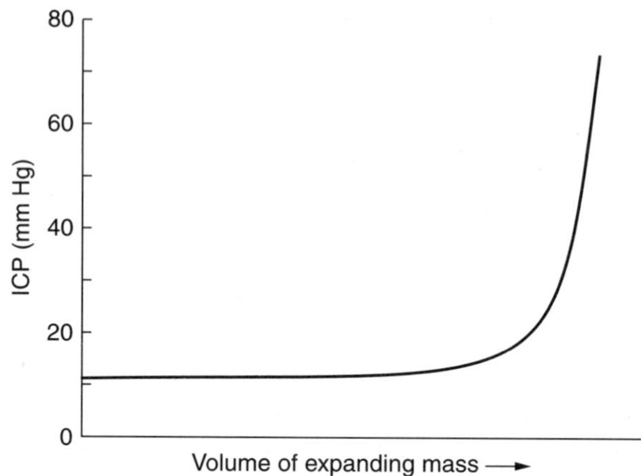

Figure 28–1. Pressure-volume compliance curve.

anesthetics. The autoregulatory curve is shifted to the right in patients with systemic hypertension. (Figure 28–2). Hypercarbia and hypoxia can increase cerebral blood flow irrespective of autoregulation.

CEREBRAL PERFUSION PRESSURE (CPP): It is the net pressure gradient between the force facilitating brain-blood flow (mean arterial pressure) and

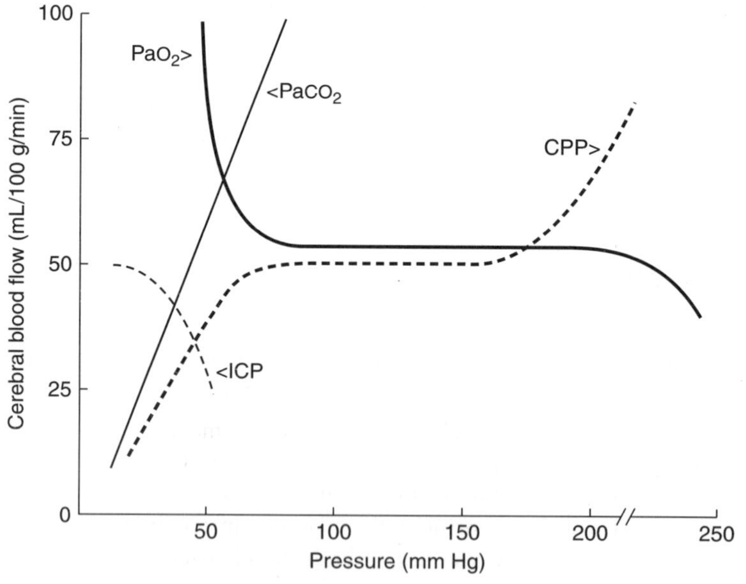

Figure 28–2. Effect of Pao_2 and $Paco_2$ on CPP and ICP.

the force impeding flow (ICP). Cerebral perfusion pressure is directly related to cerebral blood flow. CPP must be maintained within narrow limits, because too little pressure could cause brain tissue to become ischemic or too much could raise intracranial pressure (ICP). CPP is normally between 70 and 90 mm Hg in an adult human, and should not fall below 70 mm Hg for a sustained period. Some authorities, however, regard a CPP between 50 to 150 mm Hg to be within the normal range for adults since this approximates the range of autoregulation in the normal brain.

Cerebral blood flow is approximately 50 mL/100 g of brain tissue/min. It remains fairly constant over a wide range of pressures, due to autoregulation. However, outside the bounds of autoregulation, cerebral blood flow changes according to the cerebral perfusion pressure.

$CMRO_2$: Cerebral metabolic rate for oxygen is coupled with CBF. When the metabolic rate in a particular region increases, CBF to that region will also increase. Increase in $CMRO_2$ increases CBF globally. Factors that increase $CMRO_2$ are hyperthermia, seizures, and some anesthetic agents. Some inhalational agents can cause uncoupling of CBF and $CMRO_2$, that is, though they do reduce the $CMRO_2$, the CBF remains unchanged or is even increased by cerebral vasodilatation.

CLINICAL APPROACH

The SOL may cause seizures and other neurologic deficits, depending on its size and location. Often, the normal physiologic mechanisms which offset day-to-day increases in intracranial volume, such as displacing cerebrospinal fluid from the brain, will have been exhausted. Thus, patients with SOLs have a reduced intracranial compliance, meaning that even small increases in intracranial volume result in large increases in ICP. As ICP increases, the level of consciousness may be compromised, and the brain's anatomy distorted. Pressure on the brainstem can lead to herniation of the brainstem and death.

Preoperative Evaluation

In addition to the usual preoperative evaluation, patients with brain tumors warrant special examination of their neurological status. Neurological deficits may be new in onset, and/or changing. Clinical signs and symptoms of an elevated ICP are headache, vomiting, blurred vision, somnolence, and papilledema. The signs of impending brain herniation include bradyarrhythmia, hypertension, ipsilateral fixed dilated pupil (from oculomotor and abducent nerve palsy), and contralateral hemiparesis or hemiplegia.

A review of the patient's CT scan or MRI is invaluable. It gives an idea of the size and position of the tumor, the extent of cerebral edema, and the possible presence of a midline shift signaling a significantly elevated ICP. The size of the tumor, and proximity to dural venous sinuses can give an idea of possible intraoperative blood loss. Cross-matched blood should be available in the blood bank.

Management of Elevated ICP

The following strategies can be used to lower ICP:

a. **Reduction of cerebral blood volume**: Hypercarbia and hypoxia profoundly increase cerebral blood volume. So proper airway management is crucial in patients with altered intracranial compliance. Hyperventilation to a moderate hypocarbia of a $PaCO_2$ of 25 to 30 mm Hg produces cerebral vasoconstriction and is very useful in acute reduction of elevated ICP. Excessive hyperventilation should be avoided, since it can cause cerebral vasoconstriction in areas of the brain where blood flow is already compromised by cerebral edema. Hypoxia causes cerebral vasodilatation, and thus an increase in ICP. Again, meticulous attention to control of the airway and ventilation is essential. Venous drainage is facilitated by head elevation and avoiding high intrathoracic pressures.

b. **Reduction in brain tissue volume** is accomplished by diuretics and steroids. Mannitol is an osmotic diuretic administered in the dose of 0.5 to 2 g/kg body weight. It increases the serum osmolality (305-320 mOsm/L) and thus removes the excess water from the brain. Mannitol increases blood volume acutely, and can thus precipitate volume overload and even heart failure in susceptible individuals.

   Furosemide is a loop diuretic which is very effective in reducing ICP alone or when used in combination with mannitol. Furosemide reduces blood volume as well as CSF production.

   Steroids appear to be helpful in reducing the edema surrounding a SOL. They are ineffective in reducing edema due to hypoxia or hypercarbia.

c. **A reduction of CSF** can be achieved by surgical placement of a ventriculostomy catheter or a lumbar drain.

Anesthetic Management

It is ideal to have two large-bore peripheral venous accesses and an arterial line. A central line or pulmonary artery catheter is indicated based on the coexisting medical conditions, and is not an absolute requirement for supratentorial craniotomies. Excessive sedation from premedications can cause hypercarbia and hypoxia, thus elevating the ICP. Therefore, sedative premedication should be used with caution or avoided all together in patients with elevated ICP. Normal saline is the ideal maintenance fluid. Hypotonic solutions such as Ringer lactate and dextrose containing solutions should be avoided.

Routine intraoperative monitoring and invasive monitoring of arterial pressure is utilized for craniotomies. Central venous pressure monitoring is not routine, and indeed, may either expose the patient to an unnecessary risk of pneumothorax, or impede venous drainage from the neck. Moreover, placing a patient with altered intracranial compliance in Trendelenburg for line placement could also cause a dangerous increase in ICP. The one situation where a central venous catheter is indicated is during craniotomies in the sitting position, where the head is higher than the heart. In this position, there is a risk of venous air embolism potentially necessitating the aspiration of air through a central venous catheter to prevent its entry into the pulmonary circulation. The risk of venous air embolism is relatively low with supratentorial tumors, provided the tumor is not adhered to large dural venous sinuses.

Induction is typically performed with sodium thiopental, since thiopental reduces $CMRO_2$. However, propofol and etomidate are also suitable for induction. Ketamine should not be used as it increases ICP and $CMRO_2$. Following induction, hyperventilation is established to avoid hypercarbia. Either depolarizing or (more commonly) nondepolarizing muscle relaxants are used to obtain relaxation for intubation. Succinylcholine does minimally increase ICP, but when administered after an induction agent, this elevation does not appear to be clinically significant. Succinylcholine should be avoided in patients with motor deficit because of the risk of hyperkalemia from neuronal depolarization.

Narcotics do not directly affect ICP unless patients are breathing spontaneously, and they are quite useful to help blunt the response to laryngoscopy and intubation. Blunting this response is one of the crucial goals of induction, since patients with a SOL may already have a reduced intracranial compliance, and increases in arterial pressure can further increase ICP. The events that cause most intense pressor response are laryngoscopy and intubation, the placement of pins (which hold the head), the skin incision, and stimulation of the periosteum. Fentanyl, lidocaine, additional doses of the induction agent, and moderate hypocarbia aid in avoiding any rapid increases in cerebral blood flow which may result. Remifentanil, an ultrashort-acting opioid, can be also used as an infusion from induction to extubation. Long-acting opioids are best avoided. Before the dura is opened, it is essential to optimize operating conditions and to avoid a "tight" or "full" brain from cerebral edema, or an excess of cerebral blood flow. This can be accomplished by moderate hyperventilation in combination with the administration of mannitol, furosemide, and steroids.

Low concentrations of a potent inhalational agent can be added to an oxygen/nitrous oxide mixture for maintenance of anesthesia. Though nitrous oxide reduces the concentration of inhalational agents required to maintain anesthesia, recent evidence, though controversial, suggests that it increases $CMRO_2$, though this effect is blocked by hyperventilation. On the other hand, inhalational agents attenuate autoregulation, and in high concentrations increase cerebral blood flow. Ideally, after establishing moderate hypocarbia a low dose of an inhalational agent or propofol infusion are used to maintain anesthesia. Muscle relaxation and moderate hyperventilation to an end-tidal CO_2 concentration of 25 to 30 is continued during the craniotomy.

Hyperglycemia increases intracellular acidosis and facilitates cell ischemia. Therefore, hyperglycemia should be treated aggressively with insulin as required, and glucose-containing solutions should be avoided. Steroids can also contribute to hyperglycemia.

Elevations in blood pressure can cause an intracranial bleed at the surgical site requiring re-exploration. At the time of extubation, hypertension, coughing, and straining are to be avoided at all costs. Intravenous lidocaine has been used to prevent the stress responses to extubation. A short-acting opiate, such as remifentanil, can suppress the cough response and facilitates a smooth wakeup. In addition, autoregulation is impaired in areas with cerebral edema. Therefore, blood pressure is carefully controlled, the head elevated, and the patient is extubated awake.

Patients post craniotomy are monitored overnight in an intensive care setting. Periodic assessment of mental status and motor function is essential to detect any changes in neurological status, and blood pressure is meticulously controlled in the immediate postoperative period. Any acute deterioration in mental status, or a new onset neurologic deficit suggests worsening cerebral edema or an intracranial bleed and requires an immediate intervention including urgent CT scan and possible repeat craniotomy to evacuate an hematoma.

Special Considerations for a Posterior Fossa Craniotomy

Posterior fossa tumors present a special challenge. The tumors can compress the cerebellum, the lower cranial nerves, and the vasomotor and respiratory centers. Involvement of the lower cranial nerves, the glossopharyngeal and vagus can cause vasomotor instability. Indeed, surgical dissections in this area can be associated with arrhythmias and alterations in vasomotor tone. Damage to the glossopharyngeal nerve can impair gag reflex and impair a patient's ability to protect his airway. Prior to extubation, the ability to protect airway and adequacy of spontaneous breathing should be established.

The sitting position is sometimes required to access a SOL in the posterior fossa, such as an acoustic neuroma. The risk of venous air embolism is significant in sitting position, since the subdural venous pressure is much lower than the atmospheric pressure. These patients often benefit from a precordial Doppler or even a transesophageal echocardiogram as an additional monitor to detect the occurrence and/or severity of a venous air embolism (VAE). Intravascular air is suggested by sudden hemodynamic instability, or a sudden drop in the end-tidal carbon dioxide concentration. These patients benefit from placement of a multiorifice central lumen catheter, which may be used to aspirate venous air from the right atrium. As the sitting position is fraught with risks, modified supine position or prone position is preferable when possible.

Comprehension Questions

28.1. Which of the following factors increase cerebral blood flow?
  A. Hypocarbia
  B. Hyperoxia
  C. Hypercarbia
  D. Thiopental sodium

28.2. Methods to reduce an elevated ICP include which of the following?
  A. Mannitol and furosemide
  B. Hypoventilation
  C. Positioning in Trendelenburg
  D. Transfusion to increase hemoglobin-carrying capacity

28.3. Which of the following statements regarding cerebral autoregulation is accurate?
  A. In the presence of intact autoregulation, hypercarbia cannot increase cerebral blood flow.
  B. Succinylcholine impairs autoregulation.
  C. Cerebral autoregulation can be impaired in the presence of cerebral edema or extreme hypoxia.
  D. Cerebral autoregulation in a patient with long-standing systemic hypertension is no different from a normotensive individual.

ANSWERS

28.1. **C.** Hypercarbia and hypoxia increase cerebral blood flow. Hypocarbia and thiopental sodium reduce cerebral blood flow.

28.2. **A.** The head up positioning, hyperventilation to mild hypocarbia, the administration of mannitol and furosemide, and placement of a ventriculostomy or lumbar drain help in reducing elevated intracranial pressure.

28.3. **C.** Autoregulation can be impaired by cerebral edema, severe hypoxia, and long-standing systemic hypertension. In a patient with long-standing hypertension, the autoregulatory curve is shifted to the right so the mean arterial pressure needs to be higher to maintain adequate cerebral perfusion. Hypercarbia can increase cerebral blood flow even in the presence of intact autoregulation.

Clinical Pearls

- The preoperative evaluation of a patient for craniotomy should include knowledge of the size, location, vascularity, and nature of the SOL as this can influence positioning of the patient, surgical blood loss, and line placement.
- Intracranial pressure is dynamically influenced by blood pressure, $Paco_2$, and most anesthetics.
- Elevated ICP can be reduced by head elevation to 30 degrees in combination with diuretics, that is, furosemide and mannitol, moderate hyperventilation, reducing the mean arterial pressure, and in some cases by drainage of CSF.
- The goal of anesthesia for craniotomy is to maintain cerebral perfusion, reduce $CMRO_2$, preserve blood flow and hence oxygenation to "at-risk areas," and to optimize operating conditions.

REFERENCES

Cunningham AJ, Hourihan D. The sitting position in neurosurgery-unresolved hemodynamic consequences. *Can J Anesth.* 2007;54(7):497-500.

Dinsmore J. Anesthesia for elective neurosurgery. *Br J Anaesth.* 2007;99(1):68-74. Review.

Harvey M. Shapiro and John C. Drummond; Neurosurgical Anesthesia; R.D Miller Anesthesia, volume 2, 1994, NewYork: Harvey Livingstone

Pasternak JJ, Lanier WL. *J Neurosurg Anesthesiol.* 2008;20(2):78-104.

Case 29

A 76-year-old woman suffers a fall at home. She appears uninjured, but the next day becomes progressively forgetful, drowsy, and disoriented, so she is taken to the emergency room (ER) for evaluation. According to her family, the patient's only medical problem is chronic atrial fibrillation, for which she takes warfarin. Her review of symptoms is otherwise reportedly normal.

On physical examination, the patient's blood pressure is 180/110 mm Hg, HR 90 bpm, and respirations 12 breaths per minute. She opens her eyes to painful stimuli, but will neither communicate nor cooperate with a neurological examination. A CT scan of the head reveals an acute subdural hematoma (SDH), with a midline shift of 6 mm. Laboratory studies show a hematocrit of 32 and an INR of 4.3. Her ECG shows diffuse, deep, symmetrical T-wave inversions. An urgent neurosurgical consult is obtained and the patient is emergently taken to the OR for a craniotomy to evacuate the hematoma.

- ➤ What is the most important priority for an anesthesiologist in a patient with an acute subdural hematoma who has rapidly-deteriorating neurological signs?
- ➤ How should the above patient be evaluated preoperatively?
- ➤ What are the anesthetic goals for patients presenting for an evacuation of a subdural hematoma?

ANSWERS TO CASE 29:
Subdural Hematoma

Summary: This elderly, anticoagulated patient presents with an acute subdural hematoma following a fall.

- **Most important priority:** To promptly provide conditions suitable for an evacuation of the hematoma. This consideration supersedes almost all others.
- **Preoperative evaluation:** In the acute setting, there is little time to conduct a formal pre-anesthetic assessment. Moreover, the patient may not be capable of responding to questions. Knowledge of any allergies to medications, pre-existing medical conditions (which may need to be obtained from the patient's family), the circumstances of his or her injury, and a quick airway assessment may well be all that time allows.
- **Anesthetic goals:** In addition to the goals for any type of anesthetic (to maintain stability of the vital functions, provide an insensitivity to pain, prevent awareness, and optimize the surgical field), the anesthetic goals for evacuation of a subdural hematoma are to maintain adequate cerebral perfusion pressure, and to prevent or attenuate increases in ICP and cerebral edema throughout the perioperative period.

ANALYSIS

Objectives

1. Understand the etiology of subdural hemorrhage, and the characteristics of the patients most at risk.
2. Become familiar with the Glasgow coma scale and its impact on the decision for surgery.
3. Understand the concept of autoregulation, how it can be altered, and the consequences of doing so.
4. Become acquainted with the challenges of emergence following a neurosurgical procedure, and its associated risks.

Considerations

Since this patient requires emergent evacuation of the SDH, as described earlier, the preoperative assessment is abbreviated to the few questions that are absolutely necessary, and these are often asked and answered as an intravenous catheter and monitors are placed.

A quick assessment of her **"ABCs"** allows the rapid formulation of an appropriate anesthetic plan. **"Airway"** examines the potential for difficult airway management or intubation. **"Breathing"** assesses her ventilatory status

Table 29–1 GLASGOW COMA SCALE. MILD HEAD INJURY = 13-15; MODERATE 9-12; SEVERE ≤ 8

PARAMETERS	RESPONSE	SCORE
Eye opening	Spontaneously	4
	To verbal command	3
	To pain	2
	None	1
Best verbal response	Oriented, conversing	5
	Disoriented, conversing	4
	Inappropriate words	3
	Incomprehensible sounds	2
	No verbal response	1
Best motor response	Obeys verbal commands	6
	Localizes to pain	5
	Flexion/withdrawal	4
	Abnormal flexion decorticate	3
	Extension (decerebrate)	2
	No response (flaccid)	1

and oxygenation, and **"circulation"** examines her hemodynamic stability. The patient's neurological status is also categorized using the Glasgow coma scale (please see Table 29–1).

This patient requires general anesthesia with an endotracheal tube, a large bore intravenous access for aggressive fluid resuscitation, and the availability of blood products. Fresh frozen plasma and vitamin K are indicated to reverse the coagulopathy as soon as possible.

No premedication is indicated given the patient's depressed level of consciousness. Monitoring includes standard monitors (5-lead ECG, pulse oximetry, capnography, noninvasive blood pressure monitoring), urine output, body temperature, and train-of-four.

An intra-arterial blood pressure catheter is ideal, but given the acuity of the patient's neurological status, a prompt induction to allow rapid evacuation of the hematoma may take precedence. Induction is accomplished with propofol, thiopental, or etomidate. Etomidate is preferable, since significant hypotension may follow administration of the former two. In this patient with severe arterial hypertension likely reflecting a high ICP, any significant reduction in arterial pressure would rapidly reduce cerebral perfusion and thus lead to cerebral ischemia.

Paralysis is achieved with a nondepolarizing muscle relaxant, and the anesthetic is maintained with an opioid and an inhalation agent as tolerated. Postoperatively, she will most likely be kept intubated and will receive positive pressure ventilation in an intensive care unit.

APPROACH TO
Subdural Hematoma

DEFINITIONS

SUBDURAL HEMATOMA (SDH): An accumulation of blood in the subdural space between the dural and arachnoid layers of the meninges. This condition primarily occurs over the surface of a cerebral hemisphere, but may develop in the posterior fossa and spinal canal. SDH may be acute or chronic.

ACUTE SUBDURAL HEMATOMA (ACUTE SDH): Is usually caused by tearing of the bridging veins that drain from the surface of the brain to the dural sinuses. Rupture of these vessels allows for bleeding into the space between the arachnoid membranes and dura. Venous bleeding is usually arrested by the rising intracranial pressure or direct compression by the clot itself. Trauma to the cortical arteries accounts for approximately 20% to 30% of SDH cases.

GLASGOW COMA SCALE: Quantifies neurological impairment in the setting of head injury in terms of eye opening, speech, and motor function. The maximum score that can be obtained is 15, and severe head injury is determined by a score of 8 or less persisting for 6 hours or more. The numerical points assigned to patients in the Glasgow coma scale are illustrated in Table 29–1. An indication for ICP monitoring is an acute SDH with GCS score less than 9.

CEREBRAL PERFUSION PRESSURE (CPP): Is the net pressure gradient causing blood flow to the brain (brain perfusion). CPP is calculated as the difference between mean arterial pressure (MAP) and intracranial pressure (ICP).

$$\text{Cerebral Perfusion Pressure (CPP)} = \text{MAP} \quad \text{ICP or CVP}$$
$$\text{(whichever is higher)}$$

CEREBRAL AUTOREGULATION: Is a protective mechanism that maintains cerebral blood flow between mean arterial pressures (MAP) of 50 and 150 mm Hg by adjusting cerebral vascular resistance. Hypertensive patients demonstrate a shift of autoregulation to a higher blood pressure. Thus, their lower level of autoregulation could be well above 50 mm Hg, and their upper limit of autoregulation similarly increased.

Autoregulation can be abolished by trauma, hypoxia, and certain anesthetics. When blood pressure falls below the autoregulated range, cerebral ischemia can occur. When blood pressure exceeds the autoregulated range, cerebral blood flow increases markedly, thus rapidly increasing ICP, potentially disrupting the blood-brain barrier, and even causing cerebral edema. Similarly, severe intracranial hypertension can actually precipitate reflex arterial hypertension and bradycardia (Cushing triad). A rapid reduction in systemic blood pressure in these patients may precipitate cerebral ischemia by reducing cerebral perfusion pressure.

CLINICAL APPROACH

A SDH is considered acute if the patient becomes symptomatic within 72 hours of an insult or injury, subacute between 3 and 15 days, and chronic after 2 weeks. The neurological findings associated with an acute SDH may include an altered level of consciousness, a dilated or nonreactive pupil ipsilateral to the hematoma, and/or hemiparesis contralateral to the hematoma. An acute SDH typically requires a craniotomy for evacuation of the clot and decompression of the brain, while burr holes can be used to achieve the same for chronic SDH. Both subacute and chronic SDHs are usually observed in patients over 50 years of age.

Head trauma is the most common cause of SDH, with the majority of cases resulting from motor vehicle accidents, falls, and assaults. Patients with significant cerebral atrophy are particularly at risk. This category includes the elderly, those with a history of chronic alcohol abuse, and those with previous traumatic brain injury. In such patients, trivial head trauma or even whiplash injury in the absence of physical impact may produce a SDH. Similarly, the use of antithrombotic agents also increases the risk of SDH. In one series, treatment with oral anticoagulants, aspirin, or heparin at the time of hemorrhage was present in 21%, 13%, and 5% of patients with chronic SDH following head trauma.

The estimated mortality rate for patients requiring surgery for SDH is 40% to 60%. In patients who present with coma, the mortality rate approaches the higher end of that range. Age and neurological status as assessed with the Glasgow coma scale are also important prognostic indicators for patients with SDH.

The indications for surgical evacuation of SDH are:

1. SDH thickness > 10 mm, or midline shift > 5 mm on CT regardless of the GCS score
2. When SDH thickness < 10 mm or midline shift < 5 mm
   a. If the GCS starts at < 9 and deteriorates by 2 points or more
   b. Pupils are asymmetric or fixed and dilated
   c. ICP > 20 mm of Hg

Anesthetic Management of Emergent Craniotomy for Acute SDH

The principal goals of the anesthetic management for a patient with SDH are the preservation of adequate cerebral perfusion pressure and oxygen delivery, the avoidance of secondary brain damage, and the provision of optimal operating conditions.

One of the major concerns is the maintenance or reduction of ICP, particularly in the preoperative period and during induction. The volume inside the cranium is fixed, so if any of the components located in the cranial vault increase in volume, others must decrease or the ICP will increase. When the cranium is open, ICP equals atmospheric pressure, and cerebral perfusion pressure thus equals MAP. Cerebral perfusion pressure should be maintained at a minimum or 60 and 100 mm Hg systolic to prevent secondary ischemic damage.

Table 29–2 SUMMARY OF THE SPECIFIC EFFECTS OF INDIVIDUAL DRUGS ON CEREBRAL VASOMOTOR TONE AND CMR

DRUG	CBF	$CMRO_2$	ICP
Volatile anesthetics			
Isoflurane	↑/↑↑	↓↓↓	↑
Sevoflurane	No effect/↓	↓↓↓	No effect/↑
Desflurane	↑/↑↑	↓↓↓	No effect/↑
N_2O	↑/↑↑	↑/↑↑	↑/↑↑
IV anesthetics			
Barbiturates	↓↓/↓↓↓	↓↓↓	↓↓/↓↓↓
Etomidate	↓↓/↓↓↓		↓↓/↓↓↓
Propofol	↓↓/↓↓↓	↓↓↓	↓↓/↓↓↓
Benzodiazepines	↓/↓↓		No effect/↓
Opioids	No effect/ ↓	↓↓↓	No effect/↑
		↓/↓	
		No effect/↓	

The specific effects of individual drugs on cerebral vasomotor tone and cerebral metabolic rate are summarized in Table 29–2. Ensuring an adequate depth of anesthesia, controlling blood pressure to avoid hypertensive crises, maintaining cerebral perfusion, and striving for a physiological ICP are more important than the choice of any particular anesthetic drug.

The changes in CBF caused by anesthetic drugs reflect the drug's individual effects on cerebral vasomotor tone and metabolic rate. In the normal brain, a reduction in cerebral metabolic rate causes cerebral vasoconstriction and reduces CBF, counteracting the vasodilatory effect of the drug. Cerebral vasomotor tone and metabolic rate can be affected to a different extent at different concentrations. Consequently, despite the direct cerebral vasodilatory effects of volatile anesthetics, CBF remains relatively unchanged at concentrations of up to 1 MAC.

However, in patients with an acute brain injury and particularly in the presence of an increased ICP, it is advisable to avoid all anesthetic drugs that dilate cerebral vessels (ie, volatile anesthetics). Instead, agents causing vasoconstriction are preferred (ie, intravenous anesthetics except ketamine).

In the presence of an elevated ICP, thiopental is most commonly used to induce anesthesia, if the patient can tolerate the hypotension that may result. Alternative agents such as propofol or etomidate are also acceptable. In addition, lidocaine is often administered intravenously 90 seconds prior to intubation to suppress laryngeal reflexes, and esmolol may be used to reduce heart rate and blood pressure in response to laryngoscopy.

For paralysis, the possible benefits of a short-acting muscle relaxant (succinylcholine) must be weighed against the risks. Succinylcholine can transiently and modestly increase ICP, an effect which is attenuated by pretreatment with a nondepolarizer. However nondepolarizing muscle relaxants are often preferred instead.

A popular maintenance regimen for neurosurgical patients is a continuous infusion of propofol with remifentanil or fentanyl. In a hemodynamically stable patient with severe intracranial hypertension, narcotics in conjunction with a thiopental infusion (2-3 mg/kg/h) and a nondepolarizing muscle relaxant are sometimes administered with oxygen and air. However, the sedative effects of barbiturates or benzodiazepines can cause postoperative sedation, and thus impede a patient's ability to cooperate with a neurological examination. In patients with less severe intracranial hypertension, anesthesia is typically maintained with various combinations of barbiturates, narcotics, and sub-MAC concentrations of a volatile anesthetic.

Cerebral Blood Flow and $Paco_2$

Increasing arterial carbon dioxide levels cause vasodilation and an increase in cerebral blood flow. As a good rule of thumb, increasing the carbon dioxide tension from 40 to 80 mm Hg doubles cerebral blood flow; reducing the carbon dioxide from 40 to 20 mm Hg halves it. These changes are transient, and cerebral blood flow returns to normal within 6 to 8 hours even if the altered carbon dioxide levels are maintained. After induction of anesthesia, in the presence of a subarachnoid hemorrhage (SAH) care must be taken to maintain a normal $PaCO_2$. If a reduction in ICP is desired, only transient and moderate hyperventilation should be considered.

Fluid Management

The two most important principles of fluid management in the neurosurgical patient are to avoid any reductions in serum osmolality to prevent cerebral edema (ie, "keep 'em dry"), but to remember to treat the "whole" patient, and not just the patient's brain. Traumatic head injuries may be associated with other types of traumatic injuries, particularly injuries of the chest, and may be signaled by an ongoing fluid requirement.

The patient should be normovolemic, and serum osmolality normal or slightly elevated to minimize cerebral edema. Hypovolemia is associated with cerebral ischemia and perioperative neurological deficits, especially in patients with cerebral vasospasm. Dextrose containing solutions should be avoided because glucose administration increased the incidence of neurologic deficits in experimental models. Infusing large volumes of hypo-osmolar crystalloid solutions such as lactated Ringer solution may predispose to brain edema and contribute to hyponatremia. Therefore, the use of normal saline is preferable.

Central venous pressure (CVP) catheter placement can help to guide intravascular volume status, but is not the priority. Cannulation of the internal jugular vein requires the Trendelenburg position and turning of the head, both of which can critically increase ICP. A large catheter in the internal jugular vein can also impede venous drainage from the head. Patients presenting with an acute SAH are frequently coagulopathic, another relative contraindication to central venous cannulation. Most importantly, the priority is to evacuate the hematoma, and this consideration supersedes almost all others.

Serum sodium is maintained within normal limits, to help maintain serum oncotic pressure and to avoid the hyponatremia associated with cerebral salt wasting and the syndrome of inappropriate secretion of the antidiuretic hormone (SIADH). Hypertonic saline solutions can be useful for volume resuscitation because they lower ICP, increase blood pressure, and produce an osmotic diuretic effect on the brain similar to that of other hyperosmolar solutions, such as, mannitol. However, studies have shown that marked hypernatremia can result from the combination of hypertonic saline and mannitol.

Blood loss during surgery requires transfusion of cross-matched or fresh whole blood. A minimum hematocrit between 30% and 33% is recommended to maximize oxygen transport.

Brain "Relaxation" and Bulk

When the dura is opened, the brain readily demonstrates the suitability of operating conditions. On one hand, it may be bulging, almost pulsating, and appear "tense," as though it is under pressure (of course, as previously mentioned, the intracranial pressure at that time equals atmospheric pressure). On the other hand, the brain may appear "relaxed," generally indicating an absence of the signs associated with the "full" or "tense" brain.

If the brain appears "tense," the methods for reducing brain volume include hyperventilation to decrease cerebral blood flow, diuresis (usually mannitol, Lasix or hypertonic saline), the drainage of cerebrospinal fluid (by ventriculostomy or more frequently a lumbar drain), and reducing MAP (if autonomic dysregulation is present), and less frequently, suppression of the cerebral metabolic rate which also reduces cerebral blood flow (usually with barbiturates).

Emergence from Anesthesia and Surgery

Extubation is a perilous time for patients who have just undergone neurosurgery. Studies have shown the relationship between perioperative hypertension and the development of postoperative hematomas. Yet patients must also be sufficiently awake and oriented so that a neurological examination can be performed. The trick is to provide a rapid and smooth transition from the anesthetized state to being fully awake.

One significant challenge is the patient's response to the large foreign body in his trachea, namely the endotracheal tube. "Bucking" or coughing on the endotracheal tube can cause arterial hypertension and elevated ICP. Precautions to avoid coughing, straining, hypercarbia, and large swings in blood pressure include lidocaine administered before extubation, beta blockers to control blood pressure, and other antihypertensives if needed during emergence. The patient's head should be elevated by 15 to 30 degrees, but with consideration to the fact that this position increases the likelihood of aspiration.

Monitoring and Management of Intracranial Hypertension

Following the removal of an intracranial hematoma, the control of ICP is of paramount importance in the patient's recovery. It is common practice to monitor ICP in the postoperative period in these patients, since those with ICPs below 20 to 25 mm Hg tend to have significantly better outcomes than patients with elevated ICP. Various techniques are used to measure ICP including ventricular catheters, subdural and subarachnoid bolts, epidural transducers, and intraparenchymal fiberoptic devices. Table 29–3 outlines the commonly used measures to control intracranial hypertension.

Systemic Sequelae of Head Injury

In addition to the potentially devastating effects on brain tissue, the systemic effects of head injury are diverse. Many (maybe even most) patients manifest ECG changes in their ST segments and T waves following traumatic brain injury. Head injury can also result in autonomic dysfunction, even life-threatening arrhythmias. Pulmonary problems can include airway obstruction, hypoxemia, adult respiratory distress syndrome, and neurogenic pulmonary edema. Gastrointestinal problems including stress ulcers are common, and may lead to hemorrhage. Pituitary dysfunction as evidenced by diabetes insipidus, SIADH, salt wasting, and metabolic problems such as ketotic hyperosmolar syndrome and/or hyperglycemic coma, and abnormalities of temperature regulation may also occur.

But one of the most important points to remember when caring for patients with head injury is that *whatever injured the head may have also injured other parts of the body*.

Table 29–3 CLINICAL CONTROL OF INTRACRANIAL HYPERTENSION

Diuretics:	
Osmotic	Mannitol (0.25-1g/kg i.v.).
Loop	Furosemide (0.5-1mg/kg i.v. alone or 0.15-0.3 mg/kg i.v. in combination with mannitol).
Corticosteroids:	
Dexamethasone	Effective for localized cerebral edema; requires 12-36 hours for full effect
Adequate ventilation	PaO_2 ≥100 mm Hg, $PaCO_2$ 33-35 mm Hg; hyperventilation on demand.
Optimize hemodynamics	Target normotension and maintain CPP to avoid cerebral ischemia.
Fluid therapy	Target normovolemia before anesthetic induction to prevent hypotension. Use glucose free iso-osmolar crystalloid solutions to prevent increase in brain water content (from hypo-osmolality) and ischemic brain damage (from hyperglycemia).
Positioning	To improve venous return (neutral, head-up position).
Reduce $CMRO_2$	Using pharmacologic agents, eg, thiopental and propofol.
Temperature control	Avoid hyperthermia preoperatively, consider mild intraoperative hypothermia.
CSF drains	To acutely reduce brain tension.

Comprehension Questions

29.1. Which of the following is the most important indication for the surgical evacuation of a SDH?

A. A GCS score of 3
B. A recent history of fall accompanied by a change in mental status
C. Headache
D. GCS score of 10 that deteriorates to 6

29.2. Which of the following therapeutic maneuvers reduce ICP?

A. Hypotonic saline
B. An ICP drain
C. Isoflurane
D. Succinylcholine

29.3. In which of the following locations is an ICP monitor contraindicated?
A. Lumbar spinal drain
B. Subdural catheter
C. Ventriculostomy catheter
D. Intra-parenchymal catheter
E. Epidural catheter

ANSWERS

29.1. **D.** A deterioration of the GCS score or in pupillary signs are indications for surgery. A low GCS alone is not an indication for surgical evacuation of SDH. It is important to quantify any midline shift and thickness of the SDH by CT, and to measure ICP in order to triage this patient. A midline shift of 6 mm, a SDH thickness of 15 mm, a GCS score of 10 that deteriorates to 6, and an ICP of 25 mm of Hg are criteria for the evacuation of an SDH. A recent history of fall accompanied by a change in mental status may be suggestive of intracranial pathology, but in and of itself, does not indicate surgery.

29.2. **B.** Furosemide, an ICP drain, mannitol, and hypertonic saline are interventions which reduce ICP. Answer **C,** volatile anesthetics, may decrease $CMRO_2$, but they also cause a dissociation between $CMRO_2$ and CBF. Thus, their direct vasodilatory effect predominates and causes an increase in cerebral blood volume and ICP. Succinylcholine either has no effect on ICP, or reduces ICP in patients with altered intracranial compliance.

29.3. **A.** Lumbar drains are contraindicated for the same reason that spinal anesthesia is contraindicated in patients with elevated ICP: the danger of transforaminal herniation. All the other locations can be used for monitoring ICP.

Clinical Pearls

- The anesthetic goals for the evacuation of a subdural hematoma are to maintain adequate cerebral perfusion pressure, and to prevent or attenuate increases in ICP and cerebral edema throughout the perioperative period.
- While invasive arterial monitoring is desirable for anesthesia for a craniotomy, a rapidly deteriorating neurological status may take precedence.
- Traumatic head injuries may be associated with other types of traumatic injuries, particularly injuries of the chest.
- Severe intracranial hypertension can precipitate reflex arterial hypertension and bradycardia (Cushing triad). A rapid reduction in systemic blood pressure in these patients may precipitate cerebral ischemia by reducing cerebral perfusion pressure.

REFERENCES

Barash PG, Cullen BF. *Clinical Anesthesia*. 5th ed. Philadelphia, PA: Lippincott Williams & Wilkins; 2005.

Bullock MR, Chesnut R, Ghajar J, et al. Surgical management of acute subdural hematomas. *Neurosurgery*. 2006;58 (3 suppl):S16-S24; discussion si-iv.

Bullock R, Chesnut RM, Clifton G, et al. Guidelines for the management of severe head injury. Brain Trauma Foundation. *Eur Emerg Med*. 1996;3(2):109-127.

Cenic A, Bhandari M, Reddy K. Management of chronic subdural hematoma: A national survey and literature review. *Can J Neurol Sci*. 2005;32(4):501-506.

Ernestus RI, Beldzinski P, Lanfermann H, Klug N. Chronic subdural hematoma: Surgical treatment and outcome in 104 patients. *Surg Neurol*. 1997;48(3):220-225.

Gennarelli TA, Spielman GM, Langfitt TW, et al. Influence of the type of intracranial lesion on outcome from severe head injury. *J Neurosurg*. 1982;56:26.

Kotwica Z, Brzezinski J. Acute subdural haematoma in adults: An analysis of outcome in comatose patients. *Acta Neurochir (Wien)*. 1993;121:95.

Miller RD. *Miller's Anesthesia*. 6th ed. Philadelphia, PA: Elsevier Churchill Livingstone; 2005. 2-volume set.

Reymond MA, Marbet G, Radu EW, Gratzl O. Aspirin as a risk factor for hemorrhage in patients with head injuries. *Neurosurg Rev*. 1992;15:21.

Samudrala S, Cooper PR. Traumatic intracranial hematomas in neurosurgery. *Neurosurgery*. 1996;2797-2807.

Stanisic M, Lund-Johansen M, Mahesparan R. Treatment of chronic subdural hematoma by burr-hole craniostomy in adults: influence of some factors on post-operative recurrence. *Acta Neurochir (Wien)*. 2005 Dec;147(12):1249-56.

Weigel R, Krauss JK, Schmiedek P. Concepts of neurosurgical management of chronic subdural haematoma: Historical perspectives. *Br J Neurosurg*. 2004;18(1): 8-18.

Case 30

A 50-year-old woman presents for an elective ligation/clipping of an aneurysm at the bifurcation of the internal carotid artery. She recently presented to the emergency room with an unrelenting headache and neck pain. An evaluation of the headache included a CT scan and an MRI, which showed a 3-mm aneurismal dilatation at the bifurcation of the internal carotid artery and the posterior communicating artery at the circle of Willis. There was no evidence of subarachnoid hemorrhage.

The patient's past medical history is significant for systemic hypertension well controlled with atenolol. She has no known drug allergies. She has no focal neurologic deficits or cranial nerve involvement.

- ➤ What is necessary for the preoperative evaluation of this patient?
- ➤ What are the specific anesthetic goals for the clipping of an intracranial aneurysm?
- ➤ What is the management of intraoperative aneurysm rupture?
- ➤ What are the anesthetic implications of cerebral vasospasm?

ANSWERS TO CASE 30:
Anesthesia for Intracranial Aneurysm

Summary: A 50–year-old woman with a symptomatic 3-mm aneurysm of the bifurcation of the internal carotid artery presents for craniotomy and elective clipping of aneurysm.

- **Preoperative evaluation:** In a patient with an aneurysm, the evaluation includes the determination of the Hunt and Hess classification score in addition to the customary anesthesia preoperative examination. A higher score is associated with poorer preexisting neurological function, and a higher surgical risk. In addition, myocardial stress is a common occurrence after a subarachnoid bleed. Patients with preexisting heart disease need cardiac evaluation, if time permits. Remarkable ECG changes, particularly with the ST segments, occur in most patients following an intracranial bleed. These changes are associated with life-threatening arrhythmias, and a poor outcome. Autonomic dysfunction also frequently accompanies a subarachnoid hemorrhage.

- **Specific anesthetic goals for intracranial aneurismal surgery:** Carefully control systemic blood pressure to minimize the risk of intraoperative aneurysm rupture, to control intracranial pressure, and to provide optimal operating conditions.

- **Management of intraoperative aneurysm rupture:** Aneurysmal rupture can be catastrophic. The sudden, massive blood loss hinders the surgeon's ability to visualize and control the bleeding. While the overall goal is to maintain a normal blood pressure to ensure optimal collateral circulation, the rapid induction of hypotension, even to a pressure of 40 to 50 mm Hg for a short period, improves surgical visualization and can be lifesaving. A brief, manual compression of the ipsilateral carotid artery may also be helpful for this purpose. Blood transfusions may be needed to replace acute surgical blood loss.

- **Implications of cerebral vasospasm:** This is a major complication following aneurysm rupture. It usually occurs 5 to 9 days post hemorrhage. Hypotension should be avoided at this stage, since in the face of vasospasm, hypotension can be associated with reduced cerebral perfusion and a resultant neurologic deficit. Hypervolemia, hemodilution, and nimodipine, a calcium channel blocker, are used to treat cerebral vasospasm and to improve cerebral perfusion.

ANALYSIS

Objectives

1. Understand the elements of the preoperative evaluation for elective craniotomy for clipping of cerebral aneurysm, including the Hess and Hunt classification of cerebral aneurysms.
2. Discuss pharmacology of commonly used antihypertensives used for induced hypotension.
3. Briefly describe the anesthetic goals for clipping of cerebral aneurysm.
4. Know the management of intraoperative aneurysm rupture and of cerebral vasospasm.

Considerations

The preoperative evaluation of this 50-year-old patient should include an examination of the airway, the patient's mental status, and presence of any focal neurologic deficit. This patient has history of systemic hypertension, so a thorough cardiac evaluation is essential. A stress echocardiogram with radionuclide imaging provides a guide to whether the patient's myocardial blood supply is adequate to tolerate induced hypotension which is often required for aneurysm clipping. Assessment should include laboratory tests including complete blood count, coagulation profile, chemistry panel, and an electrocardiogram. The patient should be cross-matched for at least two units of packed red cells.

Anesthetic plan and technique: This patient has presented for elective clipping of an intracranial aneurysm which has not yet bled. Her symptoms are headache and nuchal rigidity, with no focal neurological or cranial nerve involvement. She falls under grade 1 in Hess and Hunt scale, and has a good prognosis from surgical clipping.

Preoperative preparation includes placement of two large-bore intravenous cannulae and an arterial line for blood pressure monitoring. The arterial transducer is positioned at the level of her external auditory canal to precisely report the arterial pressure in the head (as opposed to placing the transducers at the height of the heart, to measures pressures at heart level). This patient does not require a central venous line for this procedure.

A vasodilator or vasodilators are prepared and ready for administration prior to induction, and can profoundly affect blood pressure. Nicardipine, sodium nitroprusside (nitroprusside), and nitroglycerin are most commonly used. These drugs should also be prepared for administration as a bolus prior to starting the infusion.

The induction of anesthesia is carefully begun using sodium thiopental or propofol. Intubating doses of a nondepolarizer are used for muscle relaxation. Lidocaine, administered intravenously or locally to the trachea, as well as an opiate and/or esmolol attenuate any sudden elevations in blood pressure from laryngoscopy, intubation, or the application of surgical pins to the skull.

Anesthesia is maintained with a combination of oxygen and air, and an inhalational anesthetic. Muscle paralysis is monitored closely with a twitch monitor to prevent a patient's coughing or "bucking" while in head pins. A normal $PaCO_2$ is maintained until the dura is opened, to prevent any sudden reductions in intracranial pressure. Vasodilators are administered as necessary to control any elevations in blood pressure that occur.

Mild hypotension, such as a mean arterial pressure around 60 mm of Hg, is usually desirable to shrink the size of the aneurysm and reduce its transluminal pressures. This, in turn, improves surgical visualization and the ease with which the aneurysm can be manipulated. Mild hypotension is accomplished by increasing the level of the anesthetic and using a nicardipine infusion.

During emergence from anesthesia, surges in blood pressure, elevations in intracranial pressure, and coughing must be avoided. Remifentanil, an opiate, and lidocaine may suppress the cough reflex during emergence. A vasodilator infusion and/or esmolol provide strict blood pressure control and avoidance of tachycardia.

APPROACH TO
Anesthesia for Intracranial Aneurysm

DEFINITIONS

MEAN ARTERIAL PRESSURE = Diastolic pressure + 1/3 pulse pressure

PULSE PRESSURE = Systolic pressure Diastolic pressure

HUNT AND HESS CLASSIFICATION OF ANEURYSM: A grading scale of 1 to 5 which correlates patient symptoms on presentation with outcome (see Table 30–1).

TRANSMURAL ANEURISMAL PRESSURE: The pressure differential between the interior of the aneurismal sac and the intracranial pressure.

TRIPLE THERAPY FOR VASOSPASM: Forced hypertension, hemodilution, and hypervolemia to overcome vasospasm and preserve cerebral perfusion.

CLINICAL APPROACH

The incidence of subarachnoid hemorrhage is approximately 7 per 100,000, accounting for almost 10% of all cerebrovascular accidents. Sixteen percent of patients die within minutes of a subarachnoid hemorrhage. Of the patients who survive to be admitted to the hospital, 25% will die following admission.

Table 30–1 HUNT AND HESS CLASSIFICATION

Grade 1	Asymptomatic or minimal headache with slight nuchal rigidity
Grade 2	Moderate to severe headache, nuchal rigidity, no neurologic deficit other than cranial nerve palsy
Grade 3	Drowsiness, confusion, or mild focal deficit
Grade 4	Stupor, moderate to severe hemiparesis, possibly early decerebrate rigidity, and vegetative disturbances
Grade 5	Deep coma, decerebrate rigidity, moribund appearance

Left untreated, 50% of aneurysms will re-rupture within 6 months. The incidence of aneurismal rupture during the induction of anesthesia is between 0.5% and 6%, and carries a mortality of 75%. Only about 50% of patients recover fully. The anesthetic management of unruptured intracranial aneurysm is presented in Table 30–2

The surgery for an intracranial aneurysm may be scheduled as an elective procedure, or as an emergency, following a subarachnoid hemorrhage. The goals of the anesthetic for intracranial aneurismal surgery are: to carefully control systemic blood pressure to minimize the risk of intraoperative aneurysm rupture, to provide optimal operating conditions, and to control intracranial pressure. The risk of re-bleeding is highest between day 1 and day 4. Thus strict blood pressure control is imperative to prevent a re-bleed, especially during this period.

Before the dura is opened, any reductions in ICP can actually increase the aneurysm's transmural pressures, thus increasing the risk of rupture. For this reason, the $PaCO_2$ is maintained at a normal level. Once the dura is opened,

Table 30–2 ANESTHETIC MANAGEMENT FOR AN UNRUPTURED INTRACRANIAL ANEURYSM

- Assignment of Hunt and Hess grading of neurological status.
- Evaluation of comorbidities (emphasis on whether patient can tolerate deliberate hypotension, volume loading).
- Two large-bore i.v. access; central line/PA catheter if necessary.
- Arterial line.
- Strict control of blood pressure, possibly including deliberate hypotension .
- Risk of hypertension is highest during laryngoscopy and intubation, placement of surgical pins, craniotomy and manipulation of dura, and during emergence.
- Patient should be monitored in an intensive care setting in the postoperative period.

mild hyperventilation may be useful to improve operating conditions. Manipulation of the dura is quite painful, and can suddenly increase blood pressure, particularly in the face of light anesthesia. Anticipation of this event can minimize any changes.

The risk of vasospasm is highest between days 5 and 9. The treatment for vasospasm is forced hypertension, hemodilution, and hypervolemia, also known as triple therapy, and used to relieve vasospasm and preserve cerebral perfusion. Infusions of phenylephrine or norepinephrine are typically used to elevate blood pressure. Nimodipine, a calcium channel blocker which causes cerebral vasodilatation, is also be added to this regimen.

After hemorrhage, any blood remaining in the cisterns can contribute to the development of obstructive hydrocephalus. This may require the placement of a temporary ventricular drain or a ventriculo-peritoneal shunt.

Deliberate Hypotension

Deliberate or induced hypotension is useful in minimizing blood loss especially in orthopedic and neurological procedures. In patients with no systemic disease (including hypertension), a MAP of 50 mm of Hg can be tolerated without adverse effects. For the elderly and patients with coexisting systemic disease even in the absence of obvious end-organ damage, it is probably more appropriate to maintain MAP at 60 mm Hg or above. In patients with end-organ involvement such myocardial ischemia, impaired kidney function or those with diabetes, deliberate hypotension is relatively contraindicated. If absolutely required for the aneurysm surgery, it should be utilized cautiously and only for intermittent short periods.

The medications used for deliberate hypotension for intracranial aneurysm surgery, particularly when near the aneurysm, include:

Nicardipine, a calcium channel blocker which can be used as an infusion or as a bolus. Nicardipine dilates arteries and veins, and is not typically associated with as potent reflex tachycardia than some of the other infusions.

Nitroglycerine, a potent venodilator, reduces blood pressure by reducing venous return. It has a rapid onset and rapid offset. But as with any venodilator, nitroglycerine increases intracranial pressure. It also causes reflex tachycardia which can be treated with beta blockers. Nitroglycerine causes cerebral venodilation and increases in ICP. It is best used after the dura is opened and should be avoided in patients with poor intracranial compliance.

Sodium nitroprusside is an arterial and venodilator, which also increases intracranial pressure. Nitroprusside breaks down and releases nitric oxide which activates guanylate cyclase. This increases the concentration of cyclic guanosine monophosphate which causes smooth muscle relaxation. It has a rapid onset and rapid offset. It reduces blood pressure by reducing afterload. A major side effect is cyanide toxicity. The treatment of cyanide toxicity includes cessation of the SNP infusion and specific antidotes such as inhalation of amyl nitrate, sodium nitrate 5 mg/kg i.v., or sodium thiosulfate 150 mg/kg.

If nitroprusside is chosen as the vasodilator, it's worth noting that the sudden cessation of nitroprusside infusion can cause rebound hypertension, so nitroprusside needs to be weaned off gradually. Nitroprusside has five cyanide molecules and cyanide toxicity can occur if doses exceed > 7 mg/min. The signs of toxicity include increasing tolerance and metabolic acidosis.

Hydralazine, a direct acting vasodilator, acts independently of the adrenergic or cholinergic receptors. The peak effect is in 15 to 20 minutes and the half-life is up to 4 hours. Hydralazine causes reflex tachycardia.

Labetalol, a mixed alpha- and beta-receptor antagonist. The ratio of beta to alpha receptor blockade is 3:1 with oral administration and 7:1 with intravenous administration. Labetalol decreases the peripheral vascular resistance and reduces mean arterial pressure. It does not cause reflex tachycardia and has no effect on intracranial pressure.

Esmolol, a selective beta-1-adrenergic-receptor antagonist. Esmolol is rapidly metabolized by red cell esterases. It has a rapid onset, peak effect in 5 minutes, and a short duration of action. The half-life is 9 minutes. It is invaluable in the perioperative period due to its rapid onset and offset. It can be used even in patients with reactive airway disease.

The complications of deliberate hypotension include: myocardial ischemia, cerebral ischemia, oliguria and/or renal failure, metabolic acidosis, rebound hypertension, visual impairment (especially in the prone position and in diabetics). Deliberate hypotension is contraindicated in patients with preexisting coronary/cerebral or renal vascular insufficiencies, hypovolemia, and anemia.

Comprehension Questions

30.1. Which of the following symptoms is most closely associated with an intracranial aneurysm?

A. Headache and neck stiffness
B. Severe episodes of headache that are intermittent
C. Headache associated with photophobia
D. Headache that improves on lying down

30.2. Which of the following statements regarding "deliberate hypotension" is accurate?

A. Deliberate hypotension is a safe, effective way to reduce blood pressure in patients undergoing aneurysm surgery.
B. Deliberate hypotension can cause acute renal failure.
C. Deliberate hypotension has not been associated with visual disturbances.
D. Deliberate hypotension is a treatment for cerebral vasospasm.

30.3. Treatment of cerebral vasospasm includes which of the following?
A. Maintaining an hematocrit of 45%
B. Calcium channel blocker
C. Diuretics
D. An infusion of a local anesthetic such as lidocaine

ANSWERS

30.1. **A.** Symptoms of an intracranial aneurysm include a severe headache, neck stiffness, and changing neurological signs including hemiparesis. Headache from an aneurysm is usually relentless and constant. It is accompanied by nuchal rigidity, cranial nerve involvement, and sometimes even coma. Answer **C**, a headache accompanied by photophobia, is more characteristic of migraines. Answer **D**, a postural headache, is typical of post dural puncture headaches.

30.2. **B.** Deliberate hypotension can cause acute renal failure. It can also cause myocardial ischemia, renal failure, and visual disturbances including blindness and even stroke. The treatment of cerebral vasospasm is induced hypertension.

30.3. **B.** Nimodipine is a calcium channel blocker which has been used to treat cerebral vasospasm. Hemodilution aims for an hematocrit of 30% not 45%, and hypovolemia and intentional hypertension are part of the triple therapy used to treat vasospasm.

Clinical Pearls

- Blood pressure control is crucial in preventing rupture and re-bleed of cerebral aneurysms.
- A sudden reduction in intracranial pressure prior to the opening of the dura can increase the transluminal pressure of the aneurysm, and precipitate rupture.
- The intraoperative rupture of an aneurysm is a catastrophic event, which can occur at the induction of anesthesia. Acute management includes induced hypotension to enable surgical visualization.
- In a patient with vasospasm, even relative hypotension can be associated with neurological changes.
- Subarachnoid hemorrhage is associated with ECG changes and life-threatening arrhythmias.

REFERENCES

Cucchiara RF, et al. Anesthesia for intracranial procedures. In: Barash PG, ed. *Clinical Anesthesia*. 4th ed. Philadelphia, PA: Lippincott; 1989].

Hoff RG. Hypotension in anesthetized patients during aneurysm clipping: Not as bad as expected. Acta Anaesthesiologica *Scandinavica*. 2008;52(7):1006-1011. E pub 2008 May 20.

Newfield, Phillippa, Cottrell, James E. *Handbook of Neuroanesthesia*. 4th ed. Philadelphia, PA: Lippincott Williams and Wilkins; 2007:143-172.

Priebe HJ. Aneurismal subarachnoid hemorrhage and the anaesthetist. *Br J Anesthesiol*. 2007;99(1):102-118. E pub 2007 May 23. Review.

Case 31

A 49-year-old woman presents to preadmission testing for the removal of her sigmoid colon secondary to diverticulitis. She has a 15-year history of myasthenia gravis, and is currently receiving pyridostigmine, 800 mg/day. She was on Prednisone 10 mg/day until about a month ago for her myasthenic symptoms. But as her symptoms improved, her steroids were discontinued.

The patient's past-surgical history include a bronchoscopy and mediastinoscopy 12 years ago followed by a thymectomy a few weeks later. She reports that she was on the ventilator in the ICU afterward on both occasions.

- ➤ What preoperative information is important in the patient with myasthenia gravis?
- ➤ What is the most important point to remember when anesthetizing a patient with myasthenia gravis?
- ➤ What are the major postoperative concerns in patients with myasthenia gravis?

ANSWERS TO CASE 31: Myasthenia Gravis/Multiple Sclerosis

Summary: A 49-year-old woman presents for a sigmoid colectomy. She suffers from myasthenia gravis, and was intubated postoperatively following surgery for a thymectomy.

- **Important preoperative information:** The preoperative information important in a patient suffering from myasthenia gravis includes a history related to the severity of the disease, any related deficits, the patient's baseline activity level, and any evidence of pharyngeal muscle dysfunction. It is important to understand her medication regimen, and the need for and/or frequency of plasmapheresis. A review of any previous anesthetic records is also important, and can provide useful information as to the dosage of drugs required. Pulmonary function tests are useful to estimate the likelihood of a need for postoperative ventilation, any extra-thoracic compression of the airway caused by the thymus, and the degree of restrictive lung disease.
- **Anesthesia with myasthenia gravis:** Patients with myasthenia gravis are exquisitely sensitive to nondepolarizing neuromuscular blockers. Markedly reduced doses, perhaps even as little as 1/10 of the usual dose of a nondepolarizing muscle relaxant is commonly sufficient. However, the response to neuromuscular blockers is variable, and can be affected by pyridostigmine. Therefore, the administration of small doses of muscle relaxant to determine a patient's requirement is of paramount importance.
- **Major postoperative concerns:** The major postoperative concerns include assessing the need for prolonged ventilation, the ability to clear secretions, and optimizing the patient's medication regimen.

ANALYSIS

Objectives

1. Acquaint the learner with the items in the preoperative evaluation that are particularly important in a patient with myasthenia gravis.
2. Understand how the pathophysiology of myasthenia gravis affects anesthetic drugs and the anesthetic plan.
3. Be able to anticipate the most common postoperative concerns in the myasthenic patient.
4. Become familiar with the perioperative issues encountered in a patient with multiple sclerosis.

Considerations

This patient is suffering from myasthenia gravis which has profound implications on the conduct of anesthesia for a sigmoid colectomy. It is important to carefully study her old anesthetic records, to asses her responses to the anesthetic technique, drugs, and doses which were used. This aides the anesthesiologist in optimizing the doses of anesthetic, in an attempt to minimize the likelihood or duration of postoperative ventilation. Following her previous surgeries, she required postoperative ventilation and admission to the ICU. However, the second surgery, a thymectomy, was performed with the intent of improving her myasthenia. So in this case, the history of requiring postoperative ventilation may or may not predict her requirements following this operation.

The physical examination should focus on the neurological system. Any neurological deficits should be documented. Special attention should be paid to her ability to cough and clear secretions, since pharyngeal muscles are often involved in this disease.

Pulmonary function tests (PFTs) help delineate the degree of restrictive pulmonary disease. Both myasthenia, and its treatment can cause respiratory muscle weakness, hindering the ability to extubate the patient at the end of the procedure. Studies have shown that a preoperative vital capacity of < 2.9 L, and a reduced FEV_{25-75} of <3.0 L/sec predict a need for postoperative ventilation. In myasthenics with an intact thymus, flow volume loops may also be required to assess any extrathoracic compression to the airway.

Some poorly-controlled patients with myasthenia gravis may need preoperative plasmapheresis to reduce the patient's antibody load before surgery. Most anesthesiologists do not make any changes to the patient's medication regimen on the day of surgery, although some choose to omit pyridostigmine on the morning of the surgery to reduce the need for neuromuscular blockers.

Given the surgical procedure, a general endotracheal anesthetic is appropriate. Long-acting neuromuscular blocking agents should be minimized. A low-dose lumbar epidural technique may provide sufficient relaxation and allow nondepolarizing muscle relaxants to be avoided all together, in addition to providing postoperative analgesia. Standard monitoring utilizing ECG, pulse oximetry, urine output, and blood pressure is adequate for this patient. If however, on the basis of history and PFTs postoperative ventilation is anticipated, then an arterial line may be inserted to enable blood gas sampling as she is weaned from the ventilator.

Since her medication regimen includes steroids, providing a stress dose of perioperative steroids may be appropriate under these circumstances.

APPROACH TO
Myasthenia Gravis/Multiple Sclerosis

DEFINITIONS

DEPOLARIZING MUSCLE RELAXANTS (DMR): Depolarizing muscle relaxants act by actually binding to the acetylcholine receptors and blocking access of the drug to the receptors. In the process of binding, the receptor is activated causing depolarization that is usually visible as fasciculations or brief muscle contractions. Succinylcholine is a depolarizing muscle relaxant. The action of succinylcholine is terminated by pseudocholinesterase, an enzyme found in the blood and hence its action lasts for only a few minutes.

NONDEPOLARIZING MUSCLE RELAXANTS (NDMR): Nondepolarizing muscle relaxants bind to acetylcholine receptors in a reversible manner and act by blocking the access of acetylcholine to the receptors on the motor end plate. NDMRs do not activate the receptor in the process, so neither depolarization nor fasciculations occur.

ACETYLCHOLINESTERASE INHIBITORS: Acetylcholinesterase is an enzyme that is responsible for breaking down acetylcholine. Drugs that block this enzyme, known as cholinesterase inhibitors, result in more acetylcholine being available. This reverses the effect of the nondepolarizing muscle relaxants in a competitive manner. The most commonly used acetylcholinesterase inhibitor in anesthesia is neostigmine. Other acetylcholinesterase inhibitors include edrophonium, prostigmine, and pyridostigmine. Pyridostigmine can be taken orally and is the drug of choice in the treatment of myasthenia gravis.

CLINICAL APPROACH

Myasthenia Gravis

Anesthesiologists should consider the impact of the patient's muscular weakness on the anesthetic technique they choose. Volatile anesthetics cause some muscular weakness intraoperatively, an effect that is exaggerated in patients with myasthenia. A similar muscle-relaxing action is associated with neuraxial anesthetic technique such as epidural or spinal. Not always sufficient for surgical relaxation in normal patients, either volatile anesthetics or an epidural may provide sufficient relaxation in myasthenic patients. Allowing the nondepolarizing muscle relaxants to be used sparingly or avoided all together minimizes the possibility of prolonged paralysis associated with their use.

Regional anesthetics can also be performed without neuromuscular blocking agents, and some also provide excellent postoperative pain relief. However, it is important to take into consideration the patient's preference for remaining awake (or not) and the surgeon's comfort and speed. It is important to be cognizant that epidurals and spinals can impair respiratory effort if the motor and sensory levels rise high enough to impair the efficient working of the intercostal muscles.

Intubation is usually accomplished with succinylcholine, a depolarizing muscle relaxant. Using succinylcholine avoids the need for an intubating dose of a NDMR, and it's possible that no NDMR will be needed for the operation. The onset of succinylcholine's action may be delayed in myasthenic patients because of blockade of acetylcholine receptors by antibodies. In contrast, succinylcholine's duration of action may be prolonged since it is metabolized by plasma pseudocholinesterase, which is also inhibited by anticholinesterase medications. Preoperative plasmapheresis may also deplete plasma pseudocholinesterase levels. The bottom line: the action of succinylcholine is unpredictable, and affected by a number of factors in patients with myasthenic gravis.

In the event that the myasthenic patient is bed or wheelchair bound, or where succinylcholine would be otherwise contraindicated, it may well be possible to intubate the patient with no muscle relaxant at all, or perhaps with the aid of a volatile agent.

Neuromuscular monitoring is indicated in patients with myasthenia gravis. Before the administration of any muscle relaxants, the presence of fade in the Train of Four predicts a reduced requirement for nondepolarizing muscle relaxants (NDMR) in myasthenic patients. NDMRs normally induce a fade response, where the height of the first twitch T1 is greater than the second twitch T2 >T3 >T4. During the case, it is imperative to dose NDMRs to provide adequate surgical relaxation *without abolishing of all the twitches*. This requires that NDMRs be used sparingly if at all, and long-acting NDMRs such as pancuronium and doxacurium should absolutely be avoided. Similarly, mivacurium, although one of the shortest acting NDMRs, is relatively contraindicated because it is dependent upon plasma pseudocholinesterase for its metabolism. If required, short- and intermediate-acting NDMRs like vecuronium or cisatracurium are appropriate. Myasthenics usually require 40% to 50% of the usual dose of vecuronium. But since the individual's response can be so variable, the administration of very small doses, in succession if necessary, is appropriate.

The anesthesiologist must be aware of other drugs that may affect neuromuscular transmission. These include magnesium, corticosteroids, aminoglycoside antibiotics, lithium, and beta blockers. Similarly, some drugs inhibit pseudocholinesterase, including echothiophate eye drops and donepezil (Aricept). Many of these drugs can increase neuromuscular blockade and make matters worse for the myasthenic patient.

Extubation of myasthenic patients requires careful evaluation. First and foremost, the patient's muscle strength must support spontaneous ventilation, and he or she must be able to handle and clear secretions. This usually means that there is no fade on the Train of Four (TOF), or at least a return to the patient's baseline. The patient must be able to sustain a negative inspiratory pressure of at least 12 to 15 cm of water, able to lift his or her head off the pillow for at least 5 seconds, and obey commands prior to extubation.

On the other hand, the administration of neostigmine to reverse neuromuscular blockade, especially in patients already on large doses of pyridostigmine, can lead to a cholinergic crisis resulting from an exaggerated activation of nicotinic and muscarinic cholinergic receptors. Excessive salivation, miosis, bronchoconstriction, bradycardia, muscle weakness, jitteriness, muscle twitching, bowel cramps, nausea, urinary and bowel incontinence are some of the signs and symptoms of cholinergic crisis. The administration of anticholinergics like glycopyrrolate or atropine may mask the muscarinic actions during a cholinergic crisis, allowing nicotinic effects such as muscle weakness and twitching to predominate. Such nicotinic signs and symptoms are difficult to differentiate from an inadequate NDMR reversal, and from myasthenia itself. In order to avoid such confusion, many anesthesiologists avoid reversing residual NDMR paralysis. Instead they rely on careful dosing and the patient to remain intubated on the ventilator until all the NDMR's effects have resolved.

Multiple Sclerosis

Another neuromuscular disorder commonly encountered by anesthesiologists is multiple sclerosis (MS). MS is a demyelinating disease which affects neurons in unpredictable patterns. Because of the nature of this disorder, any neurological deficits should be carefully noted and documented preoperatively, and the patient made aware of all preexisting deficits.

The most common perioperative concern in patients with MS is the possibility of an exacerbation of the disease after surgery. Any stressful condition, such as fever/hyperpyrexia, infection, pain, or fatigue may cause an exacerbation or relapse. It is very difficult to separate the effects of these factors from the effects of the stress of the surgery itself, or the anesthetic techniques or drugs that are used. It is important that the patient must be kept at normal body temperature in the operating room, since excessive heat seems to be harmful in this group of patients.

Avoiding the stress of postoperative pain is similarly a priority. Although the rationale is not understood, epidural analgesia is thought to be associated with fewer relapses of multiple sclerosis than a spinal. An epidural catheter can be placed in the preoperative period to provide postoperative analgesia and reduce catecholamine release and pain. Amide local anesthetics like bupivacaine 0.125% with the addition of a small amount of narcotic like hydromorphone 10 µg/cc can provide excellent postoperative pain relief. Ester-based local anesthetics may also be used, bearing in mind that many of them are metabolized by pseudocholinesterase. Patients on pyridostigmine have reduced plasma pseudocholinesterase activity and hence normally short-acting ester-based local anesthetics like chloroprocaine may have an unpredictable duration of action.

Although epidural local anesthetics can cause some degree of motor weakness, bupivacaine 0.125% or 0.067% concentrations at rates of 4 to 10 cc/h should not cause appreciable motor block. It is important to titrate to analgesia and perform periodical neurological checks to ensure significant motor blocks do not set in. Alternatively, patient controlled analgesia (PCA) can also be used in the postoperative period. Use of non-opioid oral and parenteral analgesics like ketorolac, ibuprofen, acetaminophen are desirable as they offer good analgesia without appreciable postoperative nausea, vomiting, sedation, or respiratory depression.

Postoperative Management

If the patient cannot be safely extubated in the operating room, she must be transferred to an intensive care unit or PACU where close monitoring is possible and a plan to wean the patient off the ventilator in place. Prolonged postoperative ventilation is undesirable, since it is often associated with respiratory infections, resulting in more difficulties with extubation later on. Postoperatively a complete neurological examination must be performed to document any new deficits.

Comprehension Questions

31.1. A 40-year-old woman with myasthenia gravis presents for abdominal surgery. She has no other comorbidities or risk factors. Which the following tests is most likely to be useful at the pre-anesthetic visit?
A. Pulmonary function tests
B. Electrocardiogram
C. Chest x-ray
D. CBC

31.2. Which of the following is metabolized by pseudocholinesterase?
A. Cisatracurium
B. Succinylcholine
C. Pyridostigmine
D. Dexamethasone

31.3. Which of the following anesthetic management plans apply specifically to patients with multiple sclerosis?
A. Preanesthetic documentation of all neurological deficits
B. Provision of stress doses of steroids if the patient has recently abruptly stopped steroids
C. Avoidance of spinal anesthesia
D. Keeping the body temperature normal and avoiding hyperthermia

ANSWERS

31.1. **A.** Pulmonary function tests, old anesthetic records, and a complete neurological examination are useful because they give an idea of pre-existing neurological deficits and also help plan the course of the anesthetic based on previous performance and pulmonary function. An electrocardiogram, chest x-ray, and CBC in an otherwise healthy 40-year-old female is unlikely to add additional information that is helpful in the management of this patient.

31.2. **B.** Succinylcholine, is metabolized by the plasma enzyme pseudocholinesterase. Thus in patients taking cholinesterase inhibitors, the action of succinylcholine may be prolonged. Answer **A**, cisatricurium, is metabolized by Hoffmann degradation. **C**, pyridostigmine, is a drug used predominantly for the treatment of myasthenia gravis. Pyridostigmine bromide is an analogue of neostigmine that inhibits acetylcholinesterase as well as plasma pseudocholinesterase, and thus the breakdown of acetylcholine. **D**, dexamethasone, is not metabolized by pseudocholinesterase.

31.3. **D.** Higher body temperatures have been associated with an increase in neuronal demyelination and relapses. Hence, keeping normal body temperature and avoiding hyperthermia in patients with multiple sclerosis is important. Pre-anesthetic documentation of neurological deficits is important because new deficits can sometimes appear postoperatively. Stresses such as pain and anxiety have been implicated in relapses. Although there is no definitive proof that spinal anesthesia is associated with relapses and onset of new neurological deficits, most anesthesiologists would avoid spinal anesthesia in a patient with sever multiple sclerosis. Stress doses of steroids are controversial but most anesthesiologists would consider a dose of steroid in any patient who has abruptly stopped steroid medications.

Clinical Pearls

- Myasthenics are usually exquisitely sensitive to nondepolarizing muscle relaxants and these drugs should be used sparingly if at all.
- Patients suffering from myasthenia gravis have a varied and unpredictable response to nondepolarizing muscle relaxants.
- Drugs that can increase muscle weakness in myasthenics include neuromuscular blocking agents, volatile anesthetics, anticholinesterases, aminoglycoside antibiotics, beta blockers, prolonged steroid administration, lithium, magnesium, and local anesthetics.
- In patients with multiple sclerosis, minimizing surgical stress, controlling pain, fever, hemodynamic fluxes to intubation as well as maintenance of normal body temperature are goals of the anesthetic plan.

REFERENCES

Abel M, Eisenkraft JB. Anesthetic implications of myasthenia gravis. *Mt Sinai J Med.* 2002;69(1-2):31-37.

Hirsch NP. Neuromuscular junction in health and disease. *Br J Anaesthesiol.* 2007;99(1):132-138.

Miller RD. *Anesthesia.* 6th ed. vol 1. Pennsylvania: Elsevier, Churchill Livingstone; 2005.

Naguib M, el Dawlatly AA, Ashour M, Bamgboye EA. Multivariate determinants of the need for postoperative ventilation in myasthenia gravis. *Can J Anaesthesiol.* 1996;43(10):1006-1013.

Case 32

A 64-year-old man with C6 quadriplegia secondary to a spinal cord injury 1 year ago is scheduled to undergo cystoscopy for urolithiasis. Although he is insensate throughout much of his body, he still has some patchy areas of sensation, and experiences significant pain when a stone is passed. His past medical history is significant for hypertension treated with hydrochlorothiazide, and type II diabetes mellitus.

His physical examination is remarkable for atrophy of his limbs, but is otherwise normal. He is 67 in tall, and weighs 90 kg. His laboratory results, including a cardiac stress test, are normal as well. A general anesthetic is planned.

Anesthesia is induced with etomidate, the patient is paralyzed using a nondepolarizing neuromuscular agent and intubated, and surgery commences. About 30 minutes into the procedure the patient suddenly develops severe bradycardia (heart rate in the low 30's bpm range), hypertension, and diaphoresis. You ask the surgeon to stop the procedure.

- What is the most likely diagnosis?
- How can this situation be prevented?
- How should this patient be managed?
- Is it safe to continue surgery?

ANSWERS TO CASE 32: Autonomic Hyperreflexia

Summary: This is a patient with quadriplegia who has developed signs of bradycardia, hypertension, and diaphoresis following surgical manipulation of the urinary tract.

➤ **Most likely diagnosis:** Autonomic hyperreflexia (AH), which occurs in patients with high spinal cord injuries and can be precipitated by a range of stimuli including manipulation of the bladder during surgery.

➤ **Prevention:** The best way to prevent an episode of AH is to avoid the offending stimulus. The patient is often aware of the episodes, and usually knows what factors are problematic for him. If the procedure necessitates a situation which can trigger AH (such as a cystoscopy requiring bladder distension), then careful monitoring can detect the episode early in its course, and the offending stimulus removed.

➤ **Treatment:** When AH occurs during surgery, management begins with removal of the precipitating stimulus. This alone may be sufficient and blood pressure often returns back to baseline levels immediately. In addition to removing the stimulus, AH is best treated by increasing the depth of anesthesia (eg, giving a bolus of intravenous anesthetic or increasing the concentration of inspired volatile agent).

➤ **Proceed with surgery:** Surgery cannot proceed until you stabilize the patient. Most episodes of AH are brief and self-limiting. After stabilizing the patient and having increased the depth of general anesthesia, it is reasonable to allow surgery to continue whilst carefully monitoring the patient.

ANALYSIS

Objectives

1. Become familiar with the syndrome of autonomic hyperreflexia.
2. Know the precipitating factors, clinical features, and complications of autonomic hyperreflexia.
3. Understand the anesthetic options and consideration for patients with AH.
4. Review additional anesthetic issues in quadriplegics such as truncal obesity, precautions when using succinylcholine, and the possibility of sleep apnea, difficult mask airway, and difficult intubation.

Considerations

Several considerations are warranted in this patient. First, he has patchy areas of sensation which may be normal or abnormal, so he will require an anesthetic for his surgery. This is in contrast with some patients with spinal cord injuries, who are totally insensate. In insensate patients, it may be possible to perform minor procedures without any anesthesia as long as the patient does not have AH. This patient states that he does have AH, and that it is triggered by fecal impaction or urinary retention. He knows when a triggering event has occurred because he gets a severe headache.

This patient is mildly obese, and intravenous access appears to be challenging. He is also quite anxious, warranting pretreatment with a benzodiazepine. Although he has had a cervical fusion, his airway examination shows a Mallampati class 1 airway and no problems with airway management are anticipated. Like many patients with chronic spinal cord injuries, he is plagued by painful muscle spasms which he cannot control.

With the notable exception of AH and spinal cord injury, this patient is remarkably healthy, NPO, and does not have gastric reflux. Thus, following premedication with a benzodiazepine, a general anesthetic with a laryngeal mask airway is planned.

APPROACH TO Autonomic Hyperreflexia

DEFINITIONS

AUTONOMIC HYPERREFLEXIA: Autonomic hyperreflexia (AH) is a phenomenon that occurs after spinal cord transection. It is characterized by a massive and disordered autonomic response to certain stimuli below the level of the lesion.

QUADRIPLEGIA: Also known as **tetraplegia**, is a symptom in which a human experiences paralysis affecting all four limbs, although not necessarily total paralysis or loss of function. It is caused by injuries to the cervical (and occasionally thoracic) spine, and results in an impairment of limb function, bowel and bladder control, sexual function, digestion, respiration, and other autonomic functions. Sensation is usually impaired in affected areas, and can manifest as numbness, reduced sensation, or burning neuropathic pain.

CLINICAL APPROACH

What is autonomic hyperreflexia?

Autonomic hyperreflexia (AH) is a phenomenon that typically occurs after spinal cord injury. It was first recognized in 1860, and in 1917, Head and Riddoch described the effects of bladder distension on soldiers with spinal cord injury. AH is characterized by a massive and disordered autonomic response to certain stimuli below the level of the lesion. This response is thought to be due to sympathetic and parasympathetic activity, unopposed by the normal central modulatory pathways. AH can occur in up to 85% of patients with spinal cord lesions above the level of T6.

Major advances in the care of spinal cord injury patients have led to an improved survival rate, an increase in the number of spinal cord injury patients presenting for elective surgery, and thus an increase in the frequency of AH. In addition, quadriplegic patients are medically complicated due to obesity, risk of DVTs, sleep apnea, and challenges with airway management. An understanding of the relevant pathophysiology allows the anesthesiologist to provide safe perioperative care. The complications associated with spinal cord injury are listed in Table 32–1.

Clinical Features and Complications of AH

The most common clinical feature of AH is hypertension, which is typically paroxysmal and may be severe. Systolic blood pressures may exceed 260 mm Hg and diastolic pressures range from 170 to 220 mm Hg. Hypertensive crises can lead to intracranial and retinal hemorrhages, seizures, coma, myocardial ischemia, pulmonary edema, and death.

Headache is also a common feature of AH, and may be the first sign to herald the onset of an episode of AH. Profuse sweating, flushing or pallor above the level of the lesion, and reflex bradycardia are seen in the majority of cases. Other reported features include papillary changes, Horner syndrome, nausea, anxiety, and penile erections. The clinical features of AH are summarized in Table 32–2.

The neurophysiological changes in AH reflect both loss of descending inhibition from higher centers, and alterations in connections within the distal spinal cord. This results in a widespread inappropriate sympathetic response that lacks the usual descending inhibitory influences, leading to profound vasoconstriction. Circulating norepinephrine levels remain low following spinal cord transection, presumably as a result of the reduced sympathetic activity. Thus, patients post spinal cord injury are typically more sensitive to the effects of exogenous catecholamines than normal individuals.

AH occurs more frequently in the OR in patients who have experienced the syndrome in their daily lives. A range of stimuli can trigger a mass autonomic response, not just those that occur in the operating room. However, bladder

Table 32–1 COMPLICATIONS ASSOCIATED WITH SPINAL CORD INJURY

BODY SYSTEM	POTENTIAL COMPLICATIONS
Cardiovascular	• Blood volume is typically reduced in tetraplegics. • Orthostatic hypotension: head-up tilt causes a fall in stroke volume and cardiac output. Venous return is impaired and pooling of blood occurs in the lower limbs. • Elevated renin and aldosterone levels lead to salt and water retention.
Respiratory	• Obesity can cause obstructive sleep apnea and increased neck girth leading to a potentially difficult intubation. • Reduced vital capacity. • Impaired ability to cough. • Reduced respiratory drive and ventilatory response to hypercapnia. • Respiratory insufficiency: mainly due to muscle weakness (diaphragmatic, intercostals, abdominal wall and accessory muscles). Quadriplegics with central apnea due to high spinal cord lesions may potentially benefit from phrenic nerve pacing (diaphragmatic stimulators). Diaphragmatic pacing can be considered for patients who have cord lesions above the C2-C3 level since pacing of the diaphragm by phrenic nerve stimulation is possible only if the nerve cell bodies (located in the anterior horns of C3-C5) are viable.
Musculoskeletal	• In acute spinal cord injury: acetylcholine receptors proliferate over the entire muscle membrane. The use of depolarizing muscle relaxants can lead to massive ion fluxes and fatal hyperkalemia. • Spinal cord injury can lead to spasms and contractures. • Treatments include drug therapy and passive physiotherapy. • Osteoporosis due to a significant reduction in bone density below the level of the spinal cord injury is common.
Temperature regulation	• High spinal cord injuries impair normal mechanisms of thermoregulation by preventing shivering in response to cold and sweating or vasodilatation in response to heat. Patients become partially poikilothermic and body temperature reflects environmental temperature.
Skin care	• Decubitus ulcers occur in up to 60% of patients with cervical lesions. Left untreated, pressure sores can lead to chronic infection, osteomyelitis, septicemia, amyloidosis and can trigger AH.
Blood disorders	• Anemia of chronic disease is common in this patient population. • The risk of deep vein thrombosis formation is greatly increased in the early stages following a cord injury. Untreated, 80%-85% of patients will develop deep vein thrombosis.

(*Continued*)

Table 32–1 COMPLICATIONS ASSOCIATED WITH SPINAL CORD INJURY (*CONTINUED*)

BODY SYSTEM	POTENTIAL COMPLICATIONS
Genitourinary	• Spinal cord injury leads to incomplete voiding, high intravesical pressures and vesicoureteric reflux. • Urinary tract infections are common as a result of high residual volumes and the use of urethral catheters. • Renal calculi form easily.
Gastrointestinal	• Acute gastroparesis and ileus is common immediately after spinal cord injury. • Patients with spinal cord injury have residual delayed gastric emptying.
Pain	• Chronic pain may occur in up to 60% of patients with spinal cord injury and can be difficult to manage.

or bowel distension, uterine contractions, acute abdominal pathology, handling of bowel or bladder manipulations during surgery, and urinary tract infection are the most common precipitating factors. Cutaneous and proprioceptive stimuli are less commonly implicated. Thus, in patients with a high cord lesion, AH occurs most often during urological surgery, and is less common during body surface surgery. It is important to remember that these triggers may occur intraoperatively, or in the immediate postoperative period.

The Anesthetic Plan

When performing the preoperative anesthetic assessment and formulating the anesthetic plan in a cord injury patient, special consideration should be given to the following factors:

- Ask the patient whether he or she gets AH, and if so, how does he/she know?
- Sensory level, site of surgery, and completeness of lesion.

Table 32–2 CLINICAL FEATURES OF AUTONOMIC HYPERREFLEXIA

COMMON FEATURES	OTHER FEATURES
Hypertension	Nausea
Headache	Anxiety
Sweating	Pupillary changes
Pallor	Horner syndrome
Bradycardia	Penile erections

- Patient preference for anesthesia, and/or the type of anesthetic technique (general/regional/monitored anesthesia care/or no anesthesia).
- Time elapsed since spinal cord injury: The risk of a hyperkalemic response to succinylcholine is greatest from 3 days to 9 months post injury.
- Prior anesthetic history: Previous anesthetic records should be located. Many cord-injured patients have often had multiple prior procedures and may regularly undergo surgery without anesthesia.
- Airway and neck motion, which may be affected by previous cervical spine surgery.
- History of respiratory tract infections, obstructive sleep apnea, intensive care unit admissions, tracheostomy past or present, and respiratory sufficiency, or the need for respiratory enhancements such as a diaphragmatic stimulator or chronic ventilation.
- Vital capacity should be measured in all patients with lesions above C7; chest x-ray and arterial blood gases may also be indicated preoperatively.
- Cardiovascular assessment: Baseline blood pressure, heart rate, history of postural hypotension, history of prior AH.
- Musculoskeletal deformities: Spasms, contractures, pressure sores.
- Medications: Use of anticoagulants, muscle relaxants.
- Laboratory tests (complete blood count, electrolytes and renal function). Anemia is common. Electrolytes, BUN, and creatinine to exclude renal impairment.

Choice of Anesthesia

Loss of sensation below the level of the lesion following a spinal cord injury means that these patients could theoretically undergo surgery without anesthesia and without feeling pain from the operative site, as they often do. However, the decision as to whether anesthesia is required for a procedure depends on the surgery, the level of the spinal cord lesion, the completeness of the lesion and very importantly, patient preference. Patients who experience muscle spasms may require anesthesia for positioning and control during surgery, since spasms are often triggered by proprioceptive and cutaneous stimuli.

An anesthesiologist should be present, venous access secured, and standard monitoring used throughout the procedure for all operations on cord injury patients, regardless of anesthetic technique.

Premedication and i.v. Access

Patients with spinal cord injuries have typically undergone multiple surgeries and procedures since their original injury. They are also particularly susceptible to preprocedure anxiety, which should be treated with benzodiazepines.

Obesity is a secondary effect of spinal cord injury due to inactivity. The typical body habitus is that of truncal obesity with wasting of the lower limbs. The upper limbs may also display muscle wasting and fat accumulation leading to difficulties obtaining i.v. access.

The absence of reflex sympathetic activity reduces the ability to compensate for the myocardial depressant effects of anesthetic agents. Placement of a large-bore intravenous cannula is recommended and preoperative fluid loading with 500 to 1000 mL of crystalloid reduces the likelihood and severity of hypotension after induction.

General Anesthesia

Patients with spinal cord injury often have a lower blood volume with a reduced lean tissue mass secondary to muscle wasting. This leads to a smaller volume of distribution for intravenous anesthetic agents which explains the greater observed sensitivity of these patients to intravenous induction agents. Spinal cord injury is also associated with renal impairment, which may result in reduced clearance of certain drugs.

Succinylcholine may be used safely in cord injury patients within the first 72 hours of injury and after 9 months. The choice of airway technique is largely the same as for normal patients, and the use of the laryngeal mask airway in cord injured patients has been widely described. The theoretical risks of aspiration associated with the use of a laryngeal mask airway in this patient population have not been substantiated.

Positioning is of even greater importance in the in the cord injured patient compared with normal individuals due to the high incidence of pressure sores and spasmodic movements. Patients with spinal cord injuries also become poikilothermic, so the prevention of heat loss during surgery is of great importance. Passive humidifiers, fluid warming devices, hot air blankets, and operating in a warm room are all recommended in this patient population.

Regional Anesthesia

The use of regional anesthesia in cord injured patients is well established, particularly spinal anesthesia for urological surgery and epidural anesthesia for labor. The advantages of spinal anesthesia in cord injured patients are the reliable prevention of AH, and avoidance of risks associated with general anesthesia. However, disadvantages of spinal anesthesia include the inability to determine the level of the block and difficulty in determining the appropriate dose of medications to administer. In some patients, the level of the block may be determined by observing the level at which spastic paresis becomes flaccid, the disappearance of ankle or knee reflexes, temperature changes in the lower limbs, or the ability to elicit muscle spasm to ethyl chloride spray.

Placing a spinal may be technically challenging due to kyphoscoliosis, truncal obesity, prior spinal surgery, and inability to flex the spine due to spasms and bony deformities. Although spinal anesthesia can cause hypotension in normal patients, in spinal cord injured patients, spinal anesthesia is associated with cardiovascular stability, perhaps because cord injured patients have low baseline sympathetic tone. Alderson et al. recommend the use of 1.5 to 2.0 mL of hyperbaric 0.5% bupivacaine for use as a spinal anesthetic in urologic surgery.

Epidural anesthesia has been reported as being less effective in blocking AH than spinal anesthesia. Problems with epidural anesthesia in this population also include the inability to assess the block accurately, correctly verifying the effect of the test dose, the failure to block sacral spinal cord segments, and the very real possibility of missed segments due to distortion of the epidural space.

Management of AH in the OR

If AH occurs during surgery, management should begin with removal of the precipitating stimulus if at all possible. This alone may be sufficient to terminate the episode and blood pressure often returns back to baseline levels immediately. Most episodes of AH are brief and self-limiting and may not require specific treatment. During general anesthesia, AH is best treated by increasing the depth of anesthesia. Additional treatment options include calcium channel blockers, nitrates, and assumption of the upright position. If the stimulus is not obvious, bladder distension and fecal impaction should be ruled out. In the non-OR setting, a urinary catheter should be checked for blockage and urinary tract infection excluded. Tight clothing and footwear should also be loosened.

Comprehension Questions

32.1. In which of the following patients is it safe to use succinylcholine?
- A. 24 hours after a spinal cord injury
- B. 1 month after a spinal cord injury
- C. 1 week after a spinal cord injury
- D. 2 months after a spinal cord injury
- E. 6 months after this injury

32.2. A patient with C6 quadriplegia develops hypertension (BP = 240/118) under general anesthesia for laparoscopic cholecystectomy. Therapeutic maneuvers that can be initiated do not include which of the following?
- A. Increase concentration and delivery of volatile agent.
- B. Nitroglycerin infusion.
- C. Phenoxybenzamine.
- D. A propofol bolus.
- E. Nitroprusside infusion.

32.3. The patient described in question 32.2 is noted to be tachycardic with HR = 95 bpm. Which of the following is the most likely etiology?
A. Hypercarbia
B. Pheochromocytoma
C. Thyroid storm
D. Spinal dysreflexia
E. Awareness

ANSWERS

32.1. **A.** Following the development of spinal cord injuries, extra-junctional cholinergic receptors develop after 48 to 72 hours. A severe hyperkalemic response to succinylcholine may be seen up to 9 to 12 months after the injury.

32.2. **C.** Presuming that this hypertension is a result of autonomic hyperreflexia, short-acting agents should be used to correct the hypertension. Long-acting agents like phenoxybenzamine are not appropriate as they may result in prolonged hypotension following the cessation of the stimulus, particularly in a patient with low baseline sympathetic tone.

32.3. **A.** Of these syndromes, hypercarbia is both most likely, and most easily manipulated so it should be excluded from the differential first. Answer **D**, autonomic hyperreflexia, is characterized by reflex bradycardia as long as there is a functional carotid sinus. The anesthesiologist should also be careful not to miss other causes of intraoperative hypertension such as pheochromocytoma, thyroid storm, and awareness (Answers **B, C** and **E**).

Clinical Pearls

- Autonomic hyperreflexia is common in individuals with spinal cord injuries above T6.
- It is characterized by paroxysmal reflex autonomic activity in response to noxious stimuli below the level of the neurologic lesion, and can lead to pulmonary edema, myocardial ischemia, cerebral hemorrhage, and death.
- Headache, diaphoresis, flushing, bradycardia, and paroxysmal hypertension are most commonly observed.
- Bladder and bowel distention, and surgical manipulations are the most common intraoperative precipitating factors.
- Removal of the offending stimulus is key to restore the baseline autonomic activity.
- Regional anesthesia and deep general anesthesia both treat and prevent hyperreflexia.

REFERENCES

AK Karlsson. Autonomic dysreflexia. *Spinal Cord.* 1999;37:383-391.

Colachis SC. Autonomic hyperreflexia with spinal cord injury. *J Am Paraplegia Soc.* 1992;15(3):171-186.

DiMarco AF, Takaoka Y, Kowalski KE. Combined intercostal and diaphragm pacing to provide artificial ventilation in patients with tetraplegia. *Arch Phys Med Rehabil.* 2005;86:1200.

Elefteriades JA, Hogan JF, Handler A, Loke JS. Long-term follow-up of bilateral pacing of the diaphragm in quadriplegia. *N Engl J Med.* 1992;326:1433.

Hambly PR, Martin B. Anaesthesia for chronic spinal cord lesions. *Anaesthesia.* 1998;53:273-289.

Lee BY, Karmakar MG, Herz BL, Sturgill RA. Autonomic dysreflexia revisited. *J Spinal Cord Med.* 1995;18(2):75-87.

Trop CS, Bennett CJ. Autonomic dysreflexia and its urological implications: A *review. J Urol* . 1991;146(6):1461-1469.

Obstetric Patients

Case 33

A 26 year-old Gravida (G) 1 Para (P) 0 woman presents to the emergency room 26 weeks pregnant and with abdominal pain. She has received excellent prenatal care. The abdominal pain started the afternoon prior to presentation. It is diffuse in nature in the right lower quadrant, but poorly localized. She has had some loss of appetite but no nausea and vomiting since the onset of pain. Nevertheless, she ate parts of a cheeseburger and fries approximately 4 hours prior to the ER visit. The patient is otherwise healthy, and takes no medications except for a multivitamin.

She is 5 ft 8 in tall and weighs 165 pounds. Vital signs are normal, as are her laboratory values, with the exception of a WBC count of 9500/mm^3. On computerized tomography, the patient is found to have acute appendicitis and is scheduled for an urgent laparoscopic appendectomy.

- ➤ What are the anesthetic considerations in a pregnant patient?
- ➤ What is the most important goal when anesthetizing a pregnant patient undergoing nonobstetric surgery?

ANSWERS TO CASE 33: Appendectomy in the Pregnant Patient

Summary: This is a healthy woman at 26-weeks gestation, in the mid trimester of pregnancy, who presents for an urgent laparoscopic appendectomy. She may need open appendectomy if the appendix cannot be removed via laparoscopy.

- **Anesthetic concerns in pregnancy:** Physiologic changes such as airway edema and decreased gastric emptying affect intubation and increase the risk of pulmonary aspiration. The placenta acts as a sieve and all drugs delivered to the patient have potential to have effect in the baby. Choice of drugs is limited in pregnancy.
- **Most important goals:** When anesthetizing a pregnant patient for nonobstetrical surgery, the most important goals are to be vigilant and meticulous in the care of the mother, minimizing any changes in hemodynamic and acid-base parameters.

ANALYSIS

Objectives

1. Understand the nuances of nonpregnant surgery in the pregnant patient.
2. Elucidate anesthetic concerns with pregnancy in nonobstetrical surgery.
3. Review placental physiology and the concept of the uteroplacental barrier.

Considerations

This 26-year-old woman who is pregnant in the mid trimester requires general anesthesia for a laparoscopic appendectomy. She is brought to the operating room, and her uterus is displaced by placing a pillow under her lower left back to avoid potential aorto-caval compression, which would decrease venous blood flow back to the heart. Routine ASA monitors are placed, and preoxygenation is begun with 100% oxygen. A rapid sequence induction with endotracheal intubation is performed, since in both emergency cases and in pregnancy, there is an increased risk of pulmonary aspiration of gastric contents. Positive pressure ventilation is instituted following intubation to keep the $PaCO_2$ between 28 and 30 mm of Hg, which is the normal level in pregnancy. Normocarbia ensures a normal acid-base status in the mother, since maternal acidemia may lead to fetal acidemia, and maternal alkalosis may reduce uterine blood flow.

Maintenance of anesthesia is performed with a balanced combined technique consisting of appropriate doses of narcotic, inhalational agents, and muscle relaxants. Inhalation agents are useful, because they relax smooth muscle, contrary to any contractions which might occur. Nitrous oxide is commonly avoided in laparoscopic surgeries because of bowel distention. Continuous fetal heart rate monitoring while useful, may be difficult in this patient requiring an intra-abdominal procedure, and is typically not performed in this setting.

On completion of the operation, it is anticipated that the patient will be extubated just as anyone else who has undergone this procedure. An obstetrician will examine the patient in the PACU to ascertain the state of maternal and fetal well-being, and monitor for preterm labor.

APPROACH TO Appendectomy in the Pregnant Patient

PHYSIOLOGICAL CHANGES

Appendicitis is difficult to diagnose in a pregnant patient. The signs and symptoms of appendicitis may well mimic pregnancy (nausea, vomiting, constipation, abdominal pain). Moreover, the reluctance to subject a pregnant patient to radiographic exposure may further delay diagnosis. By the same token, a delayed diagnosis also leads to complications as pregnancy renders the formation of an appendiceal abscess more likely. Also, the possibility of rupture is both more plausible and more problematic. The point to remember is that ultrasonographic imaging is safe and useful in pregnancy.

The decision to proceed with laparoscopic versus open surgery is the next challenge. As in the nonpregnant patient, laparoscopic surgery is associated with improved postoperative pain control, earlier mobility, and recovery of gastrointestinal motility. The use of laparoscopy has also become very popular for appendectomies, as laparoscopy allows for an improved visualization of several intra-abdominal structures.

However, the issues with laparoscopy in the pregnant patient include:

- Carbon dioxide absorption by the fetus by placental transfer leading to fetal acidemia
- Uterine or fetal trauma
- Increased intra-abdominal pressure from the insufflation with CO_2, which could impair maternal ventilation as well as increase the possibility of aortocaval compression

If the surgery were to be performed as an "open" (nonlaparoscopic) procedure, then spinal would be the anesthetic of choice, since neuraxial techniques minimize fetal exposure to circulating drugs.

Any abdominal surgery in a pregnant patient risks fetal loss, though the risk is higher in the first trimester than in the second trimester. Unless an emergency threatens life or limb, surgery should be delayed till the second or third trimester of pregnancy.

Amniotic fluid acts can conduct electrical current to the fetus. Bipolar cautery is preferred over monopolar cautery, since the currents are more streamlined, and there is less likelihood of stray currents going through the fetus. Additionally, the grounding pad should be placed in such a way that the uterus is not in the pathway of the current.

Maternal hypotension can jeopardize uteroplacental perfusion. The most common causes of hypotension in the mother include:

- Deep levels of general anesthesia
- Aorto-caval compression by the pregnant uterus
- Sympathetic blockade from a high epidural or spinal block
- Hemorrhage
- Hypovolemia

Additional factors that affect uteroplacental perfusion include uterine vasoconstriction by vasoactive drugs such as phenylephrine and epinephrine. Indirect-acting agents such as ephedrine are preferred in pregnancy to preserve blood supply to the fetus. High levels of anxiety in the mother can also result in a catecholamine surge that may impair placental blood flow. However, benzodiazepines are contraindicated because of their teratogenic effects.

Studies of nonobstetrical surgery in the pregnant patient show an increased risk of abortion and preterm birth, especially in the first week after surgery. Prophylactic tocolysis is controversial. Monitoring the mother for uterine contractions for several days after the surgery is recommended, since in the presence of premature uterine contractions, the prompt institution of tocolysis is appropriate. Fetal monitoring is not usually performed in the operating room during the surgery, since surgery is only performed in situations with significant risk to the mother.

Comprehension Questions

33.1. What are the advantages of regional anesthesia in the gravid patient presenting for nonobstetric surgery?

A. Increased risk of aspiration due to relaxation of the lower esophageal sphincter
B. Increased risk of aspiration due to slower gastric emptying
C. Decreased placental transmission of drugs
D. Decreased risk of miscarriage

33.2. Hypotension in a gravid patient under anesthesia is most commonly the result of which of the following?

A. Aorto-caval compression
B. Hypercarbia
C. Hypervolemia
D. A "light" level of general anesthesia

ANSWERS

33.1. **D.** Regional techniques provide analgesia without exposing the fetus to a high concentration of drugs. This is possible because during a spinal anesthetic, a small amount of a local anesthetic is injected into the subarachnoid space. In contrast, general anesthesia in the gravid patient is associated with increased incidence of aspiration and difficult airway management as the result of anatomical and hormonal changes during pregnancy.

33.2. **A.** Hypotension in the supine gravid patient is most commonly a result of aorto-caval compression by the gravid uterus. Other causes include "deep" anesthesia, a sympathetic blockade during regional techniques, hemorrhage and hypovolemia are other causes of hypotension in the pregnant patient.

Clinical Pearls

- Fetal monitoring is not typically performed during nonobstetrical operations in pregnant patients during the first or second trimester.
- The pregnant uterus causes vena caval compression in the supine position, and can cause significant hypotension in both the mother and the fetus.
- The majority of drugs administered to the mother will cross the uteroplacental barrier.
- Maternal complications such as hypoxia, acidemia and hypotension are associated with the most dramatic fetal consequences.

REFERENCES

Chestnut DH. Obstetric Anesthesia: Principles and Practice. 2nd ed. Nonobstetric surgery during pregnancy. Mosby publishing.

Guidelines by the American Society for Gastrointestinal Endoscopy: Guidelines for endoscopy in pregnant and lactating women. *Gastrointest endosc*. 2005;61: 357-362.

Jackson H, Granger S, Price R, et al. Diagnosis and laparoscopic treatment of surgical diseases during pregnancy: An evidence based review. *Surg Endosc*. 2008;22:1917-1927.

Society of American Gastrointestinal and Endoscopic Surgeons: Guidelines for the diagnosis, treatment, and use of laparoscopy for surgical problems during pregnancy. *Surg Endosc*. 1998;12:189-190.

Case 34

A 23-year-old woman, Gravida (G) 2 Para (P)1 with a footling breech presentation and not in labor, presents to the labor and delivery suite for an elective cesarean section (c-section). She is in excellent physical condition, maintains a healthy lifestyle and only takes prenatal vitamins for medications. The patient is interested in discussing the options for anesthesia prior to the surgery. She has heard "bad things" about spinals. She has been fasting (NPO) since midnight, the night prior.

- ➤ What are the benefits of general versus regional anesthesia for this patient?
- ➤ What regional anesthetic techniques are available in this setting?
- ➤ What are the complications associated with regional anesthesia?

ANSWERS TO CASE 34:
Routine Cesarean Section and Local Anesthetic Toxicity

Summary: This is a healthy woman who presents for a routine, elective c-section.

- **Benefits of general versus regional anesthesia:** Regional anesthesia relieves the pain of surgery, and minimizes the concentration of drugs within the maternal circulation, which could affect the fetus. It also avoids the drowsiness seen following general anesthesia, as well as that observed postoperatively with parenteral narcotics. Less drowsiness allows for an improved interaction between the mother and the baby. In the absence of complications, paralysis and end-tracheal intubation are not required with regional anesthesia. This is desirable because the physiologic changes of pregnancy may render the airway prone to injury, or intubation difficult due to edema and increased vascularity of the glottic and supra glottic structures. If a patient has a bleeding diathesis, if especially high concentrations of oxygen need to be administered, or if a patient is unable to cooperate during the operation, or unwilling to give consent for a regional technique then a general anesthetic is indicated.
- **Types of regional anesthesia available:** Neuraxial blockade, both spinal and epidural, are types of regional anesthesia available for a routine cesarean section.
- **Complications of neuraxial blockade:** These techniques are very safe, but can cause significant morbidity. These include nerve damage, local anesthetic toxicity, high or total spinal, accidental subdural injection of local anesthetic, post-dural puncture headache (PDPH), infection from the site of injection, epidural abscess, and meningitis.

ANALYSIS

Objectives

1. Understand the changes of pregnancy and their implications regarding the choice of anesthetic.
2. Appreciate the differences in, and the indications for epidural and spinal anesthesia.
3. Understand complications of regional anesthesia as it relates to pregnancy.

Considerations

This is a healthy 23-year-old woman who presents for a c-section. She has received appropriate prenatal care, and has no other comorbidities. In discussion with the patient regarding the anesthetic plan, the advantages of regional anesthesia are emphasized, and she agrees to a spinal technique with general anesthesia as backup. A large-bore intravenous is placed; since bleeding might occur, the patient is brought to the operating room, and standard ASA monitors are applied. A spinal with bupivacaine is performed uneventfully with the patient in the sitting position, and she is asked to lie supine. Left uterine displacement is achieved by placing a pillow or "bump" under the left hip, to displace the gravid uterus from the aorta and inferior vena cava. This is an important maneuver, since aorto-caval compression is a common cause of decreased venous return and subsequent hypotension, leading to uteroplacental insufficiency.

APPROACH TO Routine Cesarean Section and Local Anesthetic Toxicity

Data suggest that use of general anesthesia with end-tracheal intubation is decreasing across the country, and the preferred anesthetic for an uncomplicated cesarean section is a "single shot" spinal. Commonly known as subarachnoid block (SAB), a spinal anesthetic is a type of neuraxial blockade that involves dural puncture with a small needle, and the injection of a small amount of local anesthetic into the subarachnoid space which contains cerebrospinal fluid. A spinal anesthetic has a quick onset, a limited duration action, and a dense sensory and motor block.

Epidural anesthesia is also a type of neuraxial blockade. It involves using a large needle to enter the epidural space, and then injecting a large volume of a dilute concentration of local anesthetic into the space. The epidural space lies outside the dura, and contains nerve roots, and blood vessels which include Batson venous plexus, engorged in pregnancy and morbid obesity. In considering the engorged venous plexus and the large needle used, an inadvertent intravascular injection of local anesthetic is a common complication of an epidural anesthetic.

An epidural block may be performed as a "single shot," whereby the epidural space is identified, the local anesthetic is injected, and the needle removed. Alternatively, a small-bore catheter can be inserted into the epidural space. This allows the periodic assessment of the adequacy of the block, and the administration of additional doses of local anesthetic once the anesthesia starts to recede. An epidural block has a slower onset, needs a greater volume of drug, and a variable duration since the catheter allows for repeated doses of local anesthetic.

Some of the nerve roots which are anesthetized by the local anesthetic during epidural anesthesia are quite large. Hence, it takes a high concentration and volume of drug, and a long time for the anesthetic to penetrate the nerve fiber and for the block to become effective. Because of this factor, as well as the unpredictable position of the catheter, which is "blindly" threaded, an epidural block is sometimes associated with a "patchy" blockade.

Yet another neuraxial technique is a "spinal/epidural." This block involves a spinal anesthetic followed by placement of an epidural catheter. This type of block has the benefits of quick onset and a dense block, as well as extended duration with the presence of a catheter. It obviously carries risks of both spinal and epidural anesthesia.

CLINICAL APPROACH

The physiologic changes of pregnancy significantly affect and alter the anesthetic plan. These changes occur as a combination of hormonal effects, mechanics of the gravid uterus, increased metabolic and nutritional demands, fetal requirements, and the placental circulation. The salient ones are mentioned below.

Cardiovascular system: There is an increase in plasma volume without an increase in red cell mass resulting in a dilutional anemia. This increased volume results in increased stroke volume and heart rate, with a resultant increase in cardiac output. There is a reduction in peripheral vascular resistance; hence there is no real change in blood pressure to accommodate the increased cardiac output.

Supine hypotension syndrome: Ten percent of parturients develop severe hypotension, and indeed, a shock state in the supine position as a result of vena caval compression by the gravid uterus. This can be avoided by positioning a pillow under the left lower back. This maneuver results in left uterine displacement and the cava is decompressed.

Respiratory system: Pregnancy is associated with an increase in both minute ventilation and work of breathing to accommodate the increased metabolic demands. Hormones, and an increase in carbon dioxide production drives the increased ventilatory demand. As the pregnancy advances, the breathing pattern becomes more diaphragmatic. Closing capacity remains unchanged, but since functional residual capacity is reduced, the small airways are more prone to collapse and atelectasis. This phenomenon manifests under anesthesia as early desaturation during induction of general anesthesia. Parturients should undergo prolonged preoxygenation (3-5 minutes) to counter the effects of small airway collapse resulting in oxygen desaturation.

Changes in the airway: Capillary engorgement of the oropharynx, vocal cords, and the airway mucosa makes tracheal intubation challenging. Minor manipulations of the airway may result in trauma and significant bleeding, producing further airway compromise.

Hematologic changes: Pregnancy induces a hypercoagulable state by increasing most of the clotting factors. An increased risk of deep vein thrombosis and pulmonary embolism result. There is a relative decrease in platelet count in the third trimester due to an increase in platelet activity. Thrombocytopenia is a relative contraindication for performing a neuraxial block.

Gastrointestinal system: There is an increased risk of pulmonary aspiration of gastric contents due to a number of hormonal and mechanical changes of pregnancy. Progesterone decreases the tone of the lower esophageal sphincter, while the gravid uterus decrease the angle of the lesser curvature and labor pain delays gastric emptying. All of these factors increase the risk of aspiration during induction of general anesthesia. All parturients are considered to be strict "full stomachs" no matter when they last ate.

Central nervous system: Pregnant women are more susceptible to the effects of both regional and general anesthetics. This is particularly true for local anesthetics. Less local anesthetic is required than the nonparturient to achieve the same anesthetic level. In addition to hormonal changes which render the parturient more susceptible, the gravid uterus also contributes by compressing the venous plexus in the epidural space. This relative reduction of the epidural space displaces epidural drugs displacement cephalad, resulting in a higher sensory level from a local anesthetic block.

The Fetoplacental Unit

The placenta is composed of intervillous tissue derived from both mother and fetus, which transmits about 80% of the uterine blood flow. Approximately 40% to 50% of the fetal cardiac output traverses the placenta. Hence, changes in uterine blood flow affect fetal circulation. Uterine blood flow lacks autoregulation, so any changes in maternal blood flow are transmitted directly to the fetus. Vasopressors such as α-adrenergic agonists (phenylephrine) cause increased uterine vascular resistance, and reduce uterine blood flow.

Local anesthetics cross membranes, including the uteroplacental membrane, in their ionized form. In the event that they cross into a fetus with acidosis, the local anesthetic becomes ionized from the H^+ circulating in the fetus, and then cannot cross back into the mother to maintain equilibrium. This syndrome is called "ion-trapping," and since local anesthetics also have general anesthetic properties, can result in an exacerbation of fetal distress.

Significant features of other drugs that cross the placenta and cause effects on the fetus are small size, high-lipid solubility, and low protein binding. Maternal drug levels and maternal and fetal pH also play a role in placental drug transfer.

Anesthetic Techniques for Cesarean Section

Table 34–1 presents the effects of neuraxial blockade. Regional anesthetic techniques result in lower circulating drug concentrations in the mother to be potentially transmitted to the fetus. In addition, physiologic changes

Table 34–1 EFFECTS OF NEURAXIAL BLOCKADE

SYSTEM	SPINAL	EPIDURAL
Cardiovascular Sympathectomy resulting in a decreased heart rate and blood pressure	With spinal the sympathectomy extends about 2-6 dermatomes above the level of sensory anesthesia.	With epidural, the sympathectomy is at the same dermatomal level as the sensory anesthesia. Also, the blood pressure drop is more gradual and of less magnitude. It also can be modified by decreasing the dose of the drug.
Respiratory Inspiratory muscles control ventilation while expiratory muscles control cough and clearing of secretions from the lung. Respiratory arrest, while rare, is usually secondary to medullary hypoperfusion rather than muscle paralysis	Decrease in vital capacity with decrease in tidal volume (usually secondary to decreased expiratory reserve volume because of abdominal muscle paralysis).	Similar to spinal, except the level is dose dependent hence can be modified with a catheter in place.
Gastrointestinal	Hyperperistalsis secondary to unopposed vagal activity usually presents as nausea during a SAB.	Protective effect on gastric mucosa in the postoperative stage, as intramucosal pH is higher with epidural than systemic analgesia.
Renal	Urinary retention may need a Foley catheter. Urinary retention usually occurs secondary to paralysis of bladder function. Lower doses of local anesthetic paralyze bladder function, than doses that paralyze lower extremity nerves.	No difference with spinal

are observed in the airway which increase the risk of pulmonary aspiration and difficult intubation. Spinal or epidurals are the most common techniques used for routine c-sections. However, there are well-documented complications of neuraxial blockade.

Post-dural puncture headache is the most common complication of a spinal block. It usually presents 24 hours to 7 days after the spinal has been administered, as a severe headache, positional in nature. Rising to sitting from laying down, or even walking to the bathroom precipitates the headache. It is not associated with signs of infection or photophobia. PDPH may be very painful. Supportive management such as hydration and bed rest helps in mild cases of PDPH. Adjuvant therapies such as caffeine and painkillers have met with varying degrees of success.

For severe cases of PDPH, a blood patch has been recommended. One hypothesis for mechanism of pain in PDPH is a continuous leakage of cerebrospinal fluid from the subarachnoid space, worsened by rising from a supine position. The blood patch uses autologous blood from a sterile venipuncture to supposedly seal off the puncture site by forming a clot. This is accomplished by epidural puncture and injecting the autologous blood. Reports have credited the blood patch with 96% success in the sure of PDPH. However, this technique remains controversial within the pain management community, since no outcome studies have been conducted to assess the true risks of this procedure.

Nerve injury is an uncommon complication of neuraxial blockade. The incidence of injury increases if the patient experiences an "electric shock" like pain during spinal or epidural place. This pain signals intraneural needle placement which could lead to nerve injury. If intraneural injection occurs, then the needle must be promptly removed and the patient questioned about continued pain. The neural injury often results in a transient paresthesia lasting up to several months, at the area of distribution of the nerve. Regrowth of the nerve results in recovery. Long-term nerve damage is very rare.

In the laboring patient under neuraxial blockade, there is no painful feedback from the possible overstretching of lumbar muscles which maybe implicated in the occurrence of back pain after spinal or epidural anesthesia. Although back pain is not uncommon, there have no reports of anatomic causes of back pain or lower back injury after neuraxial blockade.

Local anesthetic (LA) toxicity may manifest as central nervous system (CNS) or cardiovascular system (CVS) complications, usually related to an overdose of LA. Cardiovascular complications, particularly hypotension or bradycardia, are often the only manifestation of severe local anesthetic toxicity, and can even occur an hour or more after injection. In addition to progressive hypotension, bradycardia can lead to asystole. Ventricular ectopy, multiform ventricular tachycardia, and ventricular fibrillation are also indicative of cardiotoxic injury.

CNS symptoms usually lag behind CVS complications, and are often subtle at onset or absent. CNS excitation (agitation, confusion, twitching, seizure), depression (drowsiness, obtundation, coma, or apnea), or nonspecific neurologic symptoms (metallic taste, circumoral paresthesias, diplopia, tinnitus, dizziness) are each typical of LA toxicity.

An intravascular injection may present with nonspecific signs such as a metallic taste or tinnitus, and is unrelated to the dose of local anesthetic. However, if undetected, an intravascular injection can lead to the CNS and CVS complications described earlier. Indeed, to facilitate the diagnosis of possible intravascular injection with epidural, epinephrine is often added to the local anesthetic test dose. If the test does is associated with tachycardia, the injection is aborted.

Should a bloody tap or an intravascular injection occur with spinal or epidural injection, the injection should be aborted and the procedure repeated at another interspace. If these complications occur, treatment is supportive, and includes airway management and resuscitation. The arrhythmias or seizures should be treated pharmacologically as indicated.

A subdural injection of local anesthetic, or a "high" or "total" spinal is detected by the sudden, unexpected loss of consciousness, apnea, and cardiovascular collapse, sometimes accompanied by seizures. Treatment is supportive.

Comprehension Questions

34.1. A 22-year-old patient presents to the OB suite for a vaginal delivery and is interested in labor analgesia. She wants to know possible complications of a labor epidural. She claims her cousin had a labor epidural and now has long-term back pain and wants to know if she is likely to experience the same type of back injury. Back pain following an epidural is most likely due to which of the following?

A. Direct result of injury to a nerve by the needle
B. Can portend impending paralysis
C. Results from an inadvertent stretching of muscles
D. Long lasting, as experienced by her cousin

34.2. During injection of local anesthetic in the epidural space, the patient loses consciousness. You suspect which of the following?

A. Vagal reaction
B. Drug overdose
C. Subdural injection
D. Dehydration

34.3. A 28-year-old woman is wheeled into the operating room for a c-section, and placed on the operating room table. As monitors are placed, her blood pressure is 68/40 and she reports feeling dizzy. You first response is which of the following?

A. Left uterine displacement
B. Fluid administration
C. Pressor administration
D. Oxygen by nasal cannula

ANSWERS

34.1. **A.** Back pain is associated with but not caused by neuraxial blockade. A laboring patient who is free from labor pains due to a neuraxial blockade is likely to stretch muscles, leading to back pain. There is small incidence of nerve injury associated with neuraxial blockade. It usually manifests as paresthesia over the region of nerve supply, is usually temporary in duration, and may last as long as 3 months. Nerve regrowth usually causes cessation of symptoms. Paralysis is a complication of spinal cord injury, site of neuraxial blockade for labor analgesia or for c-section is at L3 to L4 level. The spinal cord ends at L1 in adults and cord injury is rare.

34.2. **C.** Subdural injection of the local anesthetic causing a total spinal with loss of consciousness. The treatment is supportive.

34.3. **A.** The hypotension is almost certainly caused by aorto-caval syndrome, secondary to compression of the aorta and/or inferior vena cava by the gravid uterus. Once left uterine displacement is performed, there is decompression and resumption of venous return and resolution of the hypotension. If the patient had recently received a local anesthetic bolus via a spinal or epidural injection, vasodilatation from the local anesthetic maybe implicated in the cause of hypotension.

Clinical Pearls

- Left uterine displacement relieves inferior vena caval and/or aortic compression and restores venous return and establishes maternal and fetal perfusion.
- General anesthesia is associated with significant maternal morbidity such as failed airway management, aspiration, inadequate ventilation, and a lower Apgar score in the fetus.
- Spinal or epidural anesthesia is the preferred anesthetic technique for caesarian section with few complications to the fetus.
- The gravid uterus causes epidural venous congestion, which may increase the spread of local anesthetic, hence drug dosing needs to be adjusted appropriately.
- Hypotension associated with neuraxial techniques can be avoided with fluid replacement and careful dosing of local anesthetic.

REFERENCES

Anesthesia for obstetrics. In: Miller RD. *Miller's Anesthesia.* 6th ed. Churchill Livingstone; 2005:Chapter 58.

Chestnut DH. Obstetric Anesthesia—Principles and Practice. 3rd ed. Elselvier Mosby.

Case 35

A 40-year-old G_3P_{2002} woman, at $38^3/_7$ weeks' gestation, was admitted in early labor. During her prenatal course, she had been diagnosed with pregnancy-induced hypertension (PIH). On admission, her BP was 155/96 mm Hg, HR 110 beats/minute (bpm), and she had +2 pedal edema. Her hemoglobin was 9.8 g/dL, platelet count was 117, 000/mm^3, and urinalysis showed 2+ proteinuria. Her laboratory tests were otherwise normal. She was started on infusions of oxytocin and magnesium.

Shortly after admission, the patient complained of a headache. Her blood pressure was noted to be 166/101 mm Hg, signs of fetal distress were noted on the monitor, and the anesthesiologist was notified of the urgent cesarean section. As the operating room team was being mobilized, the obstetrician noticed an acute change in the patient's mental status, followed shortly thereafter by a tonic-clonic seizure.

- ➤ What are the pathophysiological alterations in preeclampsia and their implications on the anesthesia for cesarean section?
- ➤ What anesthetic modalities are utilized for emergency cesarean section in PIH?
- ➤ What are the effects of the anesthetic management on PIH?

ANSWERS TO CASE 35: Pregnant Patient with Eclampsia for Emergency Cesarean Section

Summary: A 40-year-old G_3P_{2002} woman at $38^3/_7$ weeks' gestation with severe PIH and seizure requires emergency cesarean section.

- **Pathophysiological alterations with preeclampsia:** Preeclampsia can present with elevated blood pressure, proteinuria, pulmonary edema, elevated liver function tests, thrombocytopenia, and neurologic dysfunction, including seizures. These alterations may have significant impact on the anesthetic plan.
- **Anesthetic modalities in cesarean:** General and neuraxial regional anesthesia may be used for cesarean section in PIH. The choice of anesthetic technique depends on the specific patient presentation and the severity of the organ system dysfunction.
- **Effects of anesthesia:** Use of general anesthesia may be associated with rapid swings in blood pressure during airway manipulation. Additionally, the incidence of difficult airway is increased in the presence of both pregnancy and exacerbated by PIH. Use of neuraxial blockade in the presence of thrombocytopenia may be associated with epidural hematoma and neurological complications of the hematoma.

ANALYSIS

Objectives

1. Understand the pathophysiology and the clinical presentation of PIH.
2. Understand the implications of eclampsia and preeclampsia for the anesthesia management.
3. Identify the benefits and risks of general and regional anesthesia for emergency cesarean section and develop a plan for anesthesia and intraoperative monitoring.
4. Manage the perioperative complications during cesarean section of a patient with eclampsia.

Considerations

This patient's BP is well controlled with a signal agent (magnesium). Her laboratory results do not show evidence of end-organ damage which could result from her chronically elevated blood pressure. But the onset of seizures with loss of consciousness on day of presentation makes this an emergent situation requiring immediate c-section.

Given, the emergent nature of the procedure, general anesthesia with rapid-sequence intubation is the anesthetic of choice. Nevertheless, an exaggerated hypertensive response to laryngoscopy, and/or to the administration of exogenous vasopressors should be anticipated. The airway changes in pregnancy are further compounded by PIH and edema, and may result in difficulty at intubation. The patient's intravascular volume could be normal, or even markedly reduced from chronic vasoconstriction, further contributing to the considerable hemodynamic lability. Intravenous (i.v.) fluids should be administered judiciously to avoid the risks of fluid overload, congestive heart failure, and even pulmonary edema. Magnesium and beta-blockers, treatments for PIH, add to the risk of heart failure. She is receiving the definitive treatment for PIH, which is delivery of the fetus.

APPROACH TO Pregnant Patient with Eclampsia

DEFINITIONS

PIH: It includes a spectrum of disorders from isolated hypertension to hypertension associated with multiorgan dysfunction (preeclampsia) and seizures (eclampsia).

HELLP SYNDROME: It is a severe form of preeclampsia that includes *h*emolysis, *e*levated *l*iver enzymes and *l*ow *p*latelet count.

CLINICAL APPROACH

The management of PIH is individualized, and depends on the severity of the disease. Treatments range from medical treatment until the delivery for mild disease, to cesarean section for patients with major maternal complications and fetal distress. Thrombocytopenia is the most notable hematologic abnormality in PIH, increasing the risk of bleeding and thus hematoma with a neuraxial block. Thrombocytopenia in the range of 80,000 to 100,000/mm^3 does not appear to significantly increase the bleeding risk with regional anesthesia. The hypercoagulable state associated with PIH is usually less clinically significant.

Hepatic dysfunction marked by abnormal liver function can alter the clearance of anesthetic drugs. Renal dysfunction correlates with the severity of PIH. It is marked by proteinuria and oliguria and can progress to renal failure. Neurologic complications can range from visual disturbances and headache to seizures, coma, and cerebral hemorrhage. The first-line treatment is magnesium, usually administered by infusion to raise the seizure threshold. Benzodiazepines and barbiturates, particularly sodium thiopental, are used to treat seizures if they occur.

Neuraxial anesthesia is preferred in the absence of significant thrombocytopenia or coagulopathy. Neuraxial anesthesia produces a sympathectomy, with resultant drop in blood pressure. Of the neuraxial techniques, epidural anesthesia produces a more gradual sympathectomy in contrast with a subarachnoid block, useful for the judicious titration of fluids. Early epidural placement in high-risk patients provides labor analgesia thus attenuating the BP increases that occur with painful contractions, and may be used in case of an emergency cesarean section as well. However, if coagulopathies exist or are likely to develop, an epidural may not be the best choice because of the size of the needle used in the setting of engorged epidural veins. The benefits of spinal anesthesia at delivery include faster placement, more reliable blockade, and less epidural vascular trauma. Fluid administration is individualized according to the patient's needs. It can be tempting to administer fluids excessively to sympathectomized patients, since the sympathectomy increases the circulating blood volume. But excessive fluid administration can easily result in pulmonary edema.

Indications for general anesthesia include coagulopathy, hemorrhage, sepsis, or the presence of cardiovascular disorders, in which an acute reduction in the blood pressure (from sympathectomy) is detrimental. In the setting of eclampsia, general anesthesia provides control of the airway, ventilation, and seizure activity. The airway management in a patient with PIH requires careful planning and a backup intubation plan. The airway difficulties associated with pregnancy are exaggerated due to upper airway and laryngeal edema, while the coexisting coagulopathy makes the airway more friable. An awake fiberoptic intubation may provide a safer option in certain cases. Pregnancy also renders the patient at higher risk for aspiration of gastric contents during induction of general anesthesia. The need for aspiration prophylaxis should be evaluated.

The anesthetic plan must address the issue of the wide swings in BP that occur at intubation, delivery of the infant, and at emergence from general anesthesia. Magnesium, used to treat PIH, also affects anesthetic management. It causes skeletal muscle weakness, as well as potentiating the effects of the depolarizing and nondepolarizing muscle relaxants and prolonging their duration. Therefore, use of lower doses and close monitoring of muscle relaxants is indicated.

The anesthesiologist may be called for an emergency intubation to control the airway if the patient has a seizure. In this setting, sodium thiopental is the treatment of choice. It is important to remember that the goal of any treatment is to terminate the seizure. The administration of nondepolarizing muscle relaxants should be avoided, since they are longer acting, and they prevent the evaluation of reflexes, and the diagnosis of seizures should they occur.

The maintenance of anesthesia is typically achieved with a low dose of volatile anesthetic and nitrous oxide, to avoid fetal respiratory depression. Higher doses of anesthetics and supplemental opiates may be used after the fetus is delivered. Oxytocin, needed to achieve adequate uterine contraction, may also result in elevation in the blood pressure. In severe cases, invasive arterial blood pressure and central venous pressure monitoring may be indicated to guide hemodynamic control and fluid management. Prior to extubation, consideration must be given to the possibilities of persistent airway edema, blood pressure control, and the potential prolongation of the patient's neuromuscular blockade.

Comprehension Questions

35.1. A 19-year-old G_1P_0 at $39^1/_7$ estimated gestational age (EGA) is transferred from the obstetric clinic to labor and delivery with PIH for labor induction. She has no contraindication to regional anesthesia. Which of the following statements regarding the anesthesia management is accurate?

A. Platelet count should be obtained before neuraxial anesthesia is considered.
B. General anesthesia for cesarean delivery has fewer risks and is the safest option for her.
C. Her condition is likely to effect the medications used for anesthesia.
D. A vagal response to direct laryngoscopy and intubation may be encountered.

35.2. A 38-year-old G_3P_{2002} at 38 EGA is admitted in early labor. Her weight is 78 kg. BP is noted to be 151/94 and 160/96 mm Hg on two separate occasions, 6 hours apart. Mild proteinuria is noted. Which of the following is correct?

A. The seizures associated with eclampsia should be treated with magnesium only.
B. Airway difficulty is unlikely since she is not very obese.
C. Large fluid bolus should be given prior to performing regional anesthesia.
D. Platelet count of 100,000/mm^3 is not a contraindication to regional anesthesia.

35.3. A 35-year-old G_4P_2 woman at $37^1/_7$ EGA was diagnosed with severe PIH. She is treated with magnesium infusion and labor induction is started. She is noted to have acute mental status changes, followed by a seizure, and an abrupt decrease in her O_2 saturation to 85%. Which of the following is the most likely reason for her hypoxia?

A. Pulmonary edema
B. Upper airway obstruction
C. Pneumothorax
D. Pulmonary aspiration

ANSWERS

35.1. **A.** A platelet count should be obtained prior to the administration of a neuraxial block. In the absence of coagulopathy or other contraindications, regional anesthesia such as an epidural or subarachnoid block is a safer option. General anesthesia carries risks related to difficult airway management, aspiration, hemodynamic instability, prolonged drug action, and fetal depression. While the patient's condition per se does not affect the anesthetic drugs used for a general anesthetic, magnesium, which she may receive for PIH, does effect the duration of action of muscle relaxants.

35.2. **D.** A platelet count of 50,000/mm^3 (not 100,000/mm^3) represents significant thrombocytopenia, and is a contraindication to regional anesthesia. However, mild thrombocytopenia does not significantly increase the risk of bleeding with regional anesthesia. While magnesium is the drug of choice for prevention and treatment of eclampsia, other antiepileptic medications such as benzodiazepines and barbiturates may be needed to control an eclamptic seizure. Airway difficulty in pregnant women is related to multiple factors and can be exaggerated in PIH due to increased laryngeal edema. Fluid bolus prior to regional anesthesia in PIH should be determined by a patient's specific hemodynamics and given cautiously to avoid pulmonary edema.

35.3. **B.** Given the *abrupt* reduction in her SaO_2, the most likely diagnosis in this postictal patient is upper airway obstruction, which should be treated with an elevation of the mandible while oxygen is administered. Airway edema, pulmonary edema, and aspiration are all also possible causes of hypoxemia associated with eclampsia. However, the sudden desaturation makes them less likely. Spontaneous pneumothorax is much less likely in this patient.

Clinical Pearls

- In the setting of PIH, hemodynamic instability can occur with general or regional anesthesia.
- Patients typically have a significantly reduced circulating blood volume, despite the presence of pedal edema.
- Pulmonary and laryngeal edema can lead to difficult airway management and respiratory failure.
- In the absence of a coagulopathy, a regional technique is the anesthetic of choice.
- Magnesium causes muscle weakness, and prolongs the action of nondepolarizing neuromuscular blockers.
- A seizure, if it occurs, is treated with benzodiazepines and barbiturates, particularly sodium thiopental.

REFERENCES

Karumanchi SA, Lindheimer MD. Advances in the understanding of eclampsia. *Curr Hypertens Rep*. 2008;10(4):305-312.

Mandal NG, Surapaneni S. Regional anaesthesia in pre-eclampsia: advantages and disadvantages. *Drugs*. 2004;64(3):223-236.

Ramanathan J, Bennett K. Pre-eclampsia: fluids, drugs, and anesthetic management. *Anesthesiol Clin North Am*. 2003;21(1):145-163.

Tihtonen K, Kööbi T, Yli-Hankala A, Huhtala H, Uotila J. Maternal haemodynamics in pre-eclampsia compared with normal pregnancy during caesarean delivery. *BJOG*. 2006;113(6):657-663

Case 36

A 34-year-old woman (G_3P_2), 34 weeks' gestation, presents to the emergency room with a 1-day history of worsening abdominal tenderness and some dark red vaginal bleeding. She has a past medical history of smoking (15-pack-year), and sinusitis. Her prior pregnancies went to term with uneventful deliveries. She has no other significant past medical history. The patient last ate 2 hours ago. Her meal included a cheeseburger and fries with a caffeinated soda.

The patient's physical examination is remarkable for some anxiety, and significant uterine tenderness. Vital signs show a blood pressure of 99/38 mm Hg and a heart rate of 109 beats/minute (bpm). The fetal heart rate varies between 165 and 175 bpm (normal 120-160 bpm). Laboratory findings reveal a hemoglobin concentration of 9.8 g/dL, a hematocrit of 27.1%, a platelet count of 102,000/ L, and a fibrinogen level of 154 mg/dL. An urgent sonogram was obtained, and showed an anterior placenta previa, and could not rule out placental abruption. The patient is scheduled for an urgent, emergency cesarean section.

- ➤ What are the anesthetic considerations for this patient?
- ➤ What is the anesthetic of choice for this procedure and why?
- ➤ What are the complications that accompany abruptio placenta?

ANSWERS TO CASE 36: Placental Abruption

Summary: This is a 34-year-old woman, G_3P_2, at 34 weeks' gestation, with clinical signs of placental abruption.

- **Anesthetic considerations:** This patient presents for emergent surgery in the face of under-resuscitated hypovolemic shock, fetal distress, and imminent coagulopathy. Considering the nature of presentation, she has probably not observed fasting guidelines for surgery and should be considered to have a full stomach.
- **Anesthetic route of choice:** Given the emergent nature of presentation, the possibility of coagulopathy, and likelihood of massive blood loss, a general anesthesia is indicated for this case.
- **Complications of placental abruption:** Include hemorrhage, undiagnosed hypovolemia, a coagulopathy from DIC or massive blood loss, and the risks posed by factors associated with placental abruption such as pregnancy-induced hypertension and smoking.

ANALYSIS

Objectives

1. Understand pathophysiology of and major risk factors for abruption placenta.
2. Understand the risks and benefits of the different anesthetic approaches to the disorder.
3. Understand possible complications associated with placental abruption and urgent surgery.

Considerations

This patient presents with the diagnosis of placenta previa with possible imminent abruption. She has signs of hypovolemia, consumptive coagulopathy and fetal distress. This situation requires an emergent cesarean section to deliver the fetus, which is showing signs of distress. Given the signs of hypovolemia, the patient should receive immediate and aggressive fluid resuscitation. The availability of blood and blood products should be ensured, given the risk of massive blood loss. Because of the risk of DIC that accompanies placental abruption, as well as the dilutional coagulopathy that can accompany massive transfusion, general anesthesia with rapid-sequence induction and cricoid pressure is the anesthetic of choice.

Two large-bore peripheral intravenous access sites are secured and fluid resuscitation is initiated while ensuring that a sample of the patient's blood is sent for typing and screening. A urethral catheter (Foley) is placed for assessment of adequacy of fluid resuscitation. The patient should be promptly transferred to the operating room where she is positioned supine with a left hip tilt. This enables uterine displacement from the aorta and vena cava and relieves aorto-caval compression and decreased venous return. Standard monitors (for noninvasive blood pressure measurement, pulse oximetry, and 5-lead ECG display) are applied and preoxygenation is begun.

The patient is requested to take a few vital capacity breaths of 100% oxygen over the next several minutes. A hypnotic, such as etomidate, and a short-acting muscle-relaxing agent are administered in succession while an assistant holds cricoid pressure. Once muscle relaxation is confirmed, direct laryngoscopy and endotracheal intubation are performed, an endotracheal tube is placed, and its position verified with bilateral chest auscultation and presence of end-tidal CO_2. Cricoid pressure is then released, the endotracheal tube is secured, and surgery can proceed.

After delivery of the fetus, it is appropriate to administer narcotics, and an oxytocin infusion is begun to enable uterine contraction. The decision to transfuse blood and blood products is dictated by surgical blood loss, hemoglobin values, and evidence of hemodynamic instability. Depending on the site of the placental attachment, the patient may be prone to uterine atony and continued hemorrhage. Additional doses of oxytocin may be required, in addition to other contractile agents such as methylergonovine. In the rare case of refractory uterine atony and hemorrhage, a hysterectomy may be required.

As the case progresses, an arterial catheter placement may be considered to allow for quick assessment of hemoglobin and accurate hemodynamic monitoring. But in practicality, given the emergent nature of the case and the tasks that accompany transfusion, there is often simply no time for its insertion.

APPROACH TO The Patient with Placental Abruption

An abruptio placenta is the separation of a normally implanted placenta from the deciduas basalis of the uterus prior to delivery of the fetus. It occurs at an incidence of 0.42%. The risk factors associated with placental abruption include drug, alcohol, and cigarette abuse by the mother, peripartum hypertension, and placenta previa. Prenatal care plays an important role in anticipating the presentation of placental abruption.

Hypovolemia is frequently underdiagnosed and undertreated at the time of presentation to the operating room. The extent of the patient's bleeding is not necessarily evident, since some (or most) of it may remain trapped in the uterus. Once the fetus is delivered, the extent and severity of hypovolemia may well be unmasked. Active and aggressive resuscitation should be undertaken early in the course of the patient's treatment, and prior to incision so that the degree of hypovolemia may be abated. Prolonged hypotension can precipitate end-organ dysfunction.

Along with being a risk factor for abruptio placentae, smoking causes other problems in the patient requiring general anesthesia. These include bronchospasm with endotracheal intubation, increased airway mucus production, and postoperative pulmonary complications.

Disseminated intravascular coagulation (DIC) is a risk in patients with placental abruption, and may be a source of ongoing bleeding. The longer the time between the onset of bleeding and diagnosis, the longer the generation of inflammatory mediators, and the worse the DIC. DIC is associated with a falling fibrinogen level and a rising d-dimer level. Hemostasis and various blood products are used to treat the coagulopathy. Blood and blood product transfusions are guided by the regular evaluation of coagulation status, although blood products carry a risk of complications including infection, transfusion reaction, hemolysis, and acute transfusion-related lung injury.

Fetal distress is often a marker for abruption reflecting placental blood loss and poor oxygen delivery to the fetus. This calls for immediate delivery of the fetus by surgical means.

Amniotic fluid embolism is also a potential complication of placental abruption. This is a major risk, since the open maternal vessels at the deciduas basalis can absorb amniotic fluid, which can subsequently embolize in the systemic circulation. Amniotic fluid embolus usually manifests with severe maternal hypotension and hypoxia. The treatment is largely supportive, and includes airway management, mechanical ventilation, and blood pressure control with vasoactive drugs. Nevertheless, this is often a disastrous complication.

Feto-maternal transfusion is another risk in placental abruption. Special consideration is given to Rhesus-negative parturients in this situation. Prophylactic administration of Rhogam should be considered in the setting of placental abruption.

The risk of worsening hypovolemia, consumptive coagulopathy, and fetal distress make delivery by c-section an emergency. Given the emergent surgery and coagulopathy, regional anesthesia is contraindicated. Furthermore, the sympathectomy caused by regional anesthesia can significantly exaggerate any preexisting hypotension, making its correction more difficult. Similarly, the worsening coagulopathy can lead to epidural bleeding and epidural hematoma formation, and thus neurological complications.

There is only one choice of anesthetic technique for this operation: general anesthetic with rapid-sequence induction (local anesthesia is also a distant possibility). As with all cases involving pregnancy, there is a higher incidence of difficult intubation. In addition, changes in maternal physiology cause delayed gastric emptying hence making pulmonary aspiration of gastric contents a very real possibility.

Comprehension Questions

36.1. A 32-year-old woman at 34 weeks' gestation comes into the obstetrical unit for vaginal bleeding. The suspicion is placental abruption. Besides smoking and trauma, which of the following is the most significant risk factor for abruption?

A. Obesity
B. Preeclampsia
C. Prior cesarean
D. Diabetes mellitus

36.2. A 24-year-old G_1P_0 woman at 29 weeks' gestation is noted to have bright red vaginal bleeding. Her uterus is firm and tender. The BP is 140/90 mm Hg and HR 100 bpm. No fetal heart tones are able to be obtained, and ultrasound identifies fetal bradycardia in the range of 70 bpm. Which of the following is the most important anesthetic consideration in the surgical management of this patient?

A. Hypertension
B. Disseminated intravascular coagulopathy
C. Hypervolemia
D. An indication for regional anesthesia

ANSWERS

36.1. **B.** Hypertension, maternal smoking, drug, cocaine use and alcohol abuse, and placenta previa are risk factors associated with placental abruption. Obesity, diabetes, or prior cesarean delivery are not risks factor for placental abruption.

36.2. **B.** DIC. A bleeding diathesis, the presence of hemodynamic instability including hypotension (not hypertension), and inadequate volume resuscitation (hypovolemia) complicate any anesthetic. General anesthesia is required for an emergent c-section. Even in small doses, general anesthetics cause vasodilatation, and thus exacerbate any preexisting hypovolemia and hypotension. Aggressive volume resuscitation should be begun preemptively in the case of suspected abruption since bleeding is expected when the fetus is delivered and the uterine tamponade is relieved.

Clinical Pearls

- An increased maternal age, multiparity, cigarette smoking, cocaine use during pregnancy, and hypertension are amongst the highest risk factors for placental abruption.
- Anesthetic management involves adequate, large-bore intravenous access, restoration of intravascular blood volume, and correction of coagulopathy as appropriate.
- General anesthesia with tracheal intubation is indicated in patients with placental abruption.

REFERENCES

Ananth CV, Smulian JC, Srinivas N, et al. Placental abruption and perinatal mortality in the United States. *Am J Epidemiol.* 2001;153;332-337.

Oyelese Y, Ananth CV, Yeo L, et al. Placental abruption. *Obstet Gynecol.* Oct 2006; 108:1005-1016.

Sheiner E, Shoham-Vardi I, Hallak M, et al. Placental abruption in term pregnancy; clinical signs and obstetric risk factors. *J Maternal-Fetal and Neonatal Med.* Jan 2003;13:45-49.

Pediatric Patients

Case 37

A 3-year-old otherwise healthy girl is brought to her pediatrician because her parents notice that her eyes do not line up in parallel. She is referred to an ophthalmologist, who confirms that the visual axes of her eyes are indeed not parallel, and that her vision is impaired in the right eye (amblyopia). She is diagnosed with strabismus, which requires surgical repair. The patient's medical history is otherwise unremarkable. Her childhood vaccines are up-to-date, and she is not allergic to any medications. Her parents are young, and have never had surgery with the exception of the mother's receiving an epidural for delivery. She is scheduled for outpatient surgery, and arrives to the surgical suite after appropriately observing preoperative fasting guidelines.

- ➤ What are the anesthetic considerations in a pediatric patient undergoing surgical correction of strabismus?
- ➤ How can an appropriate anesthetic plan either prevent, or treat each of the above?

ANSWERS TO CASE 37: Strabismus Surgery

Summary: A 3-year-old girl presents for outpatient strabismus surgery.

- **Anesthetic considerations:** For a pediatric patient undergoing strabismus repair, the anesthetic considerations include stimulation of the oculocardiac reflex, the likelihood of postoperative nausea and vomiting, and the coexistence of malignant hyperthermia with muscle dystrophies, some of which may cause strabismus.

- **Appropriate anesthetic plan:** The treatment for oculocardiac reflex is to cease the exciting stimulus, and to use atropine if severe bradycardia persists. Postoperative nausea and vomiting is prevented by the prophylactic administration of antiemetics in combination. In addition, this patient's anesthetic must include a careful family history, as well as efforts to reduce the risk of malignant hyperthermia (MH) by avoiding triggering agents insofar as possible, and the ready availability of dantrolene sodium in preparation for its possible occurrence.

ANALYSIS

Objectives

1. Become familiar with the anesthetic issues that may be encountered during strabismus surgery.
2. Understand the oculocardiac reflex, the use of prophylactic medication, and its treatment should it occur.
3. Understand the etiology, triggering agents, and treatment for malignant hyperthermia.
4. Develop a plan of prevention and treatment of postoperative nausea and vomiting in the pediatric patient.

Considerations

This young patient has strabismus sufficiently severe as to require a surgical correction. She has no other comorbidities. However, it is possible that her strabismus may be caused by an underlying myopathy, which may place her at increased risk to MH. Strabismus surgery itself can present challenges to the anesthesiologist. Traction on the extraocular muscles can excite the oculocardiac reflex, which is associated with potentially serious cardiac dysrhythmias. Atropine or glycopyrrolate should be prepared, and the dose for this patient (given her size) determined before the case begins. Strabismus surgery also predisposes a patient to postoperative nausea and vomiting. Prevention by prophylactic medications and preparation for treatment are important aspects of the anesthetic plan.

APPROACH TO Strabismus Surgery

DEFINITIONS

STRABISMUS: A condition in which the visual axes of the eyes are not parallel and the eyes appear to be looking in different directions. Strabismus can lead to amblyopia in one eye, a form of blindness.

MALIGNANT HYPERTHERMIA: A hypermetabolic state that includes severe prolonged muscle contractions and a rapid rise in body temperature (up to or above 105°F). Susceptible patients carry an autosomal dominant gene, which has variable penetrance. The disease is caused by exposure to triggering agents (see Table 37–1).

OCULOCARDIAC REFLEX: A reflex reaction to pressure on the globe of the eye or to traction on the extraocular eye muscles that results in cardiac dysrhythmias, most commonly sinus bradycardia.

Table 37–1 ANESTHETIC MEDICATIONS AND MALIGNANT HYPERTHERMIA

TRIGGERING AGENTS	SAFE AGENTS
Succinylcholine *All volatile anesthetic agents*: Isoflurane Desflurane Sevoflurane	N_2O Benzodiazepines Propofol, etomidate, pentothal Ketamine Narcotics Local anesthetics Nondepolarizing muscle relaxants

CLINICAL APPROACH

A child arriving to the operating room for correction of strabismus presents a set of challenges for the anesthesiologist. Two of these challenges are related to the surgery itself, and the third, to the patient population in which the surgery is required.

Traction on the extraocular muscles and/or pressure on the eye can elicit the oculocardiac reflex (OCR), which can result in severe bradycardia as well as other cardiac dysrhythmias. The OCR is initiated by an afferent signal traveling along the ophthalmologic division of the trigeminal nerve to the trigeminal's sensory nucleus. Then an efferent signal travels via the vagus nerve to the heart, initiating dysrhythmias. The most common dysrhythmia is sinus bradycardia which can be severe, although a wide variety of dysrhythmias have been reported. The treatment for the OCR is to *stop the surgical stimulus*. This treatment is usually sufficient, and the heart rhythm typically returns to normal. However, if bradycardia (or other dysrhythmia) persists, atropine or another antiarrhythmic drug can be given. Since children have greater vagal tone than adults, some surgery centers routinely administer atropine prophylactically to prevent this complication.

Patients undergoing strabismus repair are also likely to experience postoperative nausea and vomiting. Traction on the extraocular muscles and or pressure on the eye is hypothesized to cause this unpleasant complication. Because the incidence of vomiting after strabismus surgery is so high (>67%), it is appropriate to treat patients undergoing strabismus repair prophylactically to prevent this response. Dexamethasone and the HT_3 antagonists such as ondansetron are the most effective prophylactic medications and should be given to all patients undergoing strabismus repair, as well as patients who have experienced postoperative nausea and vomiting following previous anesthetics. The combined use of these drugs has been shown to be more effective than either given alone, and can reduce the incidence of PONV to less than 20%.

Finally, some experts believe that children undergoing strabismus repair are at an increased risk for MH, a potentially fatal complication of exposure to some anesthetics (see Table 37–1). The incidence of MH is 1 in 15,000 anesthetics in children, and 1 in 50,000 anesthetics in adults. Every anesthesiologist needs to watch vigilantly for signs of MH in every patient, and be prepared to treat it at any time with every anesthetic given (see Table 37–2). ECG, end tidal CO_2 levels, and patient temperature are always monitored continuously.

Patients susceptible to MH carry an autosomal dominant genetic mutation leading to faulty calcium reuptake in muscle cells. This failed mechanism results in prolonged muscle contraction, rhabdomyolysis, and a dramatically increased metabolic rate. The mutation is most often silent until the patient is exposed to a triggering agent. Since patients diagnosed with a myopathy may be at an increased risk of carrying this mutation, the safest anesthetic plan is to avoid the use of all triggering agents in this setting. However it

Table 37–2 DIAGNOSIS AND TREATMENT OF MALIGNANT HYPERTHERMIA

SIGNS OF MALIGNANT HYPERTHERMIA	TREATMENT OF MALIGNANT HYPERTHERMIA
Increasing carbon dioxide production	Discontinue use of the triggering agent and stop surgery as soon as possible.
Hyperthermia (up to 2°C [35.6°F] per hour)	Apply a cooling blanket to the patient.
Rhabdomyolysis	Give intravenous fluids to maintain kidney function.
Muscle rigidity	Give dantrolene, a medication that decreases the release of calcium from the sarcoplasmic reticulum.
Increased oxygen consumption	

should be stated that the connection between strabismus and an underlying myopathy (and hence a propensity for MH) is controversial and many practitioners will not avoid triggering agents unless a family history suggests a genetic problem with anesthesia.

Succinylcholine is a depolarizing neuromuscular blocking agent that is usually avoided in young strabismus patients. First, succinylcholine is, in general, avoided in children. It has been associated with unpredictable and intractable cardiac arrest in apparently healthy children. Many of these children were ultimately shown to have an undiagnosed myopathy, as many of these diseases are not clinically apparent until past the first decade of life. Succinylcholine could cause a rapid and dangerous rise in serum potassium, causing cardiac dysrhythmias and even cardiac arrest. Second, in patients undergoing strabismus repair, succinylcholine can interfere with the surgeon's forced duction test (to evaluate muscle tone) for up to 15 minutes. Third, given the possibility that the strabismus might be associated with a myopathy, some would avoid succinylcholine in the setting of strabismus repair out of concern that it is a triggering agent for MH.

Most children scheduled for strabismus surgery are apparently otherwise healthy. Nevertheless, they are at increased risk of two serious complications: the oculocardiac reflex and malignant hyperthermia. Moreover, the likelihood that these patients will vomit warrants prophylaxis with antiemetic drugs. These factors necessitate that the anesthesiologist plan the anesthetic carefully and have a heightened awareness of potential known adverse events associated with this operation.

Comprehension Questions

37.1. A 2-year-old boy is having correction of ptosis of the right eyelid. The patient is stable during induction of anesthesia, but his heart rate drops to 50 bpm soon after the surgical incision. Which of the following is your first step in treating this patient?

A. Do nothing; his heart rate is in the normal range.
B. Give intravenous atropine.
C. Tell the surgeon to stop what he is doing.
D. Give intravenous fluids.

37.2. A 10-year-old boy requires repair of an inguinal hernia. He has no other health-related issues and has no surgical history. When asked about the surgical history of family members, his mother states she has never had surgery, but her brother (his uncle) died unexpectedly during surgery for a broken arm at age 12. Which of the following should be included in your anesthetic plan?

A. Not include the use of succinylcholine or volatile anesthetics
B. Not be altered by this information
C. Include prophylactic dosing of dantrolene
D. Include prophylactic dosing of acetaminophen

37.3. A 5-year-old girl has a history of repetitive vomiting after strabismus surgery when she was 3 years old. She is now scheduled for treatment of multiple dental caries under general anesthesia. This type of surgery is not associated with a high incidence of postoperative nausea and vomiting. Anesthesia for this young girl should include which of the following?

A. Intraoperative ondansetron for nausea and vomiting prophylaxis.
B. No prophylaxis for postoperative nausea and vomiting; this surgery doesn't cause nausea and vomiting.
C. Intraoperative dexamethasone and ondansetron for prophylaxis.
D. No general anesthesia, the patient should have her dental caries repaired under local anesthesia.

ANSWERS

37.1. **C.** The patient is having a vagal response to something the surgeon is doing on or around his eye. The first step in treating his bradycardia is to have the surgeon stop until the patient's heart rate returns to normal (110-115 bpm). If the pause in surgery does not *rapidly* return the heart rate to normal, intravenous atropine should be given.

37.2. **A.** The patient's uncle may have had malignant hyperthermia during his arm surgery, although such a story is not definitive proof of a positive family history. Since malignant hyperthermia has a 5% mortality rate, the safest approach to this patient is to avoid all triggering agents during his anesthetic. Prophylactic dosing of dantrolene does not prevent malignant hyperthermia, but may attenuate early signs of the disease and slow the initiation of proper treatment. However, dantrolene is not indicated in this case.

37.3. **C.** Although the little girl's previous strabismus surgery may have been the only cause of her postoperative vomiting, there are many other possible etiologies, and no way to be certain exactly what caused the problem. General anesthesia alone can cause some patients to have severe postoperative nausea and vomiting. The safest anesthetic plan will include the best prophylactic measures available to try to prevent vomiting. These include a multidrug regimen such as dexamethasone plus ondansetron, avoiding the use of N_2O, and being certain that the patient is well hydrated at the conclusion of surgery.

Clinical Pearls

- The oculocardiac reflex, caused by pressure on the eye or surgical traction on extraocular muscles, results in a vagal response, most often sinus bradycardia. Removal of the stimulus is the first step in treatment.
- Postoperative nausea and vomiting occurs with high incidence after strabismus surgery, indicating prophylactic treatment with a combination of antiemetic medications.
- Patients who have strabismus may have an increased risk for malignant hyperthermia. A thorough family history is important, especially in this setting.

REFERENCES

Bingham R (ed). *Hatch and Sumner's Textbook of Paediatric Anaesthesia.* 3rd ed. London, UK: Hadder Arnold;2008: 524-525.

Miller RD (ed). *Miller's Anesthesia.* 6th ed. Philadelphia, PA: Elsevier, Churchill Livingstone; 2007: 2530; 2535-2536.

Motoyama EK, Davis PJ (ed). *Smith's Anesthesia for Infants and Children.* 6th ed. Philadelphia, PA: Mosley;1996: 637-638; 641.

www.medterms.com/script/main/art.asp?articlekey=12157.

Case 38

A 3-year-old child is brought to the emergency department accompanied by his mother for complaints of coughing and wheezing. The child was laughing at a birthday party while eating some jellybeans, when he was noted to have a "choking" episode. He immediately began to cough, and wheezes could be clearly heard. He does not have asthma, and has never experienced wheezing before. His medical history is notable for sickle cell disease.

The patient is pink, and he is conversant in full sentences. He is afebrile, his oxygen saturation is 98%, his blood pressure 100/60 mm Hg, and his heart rate 89 bpm and regular. Breath sounds are reduced and wheezes are heard on the right lower lobe.

An expiratory chest radiograph shows clear lung fields with slight hyperinflation on the right. The child is immediately scheduled for a rigid bronchoscopy for removal of the foreign body.

- ➤ What is the greatest hazard facing this patient and his anesthesiologist?
- ➤ What factors are important to ascertain with regards to this patient's initiating event?
- ➤ What considerations are warranted by his sickle cell disease?

ANSWERS TO CASE 38:

Inhaled Foreign Body, Pediatric Patient with a Hemoglobinopathy

Summary: This is a 3-year-old child with a history of sickle cell disease who had a witnessed aspiration event. He is now scheduled to undergo rigid bronchoscopy for removal of the foreign body.

- **Greatest hazard:** *Complete airway obstruction.* When an aspirated foreign body is lodged in the trachea, complete airway obstruction can occur at any moment if the object shifts position. When the object is firmly lodged beyond the carina, the risk of complete airway obstruction is less. It is essential not to convert a partial proximal obstruction into a complete obstruction on induction.
- **Important factors:** *Type of object and timing of event.* Determining the type of object that was aspirated allows the provider to assess the risk of acute total airway obstruction, the potential difficulty of removal, and the potential airway damage from the object. Determining the timing of the aspiration event provides insight into how firmly the object is lodged in the airway and the potential for evolving airway or pulmonary complications. Patients with sickle cell disease should be kept warm, adequately hydrated, well oxygenated and ventilated, and any infections should be promptly treated.
- **Considerations of sickle cell disease:** Patients who have suffered an acute aspiration event should be considered to have a full stomach.

ANALYSIS

Objectives

1. Understand how to preoperatively evaluate a patient who has aspirated a tracheobronchial foreign body.
2. Become familiar with the types of induction and maintenance techniques and ventilation choices that may be used in a child who has aspirated a foreign body.
3. Understand the anesthetic considerations for a patient with sickle cell disease.

Considerations

This child's presentation is consistent with a foreign body aspiration. Not only did he have a witnessed aspiration event, but he also presents with the common symptoms of coughing and wheezing. Had his presentation been delayed, the diagnosis of the aspiration of a foreign body could have easily been mistaken for acute chest syndrome, a complication of sickle cell disease.

It is essential not to convert a partial proximal obstruction into a complete obstruction on induction. An inhalational induction has the theoretical advantage of maintaining spontaneous ventilation to prevent dislodgement of the object during induction. On the other hand, an inhalation induction poses the risk of aspiration of gastric contents in a patient with a full stomach, such as this patient who has just suffered an acute aspiration event. While spontaneous ventilation prevents the theoretical risk of pushing the foreign body further into the airway or creating a ball-valve effect with air trapping behind the foreign body, the patient will likely experience hypoventilation especially given the increased resistance of the bronchoscope. Controlled ventilation with paralysis is one way to ensure adequate oxygenation and ventilation, so important given his sickle cell disease, and to prevent coughing and bucking during rigid bronchoscopy.

In this patient, the unilateral hyperinflation seen on chest radiograph is typical of air trapping behind the foreign body. The findings on physical examination and on the chest radiograph suggest that the foreign body is in the right main stem bronchus. As this object appears to be in the bronchus, an intravenous induction is also appropriate.

Maintenance of anesthesia with either inhalational or intravenous anesthesia is effective and appropriate. However, maintaining an adequate depth of anesthesia with inhalational agents may be challenging due to a leak of anesthetic agents around the rigid bronchoscope. As with any patient with sickle cell anemia, it is important to ensure adequate oxygenation and hydration, avoid hypoventilation, and keep the patient warm.

APPROACH TO Foreign Body Aspiration

DEFINITIONS

TRACHEOBRONCHIAL FOREIGN BODY: Any material, either organic or inorganic, that is aspirated into the tracheobronchial tree.

SICKLE CELL DISEASE: An inherited hemoglobinopathy characterized by hemoglobin S, which is an abnormal hemoglobin with a single amino acid substitution in the β-globin chain.

ACUTE CHEST SYNDROME: A complication of sickle cell disease that is characterized by a lobar infiltrate on chest radiograph along with at least one clinical feature such as chest pain, pyrexia, cough, wheezing, or tachypnea.

CLINICAL APPROACH

Tracheobronchial Foreign Body

Inhaled foreign bodies are a leading cause of accidental death among children under the age of 3. Male children account for 60% of cases, whereas female children account for 40% of cases. The majority are in children less than 3 years of age with a peak incidence of about 2 years of age.

The types of foreign bodies are subdivided into two categories: organic and inorganic. Organic material accounts for 70% to 90% of inhaled foreign bodies. Typical examples include peanuts, beans, seeds, corn, and dried fruit. Inorganic material accounts for only 10% to 30% of inhaled foreign bodies. Typical examples include toys, beads, pins, stones, and pen caps.

The diagnosis of an inhaled foreign body is suggested by the history and physical examination. The initial presentation can be acute, such as when a parent witnesses a "choking" episode or aspiration event, or delayed, when an event is neither witnessed nor noticed. Children with a delayed presentation are usually treated for asthma or for a persistent pulmonary infection that does not improve with conventional treatment. Common symptoms of inhaled foreign bodies are cough and dyspnea. Stridor and cyanosis suggest that the foreign body is in the larynx, whereas wheezing and decreased breath sounds suggest that the foreign body has migrated into the bronchus.

Since only 5% to 30% of inhaled foreign bodies are radio-opaque, a chest radiograph is not always useful in making the diagnosis. In fact, 20% to 30% of children with an inhaled foreign body have a normal chest radiograph. Nonspecific findings of atelectasis or hyperinflation due to air trapping behind the object on expiratory film are suggestive of an inhaled foreign body. Bilateral decubitus films may be useful for small children who are unable to co-operate for inspiratory and expiratory films. Hyperinflation due to air trapping in the dependant lung is suggestive of an inhaled foreign body.

For children with delayed presentations, computer tomography scans using low-dose radiation protocols may be useful in assessing for other causes of airway obstruction. As history, examination, and imaging may not clearly confirm or exclude the diagnosis in selected cases, there should be a low threshold for requesting a diagnostic bronchoscopy. While rigid bronchoscopy remains the gold standard for both diagnosing and removing tracheobronchial foreign bodies, flexible bronchoscopy is becoming more popular, although it is potentially more difficult to remove some types of objects with a flexible bronchoscope.

When a child is scheduled for a rigid bronchoscopy under general anesthesia, the preoperative assessment should focus on the location and the type of the aspirated foreign body as well as the timing of the aspiration event. If the foreign body is located in the trachea, the child is at risk for complete airway obstruction and should be taken urgently to the operating room. Foreign bodies that are located in the trachea (10%) are less common than those located in the right bronchus (50%-60%) or the left bronchus (30%-40%).

The type of foreign body is also important to ascertain since certain objects are more difficult to remove. Organic materials may swell in the airways, and the organic oils from nuts can cause localized inflammation. Sharp objects can also pierce the tracheobronchial wall, or pose the potential for damage to the tracheobronchial tree or larynx as they are removed. The presence of such objects may lengthen bronchoscopy time and may require more invasive surgical removal.

The timing of the aspiration event, whether it is an acute or delayed presentation, is important to determine. Airway edema, granulation tissue, and infection may make retrieval more difficult with delayed presentations. Also, an object that has been recently aspirated may be less stable and more likely to move to a different location in the airway. Finally, the time of the child's last oral intake should be determined to assess the risk of aspiration. If the child is stable and there is little chance of the object being displaced more proximally, waiting for 6 to 8 hours from the last meal to allow gastric emptying may be appropriate. For urgent cases in which the child has recently eaten, the stomach contents can be suctioned through a gastric tube after induction, before bronchoscopy.

Once the child has been assessed, an anesthetic plan is formulated. The three main aspects of the anesthetic plan for the management of inhaled foreign bodies include the choice of induction, the choice of ventilation, and the choice of maintenance. The induction of anesthesia can be performed with either an inhalational or an intravenous agent. The choice of inhalational or intravenous induction is influenced if not determined by the position of the foreign body and the risk of converting a partial proximal obstruction into a complete obstruction. An inhalational induction has the theoretical advantage of maintaining spontaneous ventilation to prevent dislodgement of an unstable proximal object during induction. An intravenous induction that maintains spontaneous ventilation also accomplishes this goal. If the foreign body is wedged distally, the choice can be based on the child's preference and whether or not he already has intravenous access.

Both spontaneous and controlled ventilation are safe and effective during removal of inhaled foreign bodies. The advantage of spontaneous ventilation is that it prevents pushing the object further into the airway. The disadvantage of spontaneous ventilation is the risk of hypoventilation due to the increased resistance of the rigid bronchoscope. The advantage of controlled ventilation is that paralysis allows for decreased coughing and bucking and improved oxygenation. The disadvantage is that a ball-valve effect might be created with positive pressure ventilation, with air trapping behind the foreign body. A prospective study demonstrates that controlled ventilation is more effective than spontaneous ventilation and that there is not an increased incidence of dislodgement of the foreign body with controlled ventilation.

The maintenance of anesthesia can be performed with either inhalational agents or with a total intravenous anesthetic. While most studies use inhalational agents for the maintenance of anesthesia, maintaining an adequate depth of anesthesia can be challenging due to hypoventilation and leaks around the rigid bronchoscope. In contrast, an intravenous technique provides a constant level of anesthesia irrespective of ventilation. Regardless of the anesthetic technique, good communication and teamwork between the anesthesiologist and the bronchoscopist are essential to minimize complications.

One of the main intra-operative complications is dropping the foreign body back into the airway. If the foreign body returns to its previous location in the tracheobronchial tree, there is usually no untoward effect. However, if it falls into the other bronchus, there is potential for complete airway obstruction due to edema and inflammation at the original site. If the object remains in the subglottic region, there is also potential for complete airway obstruction. If this occurs, and the object cannot immediately be extracted, it is best to push the object back down into a mainstem bronchus to eliminate the proximal obstruction. Dropping the foreign body has a higher correlation with operator experience than with the mode of ventilation.

Complications can occur postoperatively from the bronchoscopy, from the anesthetic, or from the foreign body itself. Bronchoscopy complications, which occur at a rate of 3% to 20% in this setting, include tracheal laceration, desaturation with or without bradycardia, laryngeal edema, and bronchospasm. Anesthetic complications, which occur at a rate of 1% to 6%, include aspiration, airway obstruction, pneumothorax, cardiac arrest, and laryngospasm. Complications from the foreign body, which occur at a rate less than 1%, may indicate bronchotomy to the remove the object or lobectomy due to bronchiectasis or fibroatelectasis.

Sickle Cell Disease

The child's sickle cell disease adds an additional layer of complexity to the anesthetic management. Sickle cell disease is an inherited hemoglobinopathy that occurs secondary to a point mutation on the gene encoding the β-globin chain of hemoglobin A. This point mutation causes a single amino acid substitution of valine for glutamic acid. As a result, an abnormal variant, hemoglobin S, is produced that is both less stable and less soluble than hemoglobin A. The characteristics of hemoglobin S not only cause red cell deformation and "sickling," but also cause changes in red cell membrane structure and function, increased red cell dehydration, increased red cell adhesion, and hemolysis. Underlying mechanisms of the clinical features of sickle cell disease include oxidative damage to the red cell membrane and vascular endothelial inflammation.

The clinical features of sickle cell disease involve vascular damage in the kidneys, spleen, bone marrow, lungs, and central nervous system. These patients can develop chronic renal failure, splenic infarction, osteomyelitis, osteonecrosis, and hemorrhagic or ischemic stroke. The inflammatory response can lead to airway hyperreactivity and chronic lung disease. Patients with sickle cell disease are also at risk to develop a pneumonia-like complication known as acute chest syndrome. Acute chest syndrome is diagnosed by a new infiltrate involving a complete lung segment on chest radiograph with at least one of the following clinical features: chest pain, pyrexia, tachypnea, cough, or dyspnea.

Patients with sickle cell disease have a higher rate of perioperative morbidity and mortality as compared to the general population. Factors that are predictive of postoperative complications include the type of surgery, increased age, frequent recent complications, number of hospitalizations, chronic lung disease, and pre-existing infection. The preoperative assessment should focus on the frequency, severity, and pattern of any recent exacerbations of the child's sickle cell disease, and the presence of any and all organ dysfunction. Exchange transfusion to dilute hemoglobin S is typically not indicated. Transfusion to a hematocrit of 30% may improve outcome, but this practice is controversial.

Intraoperative management is similar to a child without sickle cell disease in that the patient should be kept close to pre-aspiration baselines as is feasible. As in other children, hypoxia, hypoventilation leading to atelectasis, hypothermia, and aspiration of gastric contents should be avoided. Ensuring oxygenation, avoiding acidosis from hypoventilation, ensuring adequate hydration and that the patient remains warm, and treating any infection which could result from the aspiration are all indicated in this setting. Postoperative management includes standard supportive care. Sickle cell patients are at risk for developing acute chest syndrome on postoperative days 2 to 3. If this syndrome does develop, treatment includes oxygenation, bronchodilators, incentive spirometry, chest physical therapy, and possibly antibiotics.

Comprehension Questions

38.1. A 3-year-old child undergoes rigid bronchoscopy for removal of the jellybean under general anesthesia with spontaneous ventilation. As the surgeon is using graspers to manipulate the jellybean in a distal bronchus, the child coughs several times and subsequently desaturates. Which of the following would be the initial maneuver in the anesthetic management?

A. Deepen the anesthetic and control ventilation.
B. Be certain that the bronchoscope does not move back into the trachea with coughing to prevent damage to the distal airway.
C. Ask the surgeon to remove the instruments from the bronchoscope and cap it so that adequate ventilation can be provided through the bronchoscope.
D. Perform recruitment maneuvers by providing sustained positive pressure for 10 to 30 seconds to reinflate atelectatic alveoli.

38.2. A 2-year-old child underwent an uneventful general anesthetic and the jellybean removed from his right main stem bronchus. Three days later, he develops a cough and fever. A chest radiograph demonstrates a right lower lobe infiltrate. Which is the least likely diagnosis?

A. Postoperative pneumonia
B. Pulmonary edema
C. Acute chest syndrome
D. Residual tracheobronchial foreign body

38.3. A 2-year-old child is brought to her pediatrician for follow-up of persistent wheezing. She was started on albuterol inhalers 1 month ago for asthma; however, the mother states that her symptoms have not changed. She remains afebrile, hemodynamically stable, and has adequate arterial oxygenation. Which of the following is the next appropriate step in management?

A. Admit the child to the hospital for nebulizer treatments.
B. Start the child on antibiotics for presumed pneumonia.
C. Obtain inspiratory and expiratory chest radiographs.
D. Refer the child to a pulmonologist.

ANSWERS

38.1. **A.** This child's hypoxia is likely due to a combination of increased oxygen consumption in children, hypoventilation with spontaneous ventilation through the rigid bronchoscope, and atelectasis induced by coughing. Appropriate management would include deepening the anesthetic to decrease coughing induced by airway manipulation and to allow for controlled ventilation. The surgeon should move the bronchoscope back into the trachea to prevent damage to the distal airways with coughing and should remove instruments from the airway to allow better ventilation through a capped bronchoscope. If oxygenation does not improve with these maneuvers, recruitment breaths can be performed.

38.2. **B.** Pulmonary edema, is the least likely, as it would typically present with bilateral infiltrates and not an isolated lobar infiltrate. Pyrexia, cough, and a lobar infiltrate are consistent with a diagnosis of postoperative pneumonia or with inflammation behind a retained foreign body. Since the patient definitely had a foreign body in his trachea, depending upon the type of foreign body, the possibility of retained fragments must also be considered in the diagnosis. Due to the patient's history of sickle cell disease, he is also at risk for developing acute chest syndrome 2 to 3 days postoperatively. Pyrexia, cough, and a lobar infiltrate are also typical of acute chest syndrome.

38.3. **C.** While the differential for persistent wheezing is broad, this child's history is typical for a delayed presentation of an inhaled foreign body. She is stable and is oxygenating well, so there is no need to admit her to the hospital. She is afebrile and without evidence of infection, so antibiotics are not indicated. A chest radiograph on inspiration and expiration could show a radio-opaque foreign body, atelectasis, or hyper-inflation on expiration, and is the most appropriate next step. Referring the child to a pulmonologist without further workup at this point is premature.

Clinical Pearls

- The anesthesiologist should establish where the object is lodged, what was aspirated, and when the aspiration occurred.
- The choice of induction, ventilation, and maintenance depends on an assessment of the clinical situation.
- Good teamwork and communication between the anesthesiologist and the bronchoscopist are essential.
- A basic well-conducted anesthetic is the optimal management of sickle cell disease.

REFERENCES

Aydogan LB, Tuncer U, Soylu L, Kiroglu M, Ozsahinoglu C. Rigid bronchoscopy for the suspicion of foreign body in the airway. *Int J Pediatr Otorhinolaryngol.* 2006;70:823-828.

Firth PG. Anaesthesia for peculiar cells—a century of sickle cell disease. *Br J Anesth.* 2005;95(3):287-299.

Firth PG, Head CA. Sickle cell disease and anesthesia. *Anesthesiol.* 2004;101:766-785.

Soodan A, Pawar D, Subramanium R. Anesthesia for removal of inhaled foreign bodies in children. *Pediatr Anesth.* 2004;14:947-952.

Tomaske M, Gerber AC, Weiss M. Anesthesia and periinterventional morbidity of rigid bronchoscopy for tracheobronchial foreign body diagnosis and removal. *Pediatr Anesth.* 2006;16:123-129.

Case 39

A 2-year-old 14-kg girl child presents for preoperative anesthetic evaluation in the induction area just prior to surgery for tonsillectomy. Her mother reports that she has a history of obstructive sleep apnea (OSA), though she has not had a sleep study. She has been fussy and has had a poor appetite for weeks, snores heavily, and occasionally experiences brief apneic periods during sleep. She currently has a dry cough and clear rhinorrhea. The patient's medical history is otherwise unremarkable.

- What tests are required as part of the preoperative evaluation for this patient?
- What are the anesthetic concerns for the pediatric patient with obstructive sleep apnea?
- What are the postoperative complications that follow tonsillectomy?

ANSWERS TO CASE 39:

Tonsillectomy/Sleep Apnea/Hemorrhage

Summary: A 2-year-old child with obstructive sleep apnea undergoes tonsillectomy under general endotracheal anesthesia. The child experiences postoperative somnolence and oxygen dependence.

- **Preoperative evaluation:** Children with tonsillar hypertrophy often have symptoms of an upper respiratory tract infection. It is important that their cough is not productive and that they are afebrile. The clinician should assess the severity of their sleep apnea by clinical indicators such as habitual snoring, apnea, daytime somnolence or hyperactivity, and lethargy. No further workup is required.
- **Anesthesia in patients with sleep apnea:** Children with obstructive sleep apnea are at higher risk for oxygen desaturation on induction and emergence from anesthesia. Moreover, the physiologic changes associated with OSA do not resolve immediately after surgery. It is prudent to consider the overnight observation of postoperative patients with significant OSA, especially those who are less than 3 years of age. Patients with OSA are also more sensitive to the respiratory depressant effects of narcotics. Great care must be taken not to administer a relative overdose while attempting to titrate to patient comfort, and naloxone should be readily available to reverse the narcosis if indicated.
- **Postoperative complications:** The most common postoperative complication after tonsillectomy is hemorrhage, which is life-threatening. The incidence of hemorrhage requiring reoperation for hemostasis is approximately 0.8%. Primary hemorrhage occurs within 24 hours of surgery, while secondary hemorrhage occurs later. Other rare and life-threatening complications include pulmonary edema, aspiration pneumonia, respiratory arrest, or massive hemorrhage.

ANALYSIS

Objectives

1. Review the preoperative evaluation of children for tonsillectomy.
2. Understand obstructive sleep apnea in children.
3. Understand the anesthetic considerations for pediatric tonsillectomy.
4. Discuss the significance of postoperative bleeding after tonsillectomy.

Considerations

This young child who presents for tonsillectomy with a diagnosis of OSA is at significant risk for perioperative complications. The ability to prepare for and deliver a safe anesthetic requires an understanding of the complex interplay of the pathophysiology of OSA, the intrinsic risks of airway surgery in a child, and the necessity of providing a balanced anesthetic. Every recent dataset on perioperative risk in pediatric patients highlights that airway surgeries are associated with the greatest incidence of adverse respiratory events. This child requires prompt support of the airway in the recovery room and preparation for invasive airway management including reintubation or continuous positive airway pressure (CPAP). Other causes for respiratory compromise should be excluded including post-obstructive pulmonary edema, pulmonary aspiration, or postoperative hemorrhage. It is unlikely that more systemic causes of arterial desaturation such as an occult cardiac lesion, intrapulmonary shunt, or pulmonary embolism are the cause. Children with OSA are susceptible to respiratory compromise after tonsillectomy and are potentially sensitive to opioids. This child most likely has postoperative respiratory depression due to the combination of chronic obstructive sleep apnea, residual anesthetic effect, and the relative narcosis caused by parenteral long-acting opioid. Other common anesthesia-related complications include postoperative nausea and vomiting (PONV), arterial desaturation, unplanned inpatient admissions, and airway obstruction.

APPROACH TO Tonsillectomy/Sleep Apnea/Hemorrhage

DEFINITIONS

OBSTRUCTIVE SLEEP APNEA: OSA is an obstructive breathing disorder that occurs during sleep. It is characterized by intermittent upper airway obstruction due to dysfunction in the muscles and soft tissues of the upper airway, or from obstruction resulting from tonsillar hypertrophy. Most commonly, OSA is diagnosed by the history from an observer who witnesses periods of apnea. In children, common daytime symptoms of OSA include hyperactivity, failure to thrive, poor school performance, and behavioral problems.

APNEA-HYPOPNEA INDEX: AHI is the number of apneic and hypopneic episodes per hour of sleep. The AHI estimates the severity of OSA.

PERIOPERATIVE ADVERSE RESPIRATORY EVENTS: These include laryngospasm, bronchospasm, breath holding, oxygen desaturation, and severe cough.

UPPER RESPIRATORY TRACT INFECTION: URI is a common clinical condition of childhood most often caused by infection with the rhinovirus. Children contract 4 to 6 URI infections per year and require 4 to 6 weeks to return to baseline airway reactivity.

POSTOPERATIVE NAUSEA AND VOMITING: This is a common complication of anesthesia and is known to be of significant risk after tonsillectomy. PONV is of particular concern after tonsillectomy because it not only decreases patient satisfaction but it can also delay discharge and herald significant postoperative hemorrhage where blood is swallowed, unnoticed by the patient or caregiver.

CLINICAL APPROACH

Tonsillectomy is one of the most common operations performed on children. Most commonly, it is indicated on the basis of recurrent episodes of pharyngitis and obstructive sleep apnea. Tonsillectomy is increasingly performed as an outpatient procedure. While the criteria for outpatient surgical candidates continues to expand, special consideration should be given when considering outpatient surgery in patients who are less than 3 years of age, have OSA or other breathing disorders, major heart disease, bleeding diathesis, or mental retardation. Other reasons to consider inpatient admission include "acute" tonsillectomies, as well as a patient who lives far from a treatment center or who has other social circumstances that might prevent early intervention should problems develop at home. Children with proven OSA by polysomnography have been shown to have a 23% incidence of severe postoperative respiratory compromise requiring intervention. Children with Down syndrome, cerebral palsy, mental retardation, or other congenital disorders have been shown to have a 27% incidence of major respiratory compromise. In most centers, these children would not be considered as appropriate candidates for outpatient surgery.

For pediatric tonsillectomy, a thorough preoperative evaluation determines whether the child has a history of breathing disorders including sleep apnea, asthma, allergies, and any current respiratory symptoms. Patients are also screened for any history indicating a bleeding disorder. A family history of bleeding disorder or any clinical indication of bleeding disorder such as frequent and difficult to control nosebleeds or bruise formation out of proportion to injury suggests the need for additional testing prior to surgery. Routine coagulation studies are otherwise not indicated unless there is appropriate clinical suspicion. von Willebrand disease is the most common inherited coagulopathy and is not diagnosed by a screening PT/PTT.

Children who present for tonsillectomy often also manifest symptoms of an upper respiratory infection. There may be a very narrow window of opportunity for a child to be free of respiratory symptoms at the time of presentation for surgery. Some children are almost never free of symptoms. In this situation, it is appropriate to consider proceeding with elective surgery, with the understanding that the risk of adverse respiratory complications is increased. The dependent risk factors for adverse respiratory events in children with active URIs include use of an endotracheal tube in a child less than 5 years, prematurity, reactive airway disease, parental smoking, airway surgery, copious secretions, and nasal congestion. The increase in airway reactivity may persist for several weeks after an URI.

Obstructive sleep apnea is a breathing disorder that occurs during sleep characterized by intermittent upper airway obstruction. Most commonly, the obstruction occurs at the base of the tongue or the soft palate from hypertrophic tonsils or anatomic abnormalities that narrow the aperture of the nasopharyngeal airway, allowing the tongue to be displaced posteriorly. The formal diagnosis of OSA is made by polysomnography, but for practical purposes the diagnosis is often based on clinical symptoms. Common daytime symptoms of OSA include hyperactivity, failure to thrive, poor school performance, and behavioral problems.

Children with OSA often have hypoxemia, hypercarbia, and a partial airway obstruction even while awake. Increased airway resistance secondary to hypertrophic tonsils and adenoids can cause alveolar hypoventilation. Pulmonary artery pressure progressively increases with each apneic episode, resulting in cor pulmonale and clinically significant pulmonary hypertension, followed eventually by ventricular dysfunction. ECGs may show right ventricular hypertrophy, and some patients have x-ray findings of cardiomegaly. In most cases, surgical removal of the tonsils and adenoids can reverse these progressive cardiovascular changes.

After the preoperative evaluation, consideration may be given to premedication. Pediatric patients may often receive oral midazolam (0.3-0.5 mg/kg). However, in patients for tonsillectomy, premedication is used judiciously if there is any obstruction to breathing, and it is generally avoided in patients with severe OSA. If necessary due to high levels of anxiety, patients may receive oral midazolam (0.3-0.5 mg/kg), intramuscular ketamine (5 mg/kg), or intranasal midazolam.

Because few children would not object to placement of an intravenous, induction is performed with a standard inhalational induction using sevoflurane, nitrous oxide, and oxygen. Airway obstruction should be anticipated, and alleviated with airway manipulation, an oral airway and/or administration of CPAP at 10 to 15 cm H_2O. Obese children are at increased risk of difficulty with mask ventilation. In patients with significant OSA combined with obesity or other comorbidity, an i.v. induction may be safer, albeit unpleasant for the child. An i.v. catheter allows the administration of additional anesthetic, opiates, or muscle relaxants and can thus facilitate endotracheal intubation.

An oral standard or RAE preformed endotracheal tube (ETT) is secured in the midline after placement is confirmed. However, it can become dislodged by surgical instruments, surgeon manipulation, or maneuvering of the bed.

The anesthesiologist must be vigilant to the security of the endotracheal tube at all times. A cuffed tube is preferable, since the cuff may decrease leakage of oral secretions and blood into the trachea during surgery, as well as reducing the oxygen environment at the site of electrocautery. The use of a cuffed endotracheal tube poses no additional risks in children for brief cases. Placement of the throat pack can similarly cause obstruction or kinking of the ETT. (It is also important to note and document when the throat pack is removed at the end of the case.) Maintenance is provided with standard volatile anesthetics or intravenous anesthetics such as propofol and remifentanil, which reduce postoperative nausea and vomiting as well as agitation at emergence. Muscle relaxant may or may not be necessary.

The anticipated surgical time for a tonsillectomy is 20 to 60 minutes. The surgery itself is quite stimulating, and requires a deep level of anesthetic throughout. Prior to emergence, ondansetron and dexamethasone are typically administered for vomiting prophylaxis. Metoclopramaide is no more effective than placebo for this use. Blood and secretions must be suctioned with caution prior to emergence. Keep the suction catheter in the midline to avoid the raw surgical sites on either side. The patient should be extubated either fully awake, or (rarely) at a very deep level of anesthesia with adequate respirations after throat packs have been removed. Deep extubation may avoid the coughing and bronchospasm associated with an endotracheal tube, though larygospasm can occur should secretions or blood stimulate the vocal cords. Avoidance of Valsalva maneuvers may decrease the risk of primary hemorrhage.

Common complications of tonsillectomy include hemorrhage, postoperative nausea, vomiting, and pain (sore throat with or without otalgia). Less common complications include respiratory compromise, damage to teeth, dehydration, fever, and damage to the uvula. Rare complications include velopharyngeal insufficiency, nasopharygeal stenosis, intraoperative vascular injury, subcutaneous emphysema, mediastinistis, atlantoaxial subluxation, cervical osteomyelitis, and taste disorders. Deaths are most often due to hemorrhage, unrecognized apnea, disconnection of anesthesia circuit, and drug dosing errors or reactions, and occur at a frequency of 1:1,000-27,000 cases overall.

Hemorrhage is most likely to occur within the first 24 hours following tonsillectomy, although it is not unusual for this life-threatening complication to occur 7 to 10 days postoperatively. The reported incidence of post-tonsillectomy hemorrhage varies from approximately 0.1% to 8.1%. Anesthetic risks for a "bleeding tonsil" are significant, and include the risk of hypotension with induction reflecting the patient's hypovolemia, and pulmonary aspiration from a stomach full of blood. Rapid-sequence induction (usually modified without the Sellick maneuver in children) should be used for post-tonsillectomy hemorrhage patients.

Without prophylaxis, the incidence of postoperative nausea and vomiting after tonsillectomy has been shown to exceed 70%. Postoperative vomiting can delay discharge, negatively impact patient and parent satisfaction, as well as increase the risk of bleeding, aspiration of gastric contents, dehydration, and electrolyte disturbances. A 2006 meta-analysis demonstrated that anti-serotonergic agents, including ondansetron, granisetron, and tropisetron, are clinically effective in a dose-dependent manner. The same study provided good evidence of the efficacy of dexamethasone for vomiting prophylaxis, though the optimum dose for children remains to be determined. However, recent evidence has suggested an association between post-tonsillectomy bleeding and dexamethasone at a dose of 0.5 mg/kg.

Pulmonary edema is a rare but recognized complication of tonsillectomy. It is most likely related to the presence and relief of the airway obstruction. Excess tonsillar tissue causes an obstruction and resistance to airflow with both inspiration and expiration. This resistance results in an endogenous positive end-expiratory pressure (PEEP). Pulmonary edema seems to result from the sudden release of the excess PEEP.

Tonsillectomy is known to be a painful procedure. Traditionally, opioids have been used to treat postoperative pain, with typical doses of morphine in the range of 0.05 to 0.1 mg/kg i.v. However, opioids are known to cause respiratory depression, as well as nausea and vomiting. The respiratory depression is of special concern in patients with significant OSA, because they are likely to be more sensitive to the respiratory depressant effects of the medication. When a sleep study is available, a desaturation nadir of less than 85% predicts a significant increase of opiate sensitivity. Thus, it is recommended to reduce opiate doses by approximately 50% in these children (eg, 0.05 mg/kg).

Nonsteroidal anti-inflammatory drugs (NSAIDs) such as ibuprofen are effective in the management of postoperative pain after tonsillectomy and do not appear to increase the risk of postoperative hemorrhage. However, surgical concern for this potentially lethal complication predisposes many against the use of NSAIDs in current clinical practice. Acetaminophen can be used concomitantly to increase the efficacy of opioids. Oral acetaminophen (15-20 mg/kg) can be administered preoperatively, or rectal acetaminophen (40 mg/kg, particularly useful in young children) can be administered after induction.

In uncomplicated patients, it is becoming increasingly acceptable to discharge patients on the same day as tonsillectomy. Pain is managed using a multimodal technique (a narcotic and acetaminophen), and dexamethasone is administered intraoperatively to reduce swelling (and thus pain) as well as postoperative nausea and vomiting. Tonsillar injection with local anesthetic may also improve analgesia. Lastly, surgical technique may affect pain after tonsillectomy. Tonsillectomy (eg, Coblation) seems to result in significantly lower pain scores postoperatively though with a possible increase in hemorrhage and recurrence rates.

Comprehension Questions

39.1. An 18-month-old child is scheduled for tonsillectomy due to recurrent pharyngitis and tonsillar hyperplasia. Preoperative evaluation should include which of the following apart from a complete history and physical?
A. Electrocardiogram
B. Polysomnography
C. Baseline hemoglobin
D. Chest x-ray
E. None of the above; no additional testing is needed

39.2. Which of the following is a symptom of obstructive sleep apnea more often seen in adults than children?
A. Irritability
B. Hyperactivity
C. Daytime somnolence
D. Depression

39.3. Regarding bleeding after tonsillectomy, which of the following statements is accurate?
A. The degree of hypovolemia is evident in the clinical presentation.
B. After 24 hours, the risk of significant bleeding becomes negligible.
C. Postoperative nausea and vomiting reduces gastric volume as well as the risk of aspiration.
D. Bleeding after tonsillectomy is a life-threatening situation.

39.4. The patient described at the beginning of this case undergoes an uneventful inhalation induction with sevoflurane. Her intraoperative course is unremarkable, and she receives 1.5 mg of morphine for pain management. She is extubated at the end of the surgery but in the recovery room, she remains somnolent and dependent on supplemental oxygen to maintain an arterial saturation greater than 92%. Which of the following is the most likely diagnosis and treatment?
A. Respiratory depression from pain, opiate
B. Low baseline oxygen saturation, PEEP
C. Cor pulmonale, ionotrope
D. Respiratory depression from excessive opiate, naloxone

ANSWERS

39.1. **E.** No additional testing is needed without indication from the history and physical. As described above, due to the time and financial expense of polysomnography, it is not practical to expect children to present for surgery with this data.

39.2. **C.** Adults with OSA will often exhibit daytime somnolence. Children are much more likely to be hyperactive and irritable, though sleep disturbance will often decrease scholastic function as well.

39.3. **D.** Bleeding after a tonsillectomy is a life-threatening situation. Bleeding can be quite severe, with significant hypovolemia even in a child who is not hypotensive. It is desirable that the child receives fluid resuscitation prior to induction if the situation allows. Bleeding after tonsillectomy typically occurs within hours of surgery, although a second peak in incidence occurs some 5 to 8 days later. The child with a bleeding tonsil is likely to have swallowed significant amounts of blood, warranting full-stomach precautions including a rapid-sequence intubation.

39.4. **D.** In this case, the dose of 1.5 mg of morphine is excessive in this 14-kg child and is no doubt contributing to her postoperative narcosis. Naloxone may be indicated.

Clinical Pearls

- Obstructive sleep apnea is diagnosed by a child's tendency to obstruct and remain apneic during sleep.
- Children with significant obstructive sleep apnea are more sensitive to opioids.
- The obese child with OSA undergoing tonsillectomy is at considerable risk for complications from central apnea, supraglottic obstruction, drug overdosing, and delayed emergence from volatile anesthetics.
- Hemorrhage is a life-threatening complication of tonsillectomy in children.
- The child with a bleeding tonsil can be severely hypovolemic from hemorrhage and dehydration, and is at significant risk for aspiration.

REFERENCES

Bolton CM, Myles PS, Nolan T, Sterne JA. Prophylaxis of postoperative vomiting in children undergoing tonsillectomy: a systematic review and meta-analysis. *Bri J Anesth.* 2006;97(5):593-604.

Brown KA, Laferriere AB, Lakheeram IM, Moss IR. Recurrent hypoxemia in children is associated with increased analgesic sensitivity to opiates. *Anesthesiol.* 2006;105(4):665-669.

Ferrari LR, Vassallo SA. Anesthesia for otohinolaryngology procedures. In: Coté CJ, Todres D, Ryan JF, et al. eds. *A Practice of Anesthesia for Infants and Children.* 3rd ed. Philadelphia, PA: Saunders; 2001.

McColley S, April M, Carroll J, et al. Respiratory compromise after adenotonsillectomy in children with obstructive sleep apnea. *Arch Otolaryngol Head Neck Surg.* 1992;118:940-943.

Randall DA, Hoffer ME. Complications on tonsillectomy and adenoidectomy. *Otolaryngol–Head Neck Surg.* 1998;118:61-68.

Richmond K, Wetmore R, Baranak C. Postoperative complications following tonsillectomy and adenoidectomy—who is at risk? *Int J Pediatr Otorhinolaryngol* 1987;13:117-124.

Sanders JC, King MA, Mitchell RB, Kelly JP. Perioperative complications of adenotonsillectomy in children with obstructive sleep apnea syndrome. *Anesth Analg.* 2006;103:1115-1121.

Tait AR, Malviya S, Vocpel-Lewis T, Munro HM, Siewert M, Pandit UA. Risk factors for perioperative adverse respiratory events in children with upper respiratory tract infections. *Anesthesiol.* 2001;95:299-306.

Case 40

A 4-week-old male infant is brought to the emergency room by his parents. He has been vomiting after feeding for approximately 1 week, more frequently over the last 2 days. For the past 12 hours or so the baby has been sleepy. His diapers are no longer as heavy with urine.

On physical examination, he is well nourished, but with dry mucous membranes, poor skin turgor, and sunken fontanelles. He appears lethargic. Palpation of the abdomen shows an olive-size mass just above the umbilicus, and beneath the liver's edge. A basic metabolic panel lists the Na^+ 131 mEq/L, K^+ 3.0 mEq/L, Cl^- 95 mEq/L, HCO_3^- 29 mEq/L, BUN 12 mg/dL, and creatinine (Cr) 0.6 mg/dL. Ultrasound of the abdomen reveals a pyloric muscle greater than 4 mm and longer than 16 mm, leading to a diagnosis of infantile hypertrophic pyloric stenosis. He is scheduled for a surgical correction for this problem.

- ➤ How should this patient be prepared for his surgery?
- ➤ What are the anesthetic concerns in a patient undergoing a pyloromyotomy?
- ➤ How is the airway in a neonate different from the airway in an adult?

ANSWERS TO CASE 40: Pyloric Stenosis

Summary: A 4-week-old male infant presents with persistent vomiting due to hypertrophic pyloric stenosis.

- **Preparation for surgery:** Pyloric stenosis is a medical—not surgical—emergency. This patient has a fluid deficit and electrolyte imbalances which must be corrected before surgical correction of the hypertrophic pylorus. Fluid resuscitation and correction of metabolic derangements may require 24 to 48 hours.
- **Anesthetic concerns:** Any patient who is vomiting is considered to have a full stomach. In addition, pyloric stenosis is an obstruction; therefore this patient is at increased risk of aspiration. The anesthetic plan needs to include steps to protect the patient's airway from this possibility. In addition, pyloric stenosis is a congenital anomaly and patients who have one such anomaly are at increased risk to have other anomalies, any or all of which may affect the anesthetic plan. During the period of fluid resuscitation, a workup to preclude other congenital anomalies can take place.
- **Neonatal airway:** The neonate's airway differs from an adult's in size, shape of the airway, shape of the epiglottis position of the glottis, position of the narrowest point, slanting of the vocal cords, and fixation of the mucus membranes. These characteristics combine to make intubation of the neonate's trachea much more difficult than that of an adult. (see Table 40–1).

ANALYSIS

Objectives

1. Recognize the most urgent medical issues associated with pyloric stenosis and their initial treatment.
2. Understand the anesthetic implications when caring for a neonate.
3. Describe the implications in caring for an infant with pyloric stenosis.

Table 40–1 DIFFERENCES IN THE NEONATAL AIRWAY

- Large tongue.
- Larynx is higher in the neck (C3-C4 vs C6 in the adult).
- Epiglottis is short, stubby, and angled over laryngeal inlet.
- Vocal cords slant anterior (vs transverse or slightly posterior).
- Larynx is funnel-shaped (vs cylindrical).
- Narrowest point is below cords (vs at the cords).
- Mucus membranes are loose, and susceptible to swelling.

Considerations

This young patient has presented to the emergency room with clear signs of dehydration (lethargy and low urine output) and laboratory studies showing electrolyte abnormalities. He has metabolic alkalosis, consistent with the vomiting associated with pyloric stenosis. This is a medical—not surgical—emergency. Appropriate treatment includes volume resuscitation, and stabilization of electrolyte imbalances prior to any surgical correction.

While the patient is receiving fluids, he should be examined for the presence of other congenital anomalies. Two other syndromes (among others) commonly found in the presence of pyloric stenosis are tracheoesophageal fistula and eosinophilic gastroenteritis, both of which could complicate his anesthetic care.

Once the child is euvolemic and his electrolytes repleted, he is ready for the operating room. Although the infant will not have eaten during his resuscitation, he is still considered to have a full stomach because of his hypertrophic pylorus, and the resulting obstruction which may not even allow passage of gastric secretions. Prior to the induction, the patient's stomach must be emptied. An orogastric tube is passed into the infant's stomach while he is awake and gastric contents suctioned. This process is sometimes repeated three times, with the infant first on his back, then in left lateral and right lateral positions.

Immediately after suctioning, the patient is pre-oxygenated (and denitrogenated) with 100% oxygen given by face mask. Most patients with pyloric stenosis arrive in the operating room with an intravenous in place. He is induced by a rapid-sequence induction, with cricoid pressure (some advocate intubating these patients "awake," and prior to induction). Correct placement of the endotracheal tube is confirmed by observing equal and symmetric rise of both sides of the chest when breaths are delivered. Once correct placement of the endotracheal tube has been confirmed, the cricoid pressure may be released.

Once the patient's airway is secured, general anesthesia is maintained with an anesthetic gas, and an opiate is administered for postoperative pain relief. At the end of the surgery, when the child is vigorous and awake, the endotracheal tube is removed and he is taken to the recovery room. The patient will be watched carefully over the next 12 to 24 hours as infants post-pyloromyotomy are more prone to postoperative apnea than other infants.

APPROACH TO Pyloric Stenosis

CLINICAL APPROACH

Anesthetizing a neonate is fraught with hazards and surprises, few of them pleasant. Meticulous attention to detail is imperative, since matters unimportant in the adult, such as minute amounts of air in the intravenous line, may be catastrophic in an infant. Warming devices and/or the operating room itself becomes the incubator. The neonate's airway differs significantly from the adult's, predisposing these young patients to difficulty with intubation (Table 40–1). Auscultation of bilateral breath sounds is not very useful to verify position of the endotracheal tube, as breath sounds are easily transmitted across the small chest. Similarly, tissues surrounding the airway are not firmly bound to subcutaneous tissue, predisposing to airway edema. There should be a small air leak past the endotracheal tube to help prevent damage to the patient's trachea, and no more than 15 to 20 cm of H_2O-positive pressure delivered to the lungs when giving a breath. Oxygen saturation is maintained between 93% and 95% to reduce the risk of retinopathy of prematurity. Although narcotics are tolerated, the potent inhalation agents may well not be.

The presence of pyloric stenosis, if improperly managed, adds a level of complexity to the anesthetic management of the neonate. This congenital anomaly typically presents in the first weeks of life, and occurs with a fourfold predominance in males. It is characterized by persistent, projectile, nonbilious vomiting, and a palpable hypertrophic mass (or "olive") pyloric region also visible on noninvasive imaging. Peristaltic waves are often visible in the gastrium.

The persistent vomiting that occurs in patients with pyloric stenosis leads to hypovolemia and electrolyte imbalances which progress with the degree of dehydration. The classic picture is one of dehydration with a hypokalemic, hypochloremic alkalosis, possibly accompanied by a compensatory respiratory acidosis from hypoventilation and even periods of apnea. As the child's dehydration worsens, circulatory shock may ensue, resulting in an entirely different picture: metabolic acidosis with compensatory respiratory alkalosis. Thus, the acid-base findings associated with pyloric stenosis may vary considerably, depending on the duration of the patient's vomiting. However, most patients present with hypokalemic, hypochloremic alkalosis.

Resuscitative fluids for an infant are most often 5% dextrose with either 0.9% or 0.45% normal saline. Half the patient's deficit should be given over the first 8 hours, another quarter over the second 8 hours, and the final quarter over a third 8-hour period. Maintenance fluids must be given as well. Potassium may be added to fluids once the patient has started to urinate. The patient is not ready for surgery until his serum chloride level is at least 90 mmol/L and his serum bicarbonate, no more than 26 mmol/L.

Once resuscitative fluids have been administered and any electrolyte imbalances corrected, the patient with pyloric stenosis is no different than any other neonate, with the possible exception of having a "full" stomach. Nevertheless, neonates are at a higher risk for complications than other patients. Because of the special circumstances surrounding their care, neonatal anesthesia is best performed by individuals familiar and practiced with this type of anesthesia.

Comprehension Questions

40.1. A 56-year-old man is brought to the emergency room with severe stomach pains. He has vomited four times in the last 12 hours and has had no bowel movement for 3 days. The surgeon determines that the patient needs an emergent laparotomy for a bowel obstruction. Which of the following is most appropriate to include in your anesthetic plan?

A. Medical management first with fluid resuscitation.
B. Standard induction of anesthesia with continued oxygenation after induction by delivery of positive pressure breaths before intubation.
C. Rapid-sequence induction of anesthesia.
D. Empty the patient's stomach prior to induction of anesthesia.

40.2. A 2-year-old boy is brought to the pediatrician by his parents because although he is talking, his parents cannot understand him and have noticed that his tongue doesn't move normally in his mouth. The pediatrician finds that the patient has a short frenulum which needs surgical correction. Which of the following should be included in your anesthetic plan?

A. A rapid-sequence induction because the patient had breakfast before seeing the pediatrician.
B. Ensuring that the patient has had a thorough examination for possible additional congential anomalies prior to the needed surgery.
C. Fluid resuscitation before surgery because the patient may not have been able to drink well with the restricted movement of his tongue.
D. Assume that the patient has other anomalies of the gastrointestinal tract and plan a rapid-sequence induction when surgery is scheduled.

40.3. A female neonate previously diagnosed *in utero* with gastroschisis is born early in the morning. Gastroschisis is a defect of the abdominal wall that results in exposure of the viscera which are not covered by peritoneum. The viscera are covered sterilely and the surgeon schedules surgery for the next morning. You consider your anesthetic plan and decide on which of the following?

A. The patient will need fluid resuscitation and maintenance over the next 24 hours to optimize her status in preparation for surgery.
B. She will need her stomach emptied prior to a rapid-sequence intubation.
C. The patient's surgery should be postponed for more than 24 hours in order to have time to thoroughly examine the neonate for other congenital abnormalities.
D. You approach the surgeon because you believe that the patient needs surgery more urgently by the next morning.

ANSWERS

40.1. **C.** The management of an adult with a bowel obstruction usually differs from the management of a neonate with pyloric stenosis. This patient is likely somewhat (as opposed to severely) dehydrated, but because of the possibility of perforation, his need for surgery is emergent and there is little time for fluid resuscitation. This patient has a bowel obstruction and therefore a "full stomach," and will need a rapid-sequence induction. A standard induction of anesthesia will pose a greater risk of aspirating gastric contents into his lungs before placement of the endotracheal tube. While emptying his stomach before induction of anesthesia would be optimal, adults do not tolerate this procedure as well as infants, and it is not usually done.

40.2. **B.** The patient has a problem which needs correction soon, but is definitely not emergent or urgent. His short frenulum is a congenital anomaly and the physicians caring for him have plenty of time to thoroughly examine for other anomalies prior to his surgery. Unless an anomaly of the GI tract is discovered (unlikely at this point as the patient is 2 years old), the patient can have a standard induction of anesthesia, which for a child of his age, will most likely be an inhalational induction using anesthetic gas.

40.3. **A.** Correction of gastroschisis is urgent. The viscera are exposed and severe dehydration and infection are constant threats to the life of this neonate. She needs to be euvolemic before this major surgery, and this can be accomplished over the 24 hour period before her surgery. Gastroschisis is not a bowel obstruction, and there is no need to empty the patient's stomach before induction and intubation. While this congenital anomaly should prompt a search for other anomalies in this patient, her surgery should not be postponed until such examinations are complete.

Clinical Pearls

- Pyloric stenosis is a medical emergency, not a surgical emergency. The patient is often dehydrated and has a metabolic alkalosis, both of which need correction prior to pyloromyotomy.
- The neonate's airway differs significantly from an adult's, in ways that may make intubation difficult and predispose to airway edema.
- Neonatal anesthesia is fraught with hazards and unpleasant surprises, and is best left to individuals with special expertise in this type of anesthesia.

REFERENCES

Bingham R. *Hatchard Sumner's Textbook of Paediatric Anaesthesia*. 3rd ed. London, UK: Hadder Arnold; 2008: 75-76.

Gregory George A, ed. *Pediatric Anesthesia*. 3rd ed. New York, NY: Churchill Livingston; 2001: 557-558.

Kissin I. General anesthetic action: an obsolete notion. *Anesth Analg*. 1993;76:215.

Kliegman RM, Behrman RE, Jenson HB, et al. *Nelson's Textbook of Pediatrics*. 18th ed. Philadelphia, PA: Saunders Elsevier; 2007: 1555-1557.

Part 3. “Odds and Ends”

Case 41

A 26-year-old woman presents to an outpatient surgery center for a laparoscopic excision of an ovarian cyst. The patient is very anxious and comments that she does not want to be awake. Her medical history includes asthma treated with an inhaler, and gastroesophageal reflux disease. Her only medication is albuterol, but she has not needed it for 6 months. She has no prior surgical history, no history of familial or anesthetic complications, and no allergies to medications. On examination, the patient's height is 62 in and she weighs 75 kg. Breath sounds are clear. Airway examination reveals a Mallampati 2 classification, full range of motion of the neck, and a 3-cm thyromental distance. Her hematocrit is 37. This patient's ASA physical status classification is ASA class II. Since she is a healthy patient undergoing a low-risk outpatient procedure, no further preoperative evaluation is required. The patient was taken to the operating room, and an intravenous placed. She was premedicated with bicitra, metoclopramide, and ranitidine for her gastric reflux, and midazolam for her anxiety. Standard monitors were placed, and anesthesia was induced uneventfully with propofol, cisatracurium, and fentanyl, and maintained with sevoflurane and 40% oxygen. The trachea was easily intubated and placed on the ventilator with a tidal volume of 650 mL and respiratory rate of 10 breaths/minute (bpm). She was then placed in a dorsal lithotomy and head-up position. Upon insufflation of the peritoneum, the patient's peak inspiratory pressure increased from 17 to 37 cm of water. Over the next 10 minutes, the end-tidal carbon dioxide measurement rose from 32 mm Hg to 44 mm Hg and oxygen saturation decreased from 98% to 94%. Blood pressure and heart rate remained unchanged.

- ➤ What is the differential diagnosis of hypoxia in this patient?
- ➤ What are the maneuvers to treat the complications in this patient?

ANSWERS TO CASE 41:
Complications of Laparoscopy

Summary: A healthy young woman undergoes an uneventful anesthetic induction for laparoscopic surgery. After change in patient position and insufflation, there is an increase in end-tidal carbon dioxide and hypoxia.

- **Causes of hypoxia:** Endobronchial intubation, kinking or dislodgement of the endotracheal tube, hypoventilation, pneumothorax, atelectasis, pneumoperitoneum, decreased cardiac output, gas embolism, and potential vascular injuries.

- **Corrective manuevers:** Administration of 100% oxygen, ensuring correct endotracheal tube placement, hemodynamic support with pressors or inotropes if needed, the addition of positive end-expiratory pressure (PEEP), and treating the etiology of hypoxia are the maneuvers required at this time.

ANALYSIS

Objectives

1. Identify the physiologic changes that can be encountered during laparoscopy.
2. List the possible complications of laparoscopy.
3. Describe the management of hypoxia and hypercarbia during laparoscopy.

Considerations

When an unexpected event occurs during an anesthetic, the first level of the differential diagnosis addresses the acuity of the problem. For example, is it a "little problem," or a "big problem"? In this case, the patient's hypoxemia has occurred over a 10-minute period, and her other vital signs are stable. Thus while the situation must be addressed and could be serious, it is not currently in the catastrophic category of events. Next, when hypoxemia is observed in a patient who is intubated and mechanically ventilated, it is important to differentiate an iatrogenic or mechanical cause from a patient-related medical condition. But first, the fraction of inspired oxygen is increased. Then by ventilating by hand and auscultating the breath sounds, it is possible to assess for the presence of bilateral breath sounds, the presence of wheezing, an endotracheal tube obstruction, displacement, cuff leak, and possibly, a pneumothorax. If the evaluation is unremarkable, then the ventilator and its connections should be checked. In this patient, breath sounds were clear bilaterally which implied proper endotracheal tube placement and excluded major pulmonary pathology. Oxygen saturation improved with 100% oxygen and addition of positive end-expiratory pressure (PEEP). Mechanical ventilation was resumed, with a fraction of inspired oxygen of 50% and 5 cm of water of positive end-expiratory pressure and an oxygen saturation of 98% was maintained.

Increasing the patient's minute ventilation can usually decrease the end-tidal carbon dioxide measurement. But since the pneumoperitoneum during laparoscopy often elevates peak inspiratory pressure, increasing minute ventilation is best accomplished by increasing the respiratory rate and decreasing the tidal volume for an overall increase in minute ventilation. Reducing the tidal volume may also reduce the peak inspiratory pressure, resulting in an increase in lung compliance. Increasing the respiratory rate from 10 to 16 and decreasing the tidal volume from 650 mL to 500 mL would increase the minute ventilation by 1.5 L/min, from 6.5 L/min to 8 L/min. In this case, end-tidal carbon dioxide decreased from 44 mm Hg to 40 mm Hg after the increase in minute ventilation. The procedure proceeded uneventfully, and within 20 minutes of extubation, 4 mg of ondansetron was given for prevention of post-operative nausea and vomiting.

APPROACH TO Complications of Laparoscopy

CLINICAL APPROACH

Laparoscopic surgery offers many benefits over open surgery. These include smaller incisions, less blood loss and postoperative pain, shorter hospital stay, and fewer postoperative wound infections. Performed almost exclusively by gynecologists for decades, this technique is now common for both general and genitourinary surgical procedures as well.

Laparoscopy is facilitated by insufflating gas into the abdomen. The most common gas used for insufflation is carbon dioxide, which does not support combustion as do oxygen, air, or nitrous oxide. Carbon dioxide is also more soluble than other alternatives such as helium and nitrogen, thus likely reducing the impact of a gas embolus should it occur. However, because of CO_2's solubility, there is significant absorption across the peritoneum, which often results in a mild hypercapnia.

While there are benefits to laparoscopic surgery, laparoscopy can result in profound cardiovascular and pulmonary changes in physiology. There are many factors that contribute to the hemodynamic alterations that occur during laparoscopy (Table 41–1), but the most influential are intra-abdominal pressure (IAP) and patient position. The pneumoperitoneum created for laparoscopy can compress the abdominal arterial and venous vasculature. Consequently, there is increased IAP and systemic vascular resistance (SVR)

Table 41–1 FACTORS THAT AFFECT CARDIOVASCULAR STATUS WITH PNEUMOPERITEUM

Intra-abdominal pressure
Patient position
Intravascular volume
Volume of carbon dioxide absorbed
Ventilatory technique
Surgical conditions
Anesthetic agent

and a decreased cardiac index. However, if insufflation pressure remains below 12 mm Hg, minimal hemodynamic consequences occur in healthy patients.

Changes in patient position also contribute to the hemodynamic consequences of a pneumoperitoneum. In the head-up position, there is decreased venous return and cardiac output due to venous pooling in the legs (in addition to the pneumoperitoneum), with up to a 50% reduction in cardiac index. In healthy patients, this is generally well tolerated, but hemodynamic instability can result in patients with preexisting cardiovascular disease, anemia, or hypovolemia. The head-down position is associated with a cephalad shift of the diaphragm, which decreases functional residual capacity and lung compliance, possibly leading to atelectasis, mild hypoxemia, and an increased peak airway pressure. Endobronchial intubation is also more likely to occur.

Absorption of the CO_2 used for insufflation, in addition to hypoventilation, can result in hypercarbia. Hypercarbia, in turn, stimulates the sympathetic nervous system and can increase blood pressure, heart rate, myocardial contractility, and cause arrhythmias (tachycardia is the most common). It can sensitize the myocardium to catecholamines, setting the stage for ventricular arrhythmias. Hypercarbia can typically be overcome by increasing minute ventilation. However, if it is refractory or accompanied by hypoxemia or high airway pressures, the pneumoperitoneum should be released and insufflation attempted again at a lower intra-abdominal pressure. If complications recur, it may be necessary to convert to an open procedure. For recalcitrant hypercarbia, the possibility of malignant hyperthermia should be kept in mind.

Complications of Laparoscopy

The physiological changes that accompany laparoscopy can range from the common place and almost expected to the catastrophic and fortunately, rare. The most vulnerable time for the patient is just after the induction of anesthesia, during trocar insertion and gas inflation. Trocar insertion is a blind procedure, which can result in damage to blood vessels or vital organs such as the liver. Insufflation can cause a reduction in cardiac output which may be poorly tolerated in a patient with significant comorbidities. (Perhaps ironically, the sicker the patient, the more he or she will benefit from a minimally invasive approach.) Insufflation can also be associated with the catastrophic complication of air embolus, pneumothorax, or the development of subcutaneous emphysema. Even the more minor and expected physiologic alterations, such as decreased venous return and a decrease in FRC, may be magnified because of the continued presence of anesthetic induction agents and/or the introduction of inhalation anesthetics, clouding the differential diagnosis. During this initial portion of the surgical procedure, the anesthesiologist must be especially vigilant.

Vascular injuries can occur, chiefly during insertion of the Veress needle or trocar into major vessels such as the aorta, common iliac vessels, or inferior vena cava. If this occurs, the needle or trocar should be left in place to avoid further bleeding and help identify the site of injury and a laparotomy performed. Similarly, gastrointestinal or urinary tract injuries may occur during Veress needle or trocar insertion.

Gas embolism may cause hypotension and asystole, which occur most likely during insufflation. Gas may embolize through a tear in the abdominal wall or peritoneum or directly into a vein or organ. If embolism is suspected, insufflation should be discontinued, the patient should be placed in the left lateral decubitus position and head down to allow the gas to collect in the apex of the right ventricle, and prevent entry into the pulmonary artery. Hyperventilation will facilitate the elimination of carbon dioxide. A central venous catheter can be placed in order to aspirate the gas.

Pneumothorax has been reported during laparoscopic procedures and can occur during trocar insertion, insufflation, or dissection if associated with a tear in the visceral peritoneum, parietal pleura, or rupture of preexisting bullae. The presentation of pneumothorax during laparoscopy can be insidious, or there may be an increase in peak airway pressure, a decrease in oxygen saturation, severe hypotension, and cardiac arrest. Once this diagnosis is made, the pneumoperitoneum should be released immediately. Since carbon dioxide is rapidly absorbed, there may be no need for chest tube placement unless there is cardiopulmonary compromise. With similar mechanisms, pneumomediatinum and pneumopericardium are also possible.

Pneumoperitoneum can mask blood loss, even marked blood loss exceeding 1 L. Thus, acute blood loss must be considered in the differential diagnosis of deteriorating cardiovascular function.

Bradycardia and asystole can occur during laparoscopy, and have been attributed to vagal stimulation from the stretching of the peritoneum in the face of light anesthesia, or from a more catastrophic complication, carbon dioxide embolization. (For a more complete list of the differential diagnosis of cardiovascular collapse during laparoscopy please see Table 41–2.)

Postoperative nausea and vomiting (PONV) is a common issue addressed after laparoscopic surgery. The 5-HT3 receptor antagonists, such as ondansetron, are often effective in preventing PONV when given at the end of surgery, as well as adequate hydration and pain control.

Table 41–2 CAUSES OF CARDIOVASCULAR COLLAPSE DURING LAPAROSCOPY

Acute blood loss
Cardiac tamponade
Drug-related complications
Dysrhythmia
Excessive intra-abdominal pressure
Gas embolism
Myocardial dysfunction
Respiratory acidosis
Tension pneumothorax
Vasovagal reaction

Comprehension Questions

41.1. At which point during laparoscopy are life-threatening complications most likely to occur?

A. Insertion of the trocar and insufflations of the abdomen
B. During the procedure being performed
C. After the abdomen is deflated and the CO_2 removed
D. Postoperatively, in the recovery room

41.2. A 54-year-old woman is undergoing a laparoscopic cholecystectomy procedure under general anesthesia. During the procedure, the patient's oxygen saturation decreases and peak inspiratory pressure increases. There are no breath sounds on the right side. Which of the following is the most likely diagnosis?

A. Gas embolism
B. Pneumothorax
C. Pneumomediastinum
D. Acute blood loss
E. Pulmonary aspiration

41.3. A 35-year-old woman is undergoing laparoscopy procedure for chronic pelvic pain and suspected endometriosis. During insufflation of carbon dioxide into the abdominal cavity, the patient develops hypotension and hypoxemia. Auscultation of the heart and lungs reveals a machinelike murmur. The first step in treatment for this patient should be which of the following?

A. Stop insufflating and decompress the pneumoperitoneum.
B. Place patient head up.
C. Place patient head down.
D. Place central venous catheter to aspirate gas.

ANSWERS

41.1. **A.** Most of the life-threatening complications of laparoscopy occur during insertion of the trocar and insufflation of the abdomen. This period follows closely the induction of anesthesia, and is a time when the anesthetist may be attending to charting. However, vigilance at this time is of paramount importance to the patient.

41.2. **B.** While any of the choices could result in hypoxia, the absence of breath sounds makes pneumothorax the best choice.

41.3. **A.** This patient likely has a CO_2 embolism. In the event of gas embolus, the first response to a suspected gas embolus during laparoscopy should be to stop insufflation and decompress the pneumoperitoneum. It is also advisable to place the patient in the head-down position in an attempt to prevent the embolus from entering the pulmonary artery and attempt to withdraw gas from a central venous catheter.

Clinical Pearls

- Physiologic perturbations during laparoscopy may result from the pneumoperitoneum or from surgical complications.
- Increased intra-abdominal pressure secondary to insufflation causes increased systemic vascular resistance and decreased cardiac output, which can be exacerbated by the head-up position.
- Hypercarbia, hypoxia, and atelectasis may result during laparoscopy due to a decrease in pulmonary compliance and functional residual capacity.
- Other complications of laparoscopy include arrhythmias, hemorrhage, gas embolus, tension pneumothorax, pneumomediastinum, perforation, and postoperative nausea and vomiting.

REFERENCES

Gerges FJ, Kanazi GE, Jabbour-Khoury SI. Anesthesia for laparoscopy: a review. *J Clin Anesth*. 2006;18(1):67-78.

Joshi GP. Anesthesia for laparoscopic surgery. *Can J Anesth*. 2002:49(6):R1-R5.

Joshi GP. Complications of laparoscopy. *Anesthesiol Clin North Am*. 2001:19(1):89-105.

O'Malley C, Cunningham AJ. Anesthesia for minimally invasive surgery: laparoscopy, thoracoscopy, hysteroscopy. *Anesthesiol Clin North Am*. 2001:19(1):1-19.

Case 42

A 52-year-old man presents with severe hypertension, exceptionally severe headaches, and diaphoresis. He is found to have an adrenal mass on imaging and is referred to a surgeon for excision. Before proceeding with surgery, the patient is referred to the preoperative anesthesia clinic for evaluation and management of his hypertension. He is otherwise healthy, and until the past several months, exercised regularly, and did his own yard work. His exercise tolerance has recently decreased. He has had no chest pain, no shortness of breath, but does have occasional palpitations which he states he has had for a very long time. He has not noticed any issues with mentation, speech, movement, vision, or seizure activity. The patient is quite anxious, and because of the severity of the headaches, is worried about the possibility of an intracranial aneurysm. His review of systems is otherwise negative.

The patient's family history is remarkable in that it is unremarkable. His father is 95 years old, and in good health with some signs of a senile dementia. His mother died many years ago in an automobile accident. Neither his parents nor siblings have had any problems with cardiovascular diseases, nor have experienced any type of endocrinologic problems. On physical examination, the patient's blood pressure is 220/115 mm Hg, HR 87 beats/minute, and respirations are 15 breaths/minute. He is 70 in. tall and weighs 62 kg. His physical examination is unremarkable, as is his routine blood chemistry panel. An ECG shows left ventricular hypertrophy. The patient is scheduled for surgery for his condition. Urine catecholamines are elevated.

- ➤ What other preoperative tests should be done?
- ➤ What medications would help with blood pressure control preoperatively in this patient?
- ➤ What are the likely complications following surgery?

ANSWERS TO CASE 42: Pheochromocytoma

Summary: A healthy, 52-year-old man presents with hypertension, headaches, diaphoresis, recently reduced exercise tolerance, and anxiety. An adrenal mass is discovered on imaging and scheduled for excision.

- **Preoperative tests:** Echocardiogram and cardiac stress test. In patients with evidence suggesting myocardial dysfunction, it is advisable to obtain a preoperative echocardiogram to evaluate left ventricle function. Similarly, a stress test is useful to delineate the extent of coronary artery disease, if any. In addition to the left ventricular hypertrophy seen on his ECG, pheochromocytoma can also be associated with cardiomyopathy. After initiation of alpha-receptor blockade, left ventricular function often improves dramatically. Severe, uncontrollable, intraoperative hypertension and worse outcome may result if the patient is not adequately prepared preoperatively.
- **Preoperative management:** Adrenergic receptor blockade is the hallmark of preoperative management for patients with pheochromocytomas. Alpha-receptor blockade has classically been achieved with phenoxybenzamine (nonselective alpha-1 and alpha-2 antagonist). Terazosin, prazosin, or doxazosin (selective alpha-1 blockers) may be preferable, since their half-lives are significantly shorter than phenoxybenzamine's, making persistent post-operative hypotension less likely.
- **Complications following surgery:** Following removal of a catecholamine-secreting tumor, there can be persistent postoperative hypotension. The hypotension is thought to be secondary to hypovolemia or a sluggish recovery of the vasoconstrictor mechanisms following the withdrawal of catecholamines secreted by the tumor. Generally, this type of hypotension is responsive to fluid resuscitation. Astute anesthesiologists plan ahead, and begin volume replacement (at least 1000 mL) prior to clamping of the tumor's venous drainage. It is always appropriate to consider postoperative bleeding as a possibility if postoperative hypotension is not responsive to adequate volume resuscitation.

ANALYSIS

Objectives

1. Become familiar with the issues encountered in the preoperative evaluation of a patient with pheochromocytoma.
2. Review the physiology and treatment of pheochromocytoma.
3. Understand the differential diagnosis of intraoperative hypertension.

Considerations

This patient presents with the classic signs of a pheochromocytoma: hypertension, headaches, diaphoresis, a reduced exercise tolerance, and anxiety. His decreasing exercise tolerance is suggestive of left ventricular dysfunction, particularly since he was otherwise healthy. About 10% of pheochromocytomas are of metastatic origin which could also account for the change in his exercise tolerance, but this would not obviate the need to examine his left ventricular function.

The patient is monitored closely in the days leading up to his surgical procedure. His blood pressure is well controlled, he is no longer having and PVCs, he has no ST-T wave changes on his ECG, and he does indeed have orthostatic hypotension. Nevertheless, the need for invasive monitoring is essential. Nicardipine is prepared for administration by bolus and by infusion, and nitroglycerine is in the room and ready if needed. Conversely, a phenylephrine infusion is prepared to treat hypotension, should it occur. Once the patient is brought to the operating room, a large-bore intravenous and an arterial line are placed. Approximately 500 mL of normal saline are administered to assure normovolemia. Since this is a laparoscopic procedure (and CO_2 insufflation affects CVP), central venous access is not obtained. Since this patient has noticed a decline in his exercise tolerance, etomidate is administered as an induction agent. A large dose of the opiate fentanyl is administered just prior to induction, followed by 50 mg of lidocaine to attenuate any burning on injection of etomidate and to blunt the response to tracheal intubation. The patient is induced with etomidate, paralyzed with vecuronium, and he is easily intubated. See Table 42–1.

Table 42–1 INTRAOPERATIVE MONITORING FOR RESECTION OF A PHEOCHROMOCYTOMA
Arterial line placed prior to induction
Central venous catheter (possibly prior to induction)
Standard ASA monitors
Consider PA catheter for patients with LV dysfunction

APPROACH TO
Pheochromocytoma

Pheochromocytomas are tumors of the chromaffin cells occurring in the adrenal medulla. They are found in 0.1% of the population and typically present between the third and fifth decade of life. Pheochromocytomas arise from chromaffin cells typically in the adrenal medulla. However, these tumors may also originate anywhere chromaffin cells are located throughout the neural crest including areas along the sympathetic chains, the neural tissues at the bifurcation of the aorta (the organ of Zuckerkandl), the ureters, or the urinary bladder. When located outside of the adrenal medulla, these tumors are referred to as paraganglionomas.

The atypical cells of a pheochromocytoma may produce either epinephrine or norepinephrine, or a combination. It is not surprising that the patient's symptomatology can vary with the type and amount of compound(s) produced. Symptoms can range from hypertension, tremulousness, occasional palpitations, and diaphoresis, although not all patients with pheochromocytoma are hypertensive. The most common symptoms include severe headaches, palpitations, and diaphoresis.

Biochemical markers are used when attempting to diagnose a pheochromocytoma. Plasma-free metanephrines, which are by-products of epinephrine metabolism, are considered the gold standard for biochemical testing, yielding 99% sensitivity and 89% specificity for pheochromocytoma.

A number of hereditary conditions are associated with familial pheochromocytomas and paraganglionomas. Multiple endocrine neoplasias (MEN) types II A and B are associated with pheochromocytomas, as are disorders of the neuroectoderm, such as von Hippel-Lindau syndrome, Sturge-Weber syndrome, and neurofibromatosis. MRIs are extremely sensitive for visualizing these masses, and exceed the retentivity of either CT scans, or ^{131}I-MIBG scintigraphy in localizing extra-adrenal tumors.

Classic teaching dictates that 10% of pheochromocytomas are extra-adrenal, 10% are bilateral, and 10% are malignant. Also, 10% of pheochromocytomas present in children, 10% are familial, and 10% recur after surgery.

Preoperative Care of the Patient with Pheochromocytoma

In 1987, Roizen et al proposed criteria for the preoperative management of patients with pheochromocytoma. These criteria evaluate patients for their degree of preoperative adrenergic receptor blockade. Failure to meet the Roizen criteria prior to resection of the tumor is associated with a poor outcome. These criteria are:

- No BP measurement above 160/90 mm Hg should be observed for 24 hours preoperatively.
- Orthostatic hypotension with readings of 80/45 mm Hg *should* be present.
- The ECG should have no ST changes for at least 1 week prior to surgery.
- The patient should have no more than one PVC every 5 minutes.

Adrenergic receptor blockade is imperative prior to excision of a pheochromocytoma. The treatment initially targets the alpha receptors for blockade, followed by the beta receptors (if necessary). Alpha blockers commonly used for this purpose include phenoxybenzamine, doxazosin, prazosin, and terazosin. Phenoxybenzamine is a nonselective alpha blocker and has historically been considered the gold standard. It has the potential to induce reflex tachycardia, and a very long duration of action. Selective alpha-1 blockers, including doxazosin, prazosin, and terazosin, may be more efficacious due to their specificity for the alpha-1 receptor and shorter half-lives. Generally, beta receptors are only targeted after achieving adequate alpha blockade because of the risk of inducing iatrogenic congestive heart failure.

Intraoperative Considerations

Two considerations predominate when choosing anesthetic drugs for resection of a pheochromocytoma: avoid drugs which release catecholamines, and avoid drugs which release histamine. Drugs that cause histamine release include morphine, succinylcholine, pancuronium, and atracurium. Drugs which release or potentiate catecholamines include: ketamine (releases catecholamines), ephedrine (potentiates the release of catecholamines), meperidine (causes sympathetic stimulation), and succinylcholine (fasciculations may cause release of catecholamines). Halothane is relatively contraindicated in patients with pheochromocytomas secondary to its sensitization of the myocardium to catecholamines, potentially leading to fatal arrhythmias. It deserves mentioning, however, that halothane has been used successfully in hundreds of excisions in the past. Theoretically, desflurane should not be used in patients with pheochromocytomas due to increased sympathetic discharge at high concentrations, although it too has been used successfully in numerous excisions.

Both thiopental and propofol have been safely used for induction. If LV dysfunction is present, etomidate is the preferred choice. Vecuronium is probably the nondepolarizing neuromuscular blocker of choice, since it does not cause histamine release, and sevoflurane is an ideal inhalation anesthetic when excising pheochromocytomas although isoflurane is also acceptable.

Patients with undiagnosed pheochromocytomas can have severe hypertensive reactions to anesthetics, tracheal intubation, and the surgical stimulus. There are many potential agents which can be used to treat this hypertensive response (Table 42–2).

Table 42–2 AGENTS USED TO TREAT HYPERTENSION DURING RESECTION OF PHEOCHROMOCYTOMA

AGENT	MECHANISM OF ACTION
Sodium nitroprusside	Direct vasodilator
Nitroglycerin	Direct vasodilator
Phentolamine	Alpha-1, alpha-2 antagonist
Esmolol	Beta-1 antagonist
Nicardipine	Calcium channel blocker

Surgical Considerations

Effective communication between the anesthetic and surgical teams is of utmost importance during tumor resection. During surgical manipulation of the tumor, catecholamines can be released, thus precipitating a hypertensive crisis. By communicating, the teams can help predict these hemodynamic changes and intervene appropriately.

The resection of a pheochromocytoma can be undertaken either laparoscopically or via an open approach. Laparoscopic adrenalectomy is considered to be the procedure of choice, unless the patient has a demonstrated invasive tumor or a mass larger than 15 cm. Laparoscopic resection is seemingly associated with fewer incidences of hemodynamic instability when compared to a traditional laparotomy. Conversely, there is an increase in catecholamine release during insufflation of the abdomen, but the resultant hypertension is usually transient.

Comprehension Questions

42.1. A 52-year-old man presents to the preoperative anesthesia clinic prior to excision of his pheochromocytoma for evaluation and management of his hypertension. He has significant and worsening dyspnea on exertion. An echocardiogram demonstrates an LVEF of 38% with significant ventricular wall hypertrophy. A large-bore i.v. radial arterial line, and a central line are placed preoperatively and the patient is taken to the operating room. Which of the following agents are contraindicated for the induction of anesthesia?

A. Propofol
B. Etomidate
C. Ketamine
D. Thiopental

42.2. Just prior to exposure of the pheochromocytoma, during surgical dissection of Gerota fascia, the patient's arterial pressure spikes to 220/120 mm Hg and continues to rise. Which of the following is contraindicated for the management of the hypertension in this setting?
A. Sodium nitroprusside drip
B. Esmolol drip
C. Nicardipine drip
D. Fenoldopam drip

ANSWERS

42.1. **C.** Ketamine is contraindicated in pheochromocytoma patients because ketamine indirectly releases catecholamines and can result in intractable systemic hypertension. Answers: A, B, and D, propofol, etomidate, and thiopental respectively are equally efficacious in the induction of general anesthesia with little risk of inducing a hypertensive state.

42.2. **D.** Fenoldopam is useful in inducing peripheral vasodilation via activation of the dopamine-1 receptor, but also induces diuresis. In the setting of pheochromocytomas, patients are usually hypovolemic at the time of tumor excision, and diuresis at this time is not warranted. Answers A, B, and C, sodium nitroprusside, esmolol, and nicardipine are useful to treat hypertensive crises in this setting.

Clinical Pearls

- Outcomes are improved if blood pressure is controlled, orthostatic hypotension is present, the CG has had no ST changes for the previous week, and if the patient has no more than one PVC every 5 minutes.
- Alpha blockade must be established prior to beta blockade. This should be followed by expansion of intravascular volume and normalization of myocardial performance.
- The increased blood pressure and hypermetabolism associated with pheochromocytomas may mimic other disorders including malignant hyperthermia and thyroid storm.
- Avoid drugs which stimulate or release catecholamines, and which release histamine.
- The principal postoperative complication is persistent hypotension refractory to volume replacement.

REFERENCES

Kinney MA, Narr BJ, Warner MA. Perioperative management of pheochromocytoma. *J Cardiothorac Vasc Anesth*. 2002;16(3):359-369.

Lenders J, Pacak K, Walther MM, et al. Biochemical diagnosis of pheochromocytomas. *JAMA*. 2002;287(11):1427-1434.

Roizen MF, Fleisher LA. Anesthetic implications of concurrent diseases. In: Miller RD, ed. *Miller's Anesthesia*. 6th ed. Philadelphia, PA: Elsevier Churchill Livingstone;2005: 1042-1044.

Case 43

A 27-year-old man who jumped from the second story of a burning building is brought to the emergency room with second- and third-degree burns over 50% of his body. He also has an open fracture of the left tibia. He is moaning on arrival and somewhat obtunded. Though hoarse, he is eventually able to communicate that he has no medical problems and no allergies.

On physical examination, the patient's heart rate is 50 beats/minute (with frequent premature ventricular complexes); blood pressure, 85/55 mm Hg; respiratory rate, 22 breaths/minute; SpO_2, 99%; and temperature, 34.5°C (94.1°F). Carbonaceous material is in his nares, and he has mild inspiratory and expiratory wheezes. Blood is oozing from the open tibial fracture.

The patient's hematocrit is 49%, potassium is 3.9 mEq/L, and carboxyhemoglobin level is 9%. Following the administration of 1 L of lactated Ringer solution, he is brought to the operating room for placement of an external fixation device for the tibial fracture.

- What is/are the most urgent priorities in caring for this patient?
- What is a secondary, albeit urgent issue?
- What would likely be seen at direct laryngoscopy?

ANSWERS TO CASE 43:
The Burned Patient

Summary: A 27-year-old man with severe burns and an orthopedic injury develops bleeding and dysrhythmias after undergoing emergency surgery.

- **Most urgent priorities:** Hypothermia. The patient's hypothermia is life threatening, most likely causing the disturbance in cardiac rhythm, and perhaps, a coagulopathy. His high hematocrit is suggestive of dehydration. Warmed fluid for resuscitation, radiant-air warming, and maintaining a high environmental temperature are current critical priorities.
- **Second priorities:** Once the patient is stabilized, he should be taken promptly to the operating room for fixation of the open tibial injury. Although not immediately life-threatening as are the factors above, a delay in the fixation of the open injury risks loss of limb from infection.
- **Laryngoscopic findings:** Given the patient's hoarseness and the carbonaceous material surrounding his nares, a difficult intubation should be anticipated due to swelling of the pharynx and vocal cords, potentially even obstructing the glottic opening.

ANALYSIS

Objectives

1. Become familiar with the major physiological changes after burn injuries.
2. Be able to identify the intraoperative anesthetic concerns in the burn patient.
3. Be able to recognize the potential for a difficult airway in burn patients.

Considerations

The initial 24-hour period following a significant burn is characterized by capillary leak, intravascular volume depletion, and a moderately decreased cardiac output. Fluid resuscitation using warmed crystalloid solutions is the mainstay of therapy during this period, in addition to the correction of any electrolyte abnormalities. Because of his rapidly changing fluid status, a large-bore intravenous and central venous monitoring are probably warranted. Should frequent blood gas sampling be required because of a respiratory burn, an arterial catheter may also be warranted.

The patient should be warmed and resuscitated with warm fluids to increase his body temperature and restore his intravascular volume before proceeding to the operating room. The operating room temperature should be warm to hot. Warming blankets, fluid warmers, and heated humidification are indicated in attempt to maintain the patient's body temperature.

The patient's airway may be affected by the inhalation of heated, possibly toxic substances causing airway edema and lung injury, which can be worsened by fluid loading and capillary leak. In addition to swelling and erythema, a respiratory burn may be accompanied by friable tissue in the airway, perhaps with a propensity for bleeding. Intubation, if necessary, should be performed early before the airway becomes obstructed, and appropriate equipment available in case the patient cannot be intubated using direct laryngoscopy.

APPROACH TO A Burned Patient

Major burns affect all organ systems in ways that are dynamic and sometimes contradictory. In the early phase of a burn injury, a loss of capillary integrity leads to a reduction in intravascular volume requiring fluid resuscitation, while extravascular fluid increases. The excess extravascular volume is subsequently reabsorbed, though this process is offset by evaporative losses. The net balance of these processes varies with the percentage and degree of the body burned, and from individual to individual. The later stage of a burn injury is characterized by a high cardiac output, a dramatically increased metabolic rate, and protein catabolism.

Fluid and Electrolyte Management

During the first 24 hours after a burn injury, capillary integrity to water, solutes, and plasma proteins is drastically impaired reducing intravascular volume, and increasing extravascular fluid volume. Intravascular volume is replenished with crystalloid fluid, typically lactated Ringer solution. Colloid solutions are not used because they have been linked to greater formation of pulmonary infiltrates and decreased urine output.

There are several formulas to guide early fluid requirements, the most established being the Parkland formula. This method calculates fluid requirements for the first 24 hours post burn as 4 mL/kg/% of total body surface area (TBSA) burned. Half of the calculated volume is given over the first 8 hours; the remainder, over the following 16 hours. More fluid can be given as necessary to maintain a urine output greater than 30 to 50 mL/kg/h. In certain circumstances, such as crush injuries or electric burns that produce myoglobinuria, a higher urine output may be desirable to prevent pigment nephropathy. If fluid intake is increased repeatedly without improvement in urine output, placement of a central venous catheter or pulmonary artery catheter may aid in evaluation of intravascular volume.

After 24 hours, the characteristics of the patient's vascular system change as it begins to reabsorb extravascular fluid. At the same time, burns predispose to considerable evaporative losses. During the second 24-hour period, patients with substantial burns are generally given colloid solutions equal to 0.3 to 0.5 mL/kg/% TBSA burned, supplemented with 5% dextrose in water to maintain adequate urine output. Patients with smaller burned areas (<30% TBSA) may not require colloid and can often be given standard maintenance fluids. In the postresuscitation period, the goal of fluid management is to allow the patient to mobilize, excrete fluid, and return to normal preburn weight by postburn days 8 to 10. Thus, maintenance of fluid requirements after 48 hours is calculated to allow for daily losses of 2% to 3% of maximal body weight from insensate losses.

Electrolyte disturbances are common after burn resuscitation and should be carefully monitored perioperatively. After resuscitation, patients may be slightly hyponatremic from administration of high volumes of hypotonic fluids. Hyponatremia does not typically require treatment, and is usually corrected by postresuscitation diuresis. Patients may later become hypernatremic from excessive water losses and hyperglycemia-induced diuresis. Hyperkalemia, which also is common after large burns that destroy tissue, can be exacerbated by hypoventilation and acidosis. While ionized calcium is rarely affected by burn injuries, total calcium levels may be low because levels of serum-binding proteins are low.

Cardiovascular Management

Even within half an hour following a major burn, cardiac output can decrease substantially. The decrease is disproportionate to depletion of intravascular volume, and most likely reflects other neurohumoral mechanisms. Fluid resuscitation usually results in a return of cardiac output to normal levels. However, if oliguria persists even though pulmonary artery catheterization or echocardiography indicate fluid overload, inotropes such as dopamine or dobutamine may be required to increase cardiac output.

Shortly thereafter, fluid is reabsorbed and mobilized from the extravascular space. Cardiac output increases to supranormal levels, systemic vascular resistance is low, and there is an overall increase in metabolism. This response continues until burn wounds are grafted and fully healed.

Pulmonary and Airway Management

Multiple mechanisms contribute to the respiratory failure that occurs following a burn injury. Most commonly, toxins contained in smoke injure and inflame the airway. Upper airway edema may completely obstruct the airway, and lower airway edema may close small airways and lead to pneumonia.

Patients at risk may have stridor, wheezing, hoarseness, facial burns, or carbonaceous sputum, but these signs are not always present. In many cases, fiberoptic bronchoscopy may be necessary to reveal inhalation injury.

If an inhalation injury is suspected, the airway should be secured promptly by endotracheal intubation since the development of edema is unpredictable and may worsen with fluid resuscitation. Patients are assumed to have a full stomach, indicating a rapid-sequence intubation in most cases. A small-sized endotracheal tube should be available, in case the glottis is swollen. For intubations which are predicted to be difficult because of airway swelling, atypical anatomy, or body habitus, the intubation is performed with the aid of a fiberoptic bronchoscope while the patient is breathing spontaneously. A supraglottic airway (eg, LMA) may not be useful in patients with glottic edema.

The inhalation of carbon monoxide is associated with a reduction in oxygen delivery even in the presence of normal gas exchange. Carbon monoxide binds to hemoglobin with 200 times the affinity of oxygen, shifting the oxyhemoglobin dissociation curve to the left and decreasing oxygen-carrying capacity. It is crucial to measure carboxyhemoglobin levels in patients with possible inhalation injury. Pulse oximetry and the measurement of simple arterial blood gases do not account for this effect, and may significantly overestimate oxygen delivery. Carbon monoxide poisoning should be suspected in any burn patient with confusion, loss of consciousness, or agitation, especially if the patient was burned in a closed space. A carboxyhemoglobin level greater than 10% confirms the diagnosis. Treatment consists of administration of 100% oxygen, using hyperbaric oxygen therapy if the patient is comatose or otherwise suffering from the more severe consequences of carbon monoxide poisoning.

Temperature Management

Burn patients are at high risk for hypothermia from loss of the protective barrier of the skin. This risk is proportional to the surface area burned. Hypothermia has multiple manifestations including coagulopathy, dysrhythmias, hypotension, and slow drug metabolism. The body's primary responses to hypothermia (peripheral vasoconstriction and shivering) are inhibited by anesthetics. Shivering may increase myocardial oxygen consumption.

Maintenance of normothermia relies on heating intravenous fluids, humidifying inhaled gases, using forced-air heating blankets, and raising the environmental temperature. Although effective, forced-air heating blankets are used with caution in patients with extensive burns to avoid overheating devitalized tissue.

Pharmacologic Considerations

In burn patients, the responses to medications reflect alterations in drug metabolism and receptor physiology. In the immediate postburn period, drug clearance is impaired by decreases in intravascular volume, cardiac output, and hepatic and renal blood flow. In contrast, during the hypermetabolic postresuscitation period, the clearance of drugs is typically accelerated. Drugs which are administered either intramuscularly or enterally are variably and/or poorly absorbed when cardiac output is low. Decreases in the level of plasma proteins such as albumin and increases in levels of α_1-acid glycoprotein alter drug metabolism.

Neuromuscular blocking drugs are a special concern in the burn patient. Succinylcholine can produce an exaggerated hyperkalemic response, leading to ventricular arrhythmias and cardiac arrest from the proliferation of immature extrajunctional acetylcholine receptors. The hyperkalemic response typically takes 24 to 48 hours to develop after the initial burn; its duration varies and can last years after burns have healed. Similar mechanisms may cause resistance to nondepolarizing neuromuscular blockers in burn patients. Incremental dosing with close monitoring of Train-of-Four is essential when using nondepolarizing neuromuscular blockers in this patient population. Succinylcholine is typically avoided.

The later stage of a burn injury is characterized by a high cardiac output, a dramatically increased metabolic rate, and protein catabolism. Levels of plasma proteins may be altered drastically, thus affecting plasma levels of free (not protein bound) drugs. Burn patients undergo changes in their neuromuscular junctions, which increase the requirement for nondepolarizing neuromuscular blocking agents. Depolarizing neuromuscular blockers can produce severe hyperkalemia. Management of this stage of a burn injury is multifaceted, and requires attention to nutrition, infection control, and the planning of reconstructive surgery (see Table 43–1). The surgical treatment of the burn wound is usually not the first priority, and is usually performed after the patient is stabilized and resuscitated. However, burn patients, as in the case above, may have other traumatic injuries, and these must be treated concurrently as the patient is resuscitated and stabilized.

Table 43–1

PHASE OF INJURY	CARDIAC OUTPUT	VASCULAR PERMEABILITY	METABOLISM
Early (first 48 hour)	Decreased	Increased	Normal to decreased
Late	Increased	Normal	Increased

Martyn JAJ, Abernethy DR, Greenblatt DJ. Plasma protein binding of drugs after severe burn injury. *Clin Pharmacol and Ther.* 1984;35:534-536.

Comprehension Questions

43.1. A 34-year-old woman is admitted to the intensive care unit within 24 hours after sustaining burns over 80% of her body surface area. Which of the following is most likely increased in this 24-hour period?

A. Metabolism
B. Vascular permeability
C. Oxygen tension
D. Urine output

43.2. A 67-year-old man is scheduled for surgical debridement of a leg burn suffered 5 days ago. In the preoperative holding area, he receives midazolam and fentanyl. After induction with propofol and succinylcholine, the patient's continuous electrocardiogram shows peaked T waves. Which of the following agents most likely caused the electrocardiogram changes?

A. Midazolam
B. Fentanyl
C. Propofol
D. Succinylcholine

43.3. A 19-year-old man in the emergency room has facial burns, carbonaceous sputum, and bilateral wheezing. He is agitated and confused. Abnormalities in which of the following most likely explain his neurological dysfunction?

A. Platelet count
B. Hemoglobin level
C. Carboxyhemoglobin level
D. Prothrombin time

ANSWERS

43.1. **B.** Vascular permeability increases in the initial phase after a burn injury.

43.2. **D.** The peaked T waves on ECG are suggestive of an elevated potassium level. Succinylcholine can produce an exaggerated hyperkalemic response in burn-injured patients.

43.3. **C.** Agitation and confusion are associated with carbon monoxide poisoning. Carboxyhemoglobin levels should be measured.

Clinical Pearls

- Burn injuries result in complex physiologic alterations that change over the course of the patient's recovery.
- Although most surgeries on burn patients take place after resuscitation, patients may have additional injuries that require management in the early stages of the postburn period.
- Temperature control is of paramount importance, and requires the use of warming blankets, a warm ambient room temperature, and warm fluids.
- Succinylcholine is avoided except within the first 24 to 48 hours post burn.
- Early intervention is imperative in patients with an anticipated inhalation injury.
- Carbon monoxide poisoning is not accurately reflected in the patient's Sao_2 or $Paco_2$.

REFERENCES

Goodwin CW Jr, Dorethy J, Lam V, et al. Randomized trial of efficacy of crystalloid and colloid resuscitation on hemodynamic response and lung water following thermal injury. *Ann Surg*. 1983;197:520.

Martyn JAJ, Abernethy DR, Greenblatt DJ. Plasma protein binding of drugs after severe burn injury. *Clinical Pharmacol Ther*. 1984;35:534-536.

Martyn JAJ, Richtsfeld M. Succinylcholine-induced hyperkalemia in acquired pathologic states: etiologic factors and molecular mechanisms. *Anesthesiology*. 2006;104:158-169.

Case 44

A 50-year-old man is brought to the emergency room from the scene of a 2-car motor vehicle accident. He was the restrained driver of one of the vehicles involved. He is slightly anxious and complaining of a headache, neck pain, and abdominal pain, but does not recall ever losing consciousness. His past medical history is significant only for recurring sinusitis, for which he receives antibiotics. He is not allergic to any medications.

On physical examination the patient is a thin but well-nourished middle-aged male with no obvious bruises or wounds on his body. His blood pressure is 98/31 mm Hg, heart rate is 107 beats/minute, respirations are 16 breaths/minute, and his temperature is 36.2°C (97.2°F). He has no gross neurological deficits, although he had a neck collar on. He has two large-bore peripheral intravenous cannulae in place through which fluid were being infused.

Laboratory findings include a hemoglobin level of 10.2 g/dL, a normal chest roentgenogram, and electrocardiogram. A whole body CT scan was performed to rule out aerodigestive abnormalities, major vascular injuries, and long bone fractures. A diagnostic peritoneal lavage was done at bedside and yielded aspiration of approximately 25 mL of gross blood. The patient was scheduled for an emergency exploratory laparotomy. A urethral catheter was placed and a blood sample was sent for typing and cross-matching.

- What are the anesthetic concerns for this patient?
- What are the associated injuries one should look for?
- What is the anesthetic plan?

ANSWERS TO CASE 44:
The Patient with Blunt Trauma

Summary: A 50-year-old man was involved in a motor vehicle accident and shows signs of hemodynamic instability (hypotension and tachycardia), and a peritoneal lavage positive for frank blood.

- ➤ **Anesthetic concerns:** Possibility of neck injury requiring cervical immobilization, degree of hypovolemia, and presence of associated injuries and timing of last meal.
- ➤ **Associated injuries:** Pericardial injury, tamponade, aortic dissection, aortic hematoma, rib fractures, and myocardial injury.
- ➤ **Anesthetic plan:** General anesthesia with rapid-sequence induction with cricoid pressure and intubation is the only option since this patient needs emergency surgery.

ANALYSIS

Objectives

1. Appreciate the diverse nature of injuries in blunt trauma.
2. Understand some of the different approaches to the administration of anesthesia in the presence or absence of certain injuries.

Considerations

This patient requires emergent surgery, and general anesthesia with rapid-sequence induction. While standard monitors are applied (pulse oximetry, 5-lead ECG, noninvasive blood pressure), intravascular volume repletion is continued through the existing large-bore intravenous access sites. He is asked to inspire 100% oxygen by face mask, using a few vital capacity breaths to ensure alveolar de-nitrogenation.

Since the patient is hypotensive, etomidate is chosen for induction, and succinylcholine is administered in quick succession as cricoid pressure is applied by an assistant. Laryngoscopy and endotracheal intubation are performed while a second assistant maintains stabilization of the neck. Once the endotracheal tube is secured, and its position confirmed by auscultation and capnography, the surgery may proceed.

Given the severity of the accident and possibility of associated major injuries, an arterial catheter is placed in right radial artery to achieve beat-to-beat arterial blood pressure monitoring as well as access for blood draws for continuous assessment of hemoglobin values. However, given the patient's intra-abdominal bleeding, the laparotomy is not delayed to allow placement of this line.

Once surgical exploration is begun and findings are clear, there might be a need for blood and blood product transfusion to help control surgical bleeding. A bronchoscopy and an esophagoscopy performed at the end of the procedure were negative for tracheobronchial and esophageal injuries.

APPROACH TO The Patient with Blunt Trauma

CLINICAL APPROACH

The three-point lap-shoulder seat belt is reported to reduce the risk of death or serious injury for front-seat occupants by approximately 45%. In frontal MVAs, air bags provide a reduce risk of fatality by approximately 30%. In all crashes, the reduction in the risk of death with use of seat belts has been estimated at 11%. But as the death rate declines, the number of survivors increases. Thus serious injuries following blunt trauma are on the rise. The primary survey of the Acute Trauma Life Support (ATLS) course concentrates on six immediately life-threatening injuries to the airway and the chest. The secondary survey detects another six potentially life-threatening injuries that scan the spectrum of thoracic injuries (see Table 44–1).

Many of the injuries of the thorax and abdomen result from the rapid acceleration toward the seat belt followed by subsequent, sudden deceleration. Thoracic cavity injuries occur when differential movement occurs

Table 44–1 THORACIC INJURIES IN BLUNT TRAUMA

IMMEDIATELY LIFE-THREATENING INJURIES	POTENTIALLY LIFE-THREATENING INJURIES
Airway obstruction	Simple pneumo/hemothorax
Tension pneumothorax	Aortic rupture
Open pneumothorax	Tracheobronchial rupture
Massive hemothorax	Pulmonary contusion
Flail chest	Blunt cardiac injury
Cardiac tamponade	Diaphragmatic rupture

between adjacent structures; for example the distal aorta is anchored to the thoracic spine and decelerates much more quickly than the relatively mobile aortic arch. Shear forces are generated in the aorta by the continued forward motion of the arch with respect to the distal thoracic aorta. Similar situations occur at the renal pedicles, at the junction of the cervical and thoracic spine, and also between the white and grey matter within the brain. These injuries are obviously not visible to the naked eye. Diagnostic aids include: diagnostic peritoneal lavage (DPL); focused abdominal sonography for trauma (FAST); and abdominal and pelvic computed tomography (CT). CT scans are the most useful in terms of specificity and sensitivity to aid in diagnosis.

Occult bleeding can accumulate in a closed space, since the bleeding tamponades. However, on incision, the tamponade may be suddenly relieved and hypovolemia revealed. Intraperitoneal bleeding is a common cause of hemorrhage, and most commonly results from a splenic injury. Pericardial bleeding may also manifest in hemodynamic instability. Severe pelvic fractures can also present as hypovolemic shock in the patient with blunt trauma. Repleting intravascular volume (blood and/or crystalloid) and oxygen-carrying capacity (blood) is a priority even as preparations for emergency surgery are underway. Large-bore peripheral intravenous access is required for fluid administration. The presence of a CVP line aids in both fluid resuscitation and administration of vasoactive drugs.

The presence or possibility of cervical instability precludes the routine induction of general anesthesia. If there is a high cervical vertebral fracture, awake fiberoptic intubation is indicated to prevent neurological injury from displacement of the fracture. If the stability of the neck is unclear, the neck may be immobilized during induction of general anesthesia and intubation using direct laryngoscopy.

One of the most devastating and silent injuries of the head and neck is the fracture of the larynx. Perhaps presenting only as hoarseness in the emergency room, this complication may be noted first during rapid-sequence induction. If diagnosed prior to surgery, it is, of course, an indication for an awake bronchoscopy and intubation.

Blunt trauma is associated with pneumomediastinum in approximately 10% of cases. Pneumomediastinum is usually be identified by CT scans, however in equivocal cases, bronchoscopy and esophagoscopy may be indicated. The spectrum of injuries extending into the mediastinum can range from tracheal and laryngeal displacement, to esophageal tears. The treatment depends upon extent of injury. Pneumothorax is also common in trauma patients. Positive pressure ventilation expands a pneumothorax, which will further reduce venous return and precipitate end organ hypoperfusion.

Thoracic aortic injuries are usually diagnosed by CT scan. Blood in the pericardium is suggested by nonspecific abnormalities on the ECG, and requires further evaluation such as echocardiography. The presence of a thoracic aortic dissection is obviously a surgical emergency, usually involving the cardiothoracic surgery team and perfusionists. Morbidity and mortality increase significantly if the repair of a thoracic dissection is delayed beyond 6 hours of presentation. However, approximately 85% of thoracic trauma can be managed without surgical intervention. The mainstays of management are supplemental oxygen, intercostal drainage, good physiotherapy, and pain control.

Diaphragmatic injury should be suspected in any patient who has suffered blunt trauma and is short of breath. It is diagnosed on chest x-ray by evidence of stomach herniation or misplaced nasogastric tube..

Deceleration injuries like motor vehicle accidents may be associated with hollow viscus rupture, resulting from deceleration which causes compression of gas-filled viscus. Hollow viscus rupture may be difficult to diagnose by routine tests such as DPL and CT scans. Misdiagnosed viscus injuries significantly increase the morbidity and mortality associated with blunt trauma. A high index of suspicion for hollow viscus injury should be maintained in the presence of other multiple organ injuries and in the presence of pancreatic injury with solid organ injury. An exploratory laparotomy in the face of suspected viscus injury is not unreasonable.

Spinal cord injury occurs from traction and compression of the spinal cord. Inflammatory mediators released after the injury are attributed to the phenomenon of spinal shock. Spinal cord injury is mostly managed conservatively with measures to reduce secondary injury. Steroids administered in the first 8 hours after cord injury decrease cord edema significantly. Operative intervention is reserved for cases of canal entrapment.

Comprehension Questions

44.1. A 24-year-old man is involved in a motor vehicle accident in which he veered off the road and hit a tree. In his evaluation, there are no overt bleeding sites. Which of the following findings is most likely associated with bleeding?

A. Hypertension
B. Tachycardia
C. Polyuria
D. Elevated INR

44.2. A 38-year-old man falls off a platform while cleaning a window on the second floor of building. He is suspected of having a ruptured spleen with intra-abdominal bleeding. During this surgical procedure, the surgeon notes that the abdomen is somewhat tense. He incises the peritoneum and about 750 mL of blood is rapidly suctioned from the peritoneal cavity. What else might the anesthesiologist predict to occur within that time frame?

A. Reduced anesthetic level
B. Hypercapnia
C. Hypotension
D. Hypertension

44.3. A 41-year-old woman is involved in a "head on" motor vehicle accident. She was wearing a seat belt, and the air bags deployed. An ECG is performed revealing nonspecific ST-T wave changes. Which of the following should be considered?
A. Pericarditis
B. Myocardial infarction
C. Heart failure
D. Aortic injury

ANSWERS

44.1. **B.** Tachycardia. The triad of hypotension, tachycardia, and oliguria should always evoke the suspicion of bleeding; if none is visible, occult bleeding should be high on the differential diagnosis list.

44.2. **C.** Sudden relief of tamponade is associated with hypotension secondary to hypovolemia, which is unmasked on relief of the hemoperitoneum. An appropriate action might be to reduce the level of the anesthetic.

44.3. **D.** A restrained motor vehicle accident causes acceleration and sudden deceleration which can rip the arch of the aorta from the descending portion of the aorta, causing an aortic dissection. CT angiography, transesophageal echocardiography are the diagnostic modalities of choice if there is a suspicion of aortic injuries.

Clinical Pearls

- Blunt trauma to the neck can rapidly become life-threatening due to airway compromise from a rapidly expanding hematoma or from direct disruption of the trachea or larynx. Securing an artificial airway becomes emergent in such cases.
- Pneumothorax, rib fractures (with or without flail chest), pericardial tamponade, aortic rupture, and diaphragmatic injuries are examples of devastating injuries that may result from blunt trauma.
- A low threshold for the diagnosis of pneumothorax and a chest tube or needle thoracostomy should be performed promptly.
- Blunt abdominal trauma may cause splenic and/or hepatic injury resulting in massive hemorrhage and hemoperitoneum. Hollow viscus injury should be suspected in the presence of multiple organ injury, and presence of pancreatic injury.

REFERENCES

Crosby E. Considerations for airway management for cervical spine surgery in adults. *Anesthesiol Clin*. 2007;25:3.

Donaldson VP, Heil BV, Donaldson VP, et al. The effect of airway maneuvers on the unstable C1-C2 segment. *Spine*. 1997;22(11):1215-1218.

Isenhour JL, Marx J. Advances in abdominal trauma. *Emerg Med Clin North Am*. 2007;25:3.

REFERENCES

Case 45

A 23-year-old man with no known medical history is brought to the operating room (OR) from the emergency room (ER) with a gun shot to the abdomen. The patient states that he has no medical problems, takes no medicines, and has no allergies. His last meal was lunch earlier in the day, approximately 6 hours ago.

The patient is restless and combative, though he has no signs of respiratory distress and can protect his airway. His blood pressure is 89/37 mm Hg, heart rate 112 bpm, respirations 26 breaths/min, and his Spo_2 is 100 % on 10 L by face mask. He opens his mouth well, has a full beard, and an adequate thyromental distance. His neck has not sustained any injuries that would indicate cervical immobilization. His abdomen is tense. Intravenous access consists of two 16-gauge catheters in his upper extremity.

The ER nurse informs you that he received 2 L of normal saline and 2 U of packed red blood cells in the trauma bay. His hematocrit prior to the transfusions was 24%.

- How should the airway be secured?
- What special monitors are indicated?
- What anesthetic agents should be used?
- How should the patient be resuscitated?

ANSWERS TO CASE 45: Penetrating Trauma and Massive Transfusion

Summary: A healthy, 23-year-old presents after a gunshot wound to the abdomen with signs of hypovolemic shock.

- **Securing the airway:** Rapid-sequence induction and intubation with a cuffed endotracheal tube.
- **Special monitoring:** In addition to standard American Society of Anesthesiologists (ASA) monitors, invasive arterial blood pressure monitoring and measurement of urinary output with a bladder catheter (such as a Foley) are strongly indicated. In this setting, urine output serves as a surrogate for success of resuscitation. Central venous pressure (CVP) monitoring may be helpful.
- **Anesthetic agents:** Choice of anesthetic is guided by hemodynamic parameters. While inhalational agents and opiates should ideally be given in cases of extreme hypotension, all anesthetics can worsen the shock state. In this circumstance, scopolamine may be used for its amnestic properties.
- **Resuscitation:** The treatment of choice in an acute trauma with massive blood loss is fluid replacement. A combination of packed red blood cells, fresh frozen plasma, cryoprecipitate, platelets, and balanced salt solutions are most appropriate.

ANALYSIS

Objectives

1. Highlight the differences between elective surgery and emergent trauma surgery.
2. Learn the concept of a "transfusion trigger" and massive transfusion protocol.
3. Understand the complications and consequences of massive blood transfusion.

Considerations

Any patient with a significant injury to the thorax, abdomen, or an extremity often requires emergent surgical exploration. He may have a major vascular injury, or organ damage that requires immediate surgical intervention. Adequate venous access is critical. If peripheral access is limited, a large central venous line is indicated. This patient has two large-bore intravenous lines, which are appropriate. Unless the patient is hemodynamically stable and the trip to the OR is for exploration only, invasive arterial blood pressure monitoring is usually indicated. This can be placed in ER or in the operating room, whichever is most expeditious.

If the patient is hemodynamically stable, he may have to go to radiology for imaging first to delineate the extent of injuries, followed immediately by a trip to the operating room. Given this patient's hypotension, he must go directly to the operating room.

Patients who have suffered an acute trauma will have delayed gastric emptying; this added to any recent meals mandates they be given full stomach considerations for airway management. The most common approach is rapid sequence intubation with cricoid pressure and a cuffed endotracheal tube. The management of the trauma patient's airway is sometimes more difficult than that of other emergency patients. This patient has a full beard, which sometimes camouflages a recessed chin heralding a difficult intubation. This possibility is noted, and the operating room team is prepared to perform an emergency tracheotomy if needed.

Undiagnosed hypovolemia may result from significant albeit occult bleeding, so the anesthesia team must be prepared for aggressive volume resuscitation.

APPROACH TO
Acute Penetrating Trauma

A gun shot or stab wound to the thorax or abdomen is a life-threatening emergency until proven otherwise. Penetrating chest wounds may require anything from a chest tube to a thoracotomy with cross-clamping of the aorta. Abdominal or extremity injuries that are not associated with hemodynamic instability may permit a CT scan for a more complete evaluation before surgery. Yet many injuries can be managed by the trauma team without proceeding to the operating room.

When the patient first arrives to the OR, the anesthesiologist should perform a quick assessment of the patient. The surgical staff can provide information on mechanism of injury or suspected injuries. Simply knowing the locations of entry and exit wounds can give one an idea of what structure(s) may be injured (vasculature, spine, liver, bowl, etc). The surgeons and any accompanying emergency room staff should be able to detail line placement and resuscitative measures. A quick assessment of the airway is critical.

The airway is often more difficult to manage in a trauma patient than in a patient presenting for another type of emergency surgery. The trauma patient may be intoxicated or unable to cooperate with an airway examination. A deforming injury to the face or neck, or a previously undiagnosed occult injury may complicate laryngoscopy. Hemorrhage from the nose, pharynx, or mouth can obscure a view of the vocal cords. Trauma patients may vomit before or during induction. An experienced anesthesiologist can learn a lot by assessing external factors like thyromental distance, neck circumference, and tongue size.

If airway management will likely be difficult, the decision must be made to either proceed with induction and laryngoscopy, or to take extra time to perform an awake intubation or tracheostomy. The patient's injuries, hemodynamic status, and ability to cooperate determine which direction to take. If the decision to proceed with induction and laryngoscopy is made, a rapid-sequence induction with cricoid pressure should be performed. The patient may have recently eaten, and acute trauma decreases gastric emptying. Ordinarily, a rapid-sequence induction is performed with succinylcholine, so if the patient cannot be intubated, he is allowed to emerge, and an awake fiberoptic intubation is performed. Trauma victims with burns or denervation injuries can safely receive succinylcholine if the injury occurred less than 24 hours previously: the risk of hyperkalemia is not increased immediately after such injuries. Rocuronium at 1.2 mg/kg or vecuronium 0.2 mg/kg can also provide rapid intubating conditions if a nondepolarizing agent is preferred. Following the administration of nondepolarizers, a failed intubation leads to a surgical airway. Similarly, if a patient is unstable and surgery must proceed, allowing a patient to emerge from anesthesia after a failed intubation is not a reasonable option and a cricothyroidotomy is performed.

Cervical collars make positioning for intubation difficult. The patient's neck must be kept in a neutral position, with care made not to extend the head during laryngoscopy. Alternatively, the cervical collar is removed, and the neck is stabilized by an assistant throughout airway manipulation. Indeed, this technique of laryngoscopy with proper in-line stabilization is as effective as an awake fiberoptic intubation at protecting the patient from further c-spine injury.

Hemorrhage and/or hypotension favor using an induction agent associated with hemodynamic stability such as etomidate. Ketamine may also be a good choice, as it causes release of endogenous catecholamines. However, it should be remembered that ketamine is a direct myocardial depressant, and in someone whose sympathetic response is already blunted (eg, an individual on beta-blockers), ketamine can result in a precipitous drop in blood pressure.

A patient who is severely hypovolemic may not tolerate the induction of anesthesia. In extreme cases, it may be necessary to intubate with succinylcholine alone. Preservation of life trumps the possibility of intraoperative recall, an inherent risk of trauma surgery. Fortunately, cognitive impairment secondary to hypotension, intoxication, or traumatic brain injury helps decrease this risk. Scopolamine 0.2 to 0.4 mg i.v. can decrease the risk of awareness or recall by causing central anticholinergic confusion. These patients often already have rapid heart rates from pain, sympathetic surge from their injuries, and from hypovolemia; so scopolamine often does not further increase heart rate. One troublesome effect of scopolamine is papillary dilatation, which can confound efforts to assess neurological status in the patient who is intubated and paralyzed. Once bleeding is controlled and volume replacement has been given, patients will often tolerate a volatile anesthetic and narcotics.

Resuscitation is accomplished by a combination of crystalloid and colloid administration. Crystalloid balanced salt solutions, such as normal saline, Plasmalyte, and lactated Ringers, are inexpensive and easy to obtain. They are often chosen for initial volume replacement. If the source of bleeding is easily diagnosed and quickly controlled, crystalloids may be all that a patient requires. In patients with hemoglobin values above 7gm/dL but mild hypovolemia, colloids such as albumin or hetastarch (Hespan) may be administered.

However, penetrating trauma frequently involves significant and extensive bleeding that necessitates blood and blood product transfusion. Packed red blood cells (PRBCs) may constitute much of the fluids given. Trauma centers will often have uncross-matched O-negative blood available on hand for immediate use; a blood sample should be sent as soon as possible so the blood bank can prepare type-specific, cross-matched blood products. As long as the patient has received PRBC and not whole blood, cross-matched blood products can be given as soon as they are available. If the blood bank's supply of O-negative blood is critically low, a male patient can usually be given O-positive blood without suffering an acute transfusion reaction. Transfusion of Rh-incompatible blood results in delayed reactions that are not usually life threatening and can be followed later. Rh-negative women of reproductive age should be given Rh-immune globulin (Rhogam) prophylaxis until their blood type is known.

Massive transfusion, the replacement of more than one blood volume in a patient in less than 24 hours, carries special risks. Potassium increases in PRBCs, particularly as their unit ages. Potassium from this source can materially increase serum potassium levels, especially in the patient who is acidotic. Stored blood also contains citrate as an anticoagulant, which binds serum calcium. While the liver rapidly metabolizes citrate, rapid transfusion of large volumes of blood products can result in hypocalcemia. Hypocalcemia can in turn exacerbate both the hypotension and the coagulopathy, worsening the situation in the trauma patient. Blood is also cold: it is stored in the blood bank at 4°C (39.2°F). Thus a fluid warming device should be used for all cases where blood products are administered rapidly to prevent hypothermia (which can also worsen a coagulopathy). Lactate from anaerobic metabolism of red blood cells in PRBC can cause or worsen metabolic acidosis. Electrolytes and arterial blood gasses should be checked periodically, and metabolic abnormalities corrected accordingly. Levels of 2,3-DPG are reduced in red cells that have been stored a long time, causing a left shift of the oxygen-hemoglobin dissociation curve. This left shift may be offset by local tissue acidosis in the hypoperfused patient.

Dilutional coagulopathies follow the infusion of large volumes of PRBC and crystalloids. Current recommendations for massive transfusion are to transfuse 1 U of FFP for every unit of PRBC transfused. The FFP is given empirically, rather than waiting for coagulation laboratory results. The factor that reaches low levels the earliest is often fibrinogen. While FFP usually contains adequate fibrinogen, cryoprecipitate may occasionally be a useful adjuvant as it is rich in fibrinogen. Both FFP and cryoprecipitate need to be given through a fluid warmer. Massively transfused patients can also develop a dilutional thrombocytopenia. Low platelet levels can result in microvasular bleeding that can be almost impossible to control without transfusion. Platelets do not need to be warmed, as they are stored at warmer temperatures. Platelets should be given more slowly than other fluids. The rapid administration of platelets can cause platelet rupture, the release of vasoactive metabolites, and hypotension.

Comprehension Questions

45.1. A 19-year-old man comes to the operating room for exploratory laparotomy after sustaining stab wounds to the chest and abdomen. His breathing is labored; the only intervention in the emergency room was administration of 1 L of normal saline. After rapid-sequence induction and intubation, peak airway pressures are 51 and delivered tidal volumes are 110 mL. After intubation, HR increases from 111 to 132; BP drops from 97/50 to 81/36. Which of the following is the next appropriate step?

A. Rapid infusion of 2 L of normal saline.
B. Check the endotracheal tube placement.
C. Immediate chest tube placement on the side of the injury.
D. Lighten the anesthetic.

45.2. A 32-year-old man is brought to the OR for surgical exploration of a stab wound to the neck. The entrance wound is just below the angle of the mandible in the mid-cervical spine. He was intubated in the ER. There is only a small hematoma, and bleeding is mild. His blood pressure is 68/32 mm Hg with a heart rate of 47 bpm. There are no other injuries. How should the patient be resuscitated?

A. Infusion of PRBC and normal saline in a 1:1 ratio
B. Infusion of epinephrine and normal saline
C. Rapid infusion of 3 L of normal saline
D. Infusion of isoproterenol and PRBC

45.3. A 24-year-old is in the OR after a gunshot to the abdomen. The surgeons are repairing a perforation in the small bowl. The patient has been stable for about an hour, and the urine output is 1 cc/kg/h. The patient suddenly becomes hypotensive after they accidentally cut the inferior vena cava. The patient loses 1500 cc of blood before the bleeding is brought under control. Using a rapid infuser, you infuse 5 U of PRBC (about 1500 cc) in 5 minutes. The patient is still hypotensive. Which of the following is your best option?

A. Give calcium chloride.
B. Give three more units of PRBC.
C. Give 2 L of normal saline.
D. Start a vasopressin infusion.

ANSWERS

45.1. **C.** The patient has a tension pneumothorax and requires immediate decompression. There is an injury to the lung. While the patient was breathing spontaneously, a pneumothorax may have been slowly enlarging. When positive pressure ventilation was initiated after intubation, however, the pneumothorax rapidly expanded. A tension pneumothorax can be recognized by hypotension (inadequate venous return from high intrathoracic pressures resulting in decreased preload), high airway pressures/inadequate ventilation, a shift of the trachea away from the injured side, and decreased breath sounds on the side of the injury.

45.2. **B.** This patient is suffering from spinal shock secondary to transaction of the spinal cord. Significant lesions high in the spinal column can cause a massive sympathectomy, with resultant vasodilatation and venodilatation in most of the vascular beds of the body. This leads to venous pooling (decreasing preload) and a very low systemic vascular resistance. Additionally, the cardioaccelerator fibers that innervate the heart (T1-T4 innervation) have been lost. This limits the body's ability to compensate with a tachycardia and increased contractility. The treatment of choice is pharmacologic replacement of the sympathetic nervous system. In the absence of significant bleeding, concurrent administration of a balanced salt solution to correct the new relative hypovolemia is appropriate. Spinal shock typically resolves after several weeks as the patient develops a new homeostatic equilibrium.

45.3. **A.** This patient has hypocalcemia. Rapid infusion of large amounts of blood products can result in citrate toxicity. Citrate is used as an anticoagulant in stored blood products. When given more slowly, it is rapidly cleared by the liver. In massive transfusion situations, however, citrate levels can be critically low. The hypocalcemia can cause hypotension and a coagulopathy.

Clinical Pearls

- Trauma patients come to the OR with significant physiologic derangements including hypotension, hypovolemia, academia, and anemia. Anesthetic care may be directed entirely at resuscitation for several hours until surgical stabilization of injuries has occurred.
- Injuries can complicate airway management in a situation where performing a controlled, awake intubation is not an option.
- PRBCs may cause hypothermia, hyperkalemia, hypocalcemia, acidosis, and a shift to the left of the hemoglobin dissociation curve.
- If massive transfusion of PRBC is performed, FFP should be given empirically in a 1:1 ratio to prevent a dilutional coagulopathy. Dilutional thrombocytopenia must also be treated.

REFERENCES

Dutton RP, McCunn M. Anesthesia for trauma. In: Miller RD, ed. *Anesthesia.* 6th ed. Philadelphia, PA:Elsevier; 2005: 2451-2495.

Perkins JG, Cap AP, Weiss BM, Reid TJ, Bolan CE. Massive transfusion and nonsurgical hemostatic agents. *Crit Care Med.* 2008;36 (suppl. 7):S325-S339.

Case 46

You are scheduled to provide anesthesia for three cases outside the operating room. The first case is a 4-year-old child for an MRI, the second case is an endoscopic retrograde cholangiopancreatography (ERCP) in an adult, and the third case of the day is an electro-convulsive therapy (ECT) for an adult. These cases will all likely be general anesthetics, and all require consideration about the site of anesthesia delivery.

➤ What three factors are common to all cases performed outside the operating room?

ANSWER TO CASE 46:
Cases Outside the Operating Room

Summary: You are asked to provide anesthesia for three very different patients undergoing three different types of procedures in three different locations—radiology, GI, and the induction room (or ECT suite).

➤ **Three common factors:** (1) Need for equipment and drugs must be anticipated, since these items are not likely to be readily available in the remote site; (2) inexperienced health care personnel unfamiliar with the "ways of the operating room" to be able to provide effective assistance in an emergency; (3) absence of essential equipment such as "piped" oxygen, and sometimes even wall suction.

ANALYSIS

Objectives

1. Understand the unique environment of out of OR cases.
2. Become acquainted with how some of these challenges are met.
3. Understand the unique equipment challenges of MRI anesthesia.

Considerations

Since an MRI can be performed under sedation, if anesthesia services are requested, then there is usually an indication for general anesthesia. Children who are unable to cooperate represent just such an indication. The safest way to care for this child is to provide a general anesthetic using an ETT and an MRI-compatible machine. The child is kept NPO for a suitable period depending on his age, and standard monitors are applied (BP, pulse oximetry, capnography, ECG, and temperature) and must be compatible with the MRI environment. The MRI room is usually cold, but the scanner itself produces heat, so hypothermia is generally not as problematic as in the operating room.

ERCP is a fairly invasive and painful procedure usually performed under general anesthesia. The prone position involves turning the patient after induction, as well as turning the patient's head to one side to allow entry of the endoscope. Preoperative assessment of neck sideway range of motion is important in anticipation of this positioning.

ECTs are performed in a wide variety of patients using general anesthesia with mask ventilation. Since antidepressant drugs may have some synergies with anesthetic drugs, doses are minimized and reduced on subsequent treatments if possible.

APPROACH TO
Cases Outside the Operating Room

Providing anesthesia outside the operating room suite is challenging for many reasons. The equipment to perform the anesthetic and treat complications must be anticipated, and transported to the distant site. Generally, each institution will set up equipment carts to accomplish this task efficiently. These carts have limited capacity, however, so compromises are made and one doesn't have all the equipment necessary to deal with any and all potential anesthetic scenarios.

Another challenge is the remote location away from other anesthesia personnel. In an emergency situation having help and equipment is important, so it is easy to see the challenge when those resources are not available. Also, the personnel at the locations away from the operating room may not be familiar with anesthesia services. There may be limited room for equipment in the procedure room and there may be limited understanding of the sequence and timing of events during anesthesia delivery. Communication can help bridging this disconnect, but in the emergency situation the anesthesia provider can be left feeling very much alone.

The MRI Scanner

The magnet in an MRI scanner is a remarkably powerful device. All equipment inside the room housing the MRI must be nonmagnetic (this includes implants within the patient). Stories of intubating stylets hurling as projectiles across the room, or even a metal anesthesia cart with a resident holding on to it are not unheard of. (The resident's nose was broken, the cart had minor damage, but the MRI was out of service for several months). A second consideration is that the scanner is a long narrow tube. The patient's airway is inaccessible inside the scanner. Moreover, sudden patient movement can result in injury to the patient.

The anesthetic procedure is dictated largely by the availability (or lack of) equipment compatible with the MRI within a given institution. If the anesthesia machine is not MRI compatible, then it must remain outside the scanner and long breathing circuit tubing will be needed to connect the patient to the machine. First, a choice must be made as to whether to induce the patient on a stretcher outside the MRI room and transfer him/her into the MRI machine while anesthetized, or whether MRI-compatible equipment is available which can allow induction with the patient lying on the MRI. Most institutions currently have devices capable of measuring blood pressure, ECG (including ECG patches), and pulse oximetry probes and devices that are

MRI compatible. However, the pulse oximetry devices used in the operating room interfere with the imaging process, and the imaging process interferes with the pulse oximetry.

Securing the airway in the MRI scanner must be done with MRI-compatible laryngoscopes or the patient has to be outside the MRI scanner for intubation. Some institutions have anesthesia machines that are MRI compatible. The presence or absence of an MRI-compatible anesthesia machine is particularly important with respect to ventilatory dead space. Some centers have MRI-compatible machines and therefore the circle system dead space is identical to that in the operating room. However, if there is no MRI-compatible machine, then the anesthesia machine is placed outside the MRI scanner. Dead space ventilation is the space occurring beyond the y-piece of a circle system, so the extensive tubing required to reach from outside to inside the scanner increases dead space ventilation and leads to inaccurate tidal volume measurements. Most Ambu bags are MRI compatible, however don't forget to have long enough oxygen tubing to reach an oxygen source (which could be an oxygen E-cylinder located outside the MRI) if providing positive pressure breaths inside the scanner. If relying on spontaneous ventilation, there must be some assessment of adequacy of ventilation (ET CO_2 monitoring) as well as a plan for positive pressure ventilation if that becomes necessary.

The issue of an MRI-compatible machine is a particular issue when taking care of a child with a small tidal volume. Because the child's tidal volume is small, any inaccuracies in its measurement represent a larger percentage of the child's tidal volume. Another option is to use Mapleson circuits (provided the circuit has no magnetic metal) or to provide oxygen by cannula or mask and have the patient spontaneously ventilate.

The GI Suite

Anesthesia services are most often requested in the GI suite because of patient intolerance to sedation, extensive comorbid diseases, or an anticipated painful or long ERCP. General anesthesia is most often performed for ERCP using standard monitors. The patient may be prone or supine, depending on the preferences of the gastroenterologist. The prone position involves turning the patient after induction as well as turning the patient's head to one side to allow entry of the endoscope. Preoperative assessment of neck sideway range of motion is important in anticipation of this positioning. The placement and removal of the endoscope can also dislodge the ETT, so careful observation and monitoring for continued ventilation is imperative. An ERCP produces only minor postoperative pain in comparison to other surgeries (if sphincterotomy is performed at the sphincter of Oddi then expect more pain). However, the gas insufflation will often lead to bloating and discomfort post procedure despite the gastroenterologist's attempts to decompress the stomach. At the conclusion of the procedure, the prone patient is turned supine and then ETT removed when extubation criteria are met.

Anesthesia for Electroconvulsive Therapy

ECTs are performed under general anesthesia with ventilation by mask. Premedication is limited to an antisialagogue (glycopyrrolate), atropine, analgesics, or antihypertesives if appropriate. Caffeine is sometimes administered as a premed to promote longer seizure duration. Benzodiazepines are avoided, because they raise the seizure threshold. If the patient is on chronic benzodiazepines, then flumazenil may be requested by the psychiatrist to reverse their effects (with the caveat that a benzodiazepine will be given before emergence to prevent excessive patient anxiety). The patient is positioned on the procedure table with standard monitors and an extra BP cuff on the arm opposite the intravenous or on the leg. Sometimes the procedure is performed in the patient's stretcher.

After preoxygenation, anesthesia is induced with methohexital. The dose of methohexital is titrated so that unconsciousness is attained at the lowest possible dose so as to minimize any elevation of seizure threshold. The dose is often determined by that administered at the previous ECT treatment, or it is reduced if at all possible. Once the patient is unresponsive, the BP cuff on the arm or leg is inflated to a sustained pressure to cut off blood flow and prevent muscle relaxant from paralyzing that limb. A bite block is placed to protect the patient's teeth and the patient is hyperventilated to lower the seizure threshold. Succinylcholine is given and twitches monitored. Once there are no twitches an electrical stimulus is applied to the head and a seizure ensues.

The peripheral seizure activity is monitored in the leg with the BP cuff and the central seizure is monitored by EEG strip on the ECT machine. The initial tonic phase of the seizure is accompanied by a parasympathetic surge that usually manifests as bradycardia. The clonic phase follows shortly thereafter. It is conversely accompanied by a sympathetic surge resulting in tachycardia and hypertension. Pharmacologic treatment of these two phases can be employed depending on the comorbidities of the patient. Since the parasympathetic surge is very brief, treatment generally focuses on lessening the sympathetic surge by beta blockers or i.v. antihypertensives.

Once the seizure activity has abated, the patient's airway is supported until emergence. Analgesics are sometimes given to lessen any myalgias associated with succinlycholine-induced fasciculations. Once the patient is awake and supporting their airway they are transported to recovery.

Comprehension Questions

46.1. Which of the following statements best describes the difference between delivering anesthesia in the OR versus outside the OR?
A. Endotracheal tubes are not used for anesthetics in remote locations.
B. There are always extra personnel to help in remote locations.
C. Equipment must be transported to these locations.
D. Most out of OR procedures can be completed with a regional anesthetic technique

46.2. Which of the following is accurate for anesthesia in the MRI scanner?
A. Standard monitoring equipment will work in the scanner.
B. Hypothermia in the MRI scanner is uncommon.
C. The anesthesia machine is never located outside the scanner.
D. General anesthesia is contraindicated during an MRI.

46.3. Which of the following statements is most accurate regarding ERCP?
A. They are all performed in the supine position.
B. Accidental extubation is uncommon.
C. Patient neck range of motion is only important for intubation.
D. The procedure is painful.

46.4. Which of the following hemodynamic changes are seen with ECT?
A. Hypertension during the tonic phase
B. Tachycardia during the clonic phase
C. Tachypnea during the clonic phase
D. Tachycardia during the tonic and clonic phases

ANSWERS

46.1. **C.** The need for equipment must be anticipated, and then transported to the appropriate site. Help is not as readily available. The space may be insufficient for the amount of equipment required. The personnel may not be familiar with anesthesia services.

46.2. **B.** The MRI scanner gets warm during a scan. Special MRI-compatible monitors must be used near the MRI scanner. The anesthesia machine is often located outside the scanner (unless it is a special MRI-compatible machine). General anesthetics are common for MRI scans when anesthesia services are requested.

46.3. **D.** An ERCP can be performed under sedation, but because it is painful, general anesthesia is often chosen. Movement of the endoscope out of the esophagus can dislodge the ETT. Patient neck range of motion is important for intubation, but in ERCP it is also important to assess because if done in the prone position the head will be turned to the side.

46.4. **B.** When the electrical stimulus is applied for an ECT, there is an initial parasympathetic discharge manifested by bradycardia during the tonic phase. Upon initiation of the clonic phase, there is a sympathetic discharge manifested by tachycardia and hypertension. The patient is paralyzed and apneic during for the application of electrical stimulus and seizure, and cannot thus become tachypneic.

Clinical Pearls

- Anesthesia outside the operating rooms is challenged by the remote location and unique setup of each site.
- When giving anesthesia outside the OR, equipment must be transported, and one must be cognizant that the personnel and amount of equipment is limited.
- Providing anesthesia in the MRI area presents unique challenges including ensuring that the equipment and monitoring devices are MRI compatible.
- ECT is a wonderful opportunity to provide mask general anesthetics.

REFERENCES

Gross WL, Gold B. Anesthesia outside the operating room, an issue of anesthesiology clinics. *Anesthesiol Clin* 2009;27(1). Elsevier Health Sciences.

Case 47

While taking call on the Labor and Delivery unit, you are called emergently to see a 28-year-old woman G_1P_0 with fetal distress for an emergent cesarean section. The patient is 5 ft 2 in, weighs 90 kg, and is otherwise healthy. Fetal heart tones show poor variability and a rate of 90 bpm. The patient has had an uneventful general anesthetic previously for an appendectomy.

Considering the emergent nature of the surgery, a general anesthetic is performed with a rapid-sequence induction utilizing propofol and succinylcholine. After a successful endotracheal intubation, 2% sevoflorane in 100% oxygen is started. Approximately 4 minutes after induction, a 7 lb 8 oz female infant is born with Apgar scores of 4 and 9. The baby does well and the rest of the anesthetic is uneventful.

During the postoperative anesthesia visit on the day following surgery, the patient reports to you that she recalls events that occurred during her procedure and felt that she was in pain but was unable to move.

➤ What is the most likely diagnosis?

➤ What are the next steps in caring for this patient?

ANSWERS TO CASE 47:
The Patient with Intraoperative Awareness

Summary: A 28-year-old female patient reports recall after general anesthesia for an emergency caesarean section.

- **Most likely diagnosis:** Awareness or recall during anesthesia, which can be of two types
  - A. Explicit recall which is conscious recall of events occurring during surgery and may or may not be associated with a sensation of pain and the inability to move.
  - B. Implicit recall which is nonspecific recognition of events occurring during surgery or a vague awareness of events occurring during surgery.
- **Next steps:** This patient requires a thorough evaluation of the extent of her recall and may need additional consultative services such as psychiatry or counseling to deal with the emotional consequences of recall during surgery.

ANALYSIS

Objectives

1. Review the incidence and factors associated with intraoperative awareness.
2. Describe why certain procedures may be associated with an increased incidence of intraoperative awareness.
3. Understand the steps in evaluating the patient who reports intraoperative awareness.

Considerations

This particular patient has undergone an anesthetic and surgery that is associated with a higher than normal incidence of intraoperative awareness. Emergent caesarean section for fetal distress, particularly in a parturient who is hypotensive and bleeding, is one of the most complicated and difficult anesthetics to perform. The need for urgent delivery of the hypoxic fetus and to anesthetize a mother who is hypotensive demands that doses of anesthetic induction agents and inhalation agents be limited to avoid additional maternal hypotension and fetal hypoxia.

It is essential that this patient receives an honest and thorough postoperative visit. It is important to determine the extent of her recall, and to elicit whether the recall of intraoperative events is disturbing to her. Occasionally, patients experience recall of intraoperative events during emergency surgery, but are not particularly disturbed by the experience. Other patients are markedly traumatized by the recall of intraoperative events. Once the experience has been documented, the patient should be offered a variety of services to deal with any posttraumatic stress they may be experiencing because of recall. These services can include counseling and psychiatric services and in some instances may require medication. It is essential that the patient's feelings regarding intraoperative recall are not dismissed.

APPROACH TO
The Patient with Recall

DEFINITIONS

INTRAOPERATIVE AWARENESS: Recall (either explicit or implicit) of events occurring during general anesthesia in the operating room.

EXPLICIT RECALL: Remembering exact events that occurred with or without pain during the operation.

IMPLICIT RECALL: Recognition but not specific recall of events happening in the operating room during general anesthesia.

BISPECTRAL INDEX OR BIS MONITOR: A processed or spectral EEG which represents activity of the cerebral cortex. The EEG is very active when patients are awake but relatively quiet during anesthesia or natural sleep. The monitor processes the EEG signals into a single number with 100 representing fully awake and 0 representing electrical silence.

CLINICAL APPROACH

Intraoperative awareness is reported to occur in approximately 0.0068% to 0.13% of general anesthetics performed in the United States. Despite the somewhat rare nature of recall, it is one of the most feared complications of general anesthesia and surgery. In contrast to the increasing public interest, awareness, and discussion of the incidence of intraoperative awareness, the American Society of Anesthesiologist Closed Claims database of malpractice claims indicates that there has been no substantial change in the liability associated with recall during anesthesia in the 1990s compared to previous reporting periods. It is possible, however, that there has been an increase in claims and judgments awarded that have not yet been detected by this database (see Table 47–1).

Despite the inability to predict precisely which patients may experience intraoperative recall, it is possible to suggest which patients may be at higher risk. Grouped by procedure, those at highest risks include patients undergoing coronary artery bypass grafting surgery, cesarean section, and emergency or trauma surgery performed at night. Grouped by patient characteristics, those at highest risks include patients of a younger age, an increased body weight,

Table 47–1 INFLATION-ADJUSTED PAYMENTS FOR AWARENESS OVER THREE DECADES

	1970s	1980s	1990s
Claims for awareness	7 (1%)	57 (2%)	65 (2%)
Payment made	4 (67%)	32 (62%)	31 (52%)
Median payment amount in 1999 dollars	$32,060	$21,455	$33,599

smokers, patients who are critically ill, and those who may have increased tolerance because of long-term use of alcohol, opiates, or amphetamines. Patients who primarily receive an opioid-based anesthetic rather than an inhalation anesthetic are also at higher risk for recall, as are patients who receive muscle relaxants during surgery.

Differing states of wakefulness and recall may be reported by different patients. The smallest group of patients experiencing recall (0.03%) report conscious awareness and pain during surgery, and a desire "to scream during surgery but not being able to move." It is this group of patients that is most likely to experience symptoms of posttraumatic stress secondary to recall during surgery. A higher percentage of patients (0.1%-0.2%) may report nonpainful but explicit recall of intraoperative events. These patients may be able to report verbatim conversations that occurred in the operating room during surgery, but do not report concomitant feelings of pain. The final group of patients may report nonspecific or amnesic awareness during surgery. These patients do not recall specific events or conversations that occur during surgery, but may have recognition recall of intraoperative events (Table 47–2).

Table 47–2 CHARACTERISTICS ASSOCIATED WITH INCREASED INCIDENCE OF INTRAOPERATIVE AWARENESS

FACTORS ASSOCIATED WITH INCREASED AWARENESS	
Patient characteristics	Younger age, increased weight, smokers, long-term use of EtOH, opiates, or amphetamines
Types of surgery	Cesarean section, coronary artery bypass grafting, emergency surgery at night, trauma surgery
Anesthetic techniques	Muscle relaxants, narcotic-based techniques, inadequate dosing, equipment malfunctions such as empty vaporizers

Table 47–3 BISPECTRAL INDEX SCORES

BIS NUMBER	CLINICAL CORRELATION
100	Patient awake and fully alert
40-60	Patient anesthetized or natural sleep
0	Electrical silence, no cerebral activity

Manufacturers of processed EEG monitors have speculated that these monitors can reduce the incidence of intraoperative awareness. The company's formula for arriving at the bispectral index (BIS) number is proprietary but is predominantly determined by the patient's EEG. Manufacturers suggest that the ideal range for anesthetic management and decreased intraoperative awareness is a BIS level of 40 to 60. Recent large randomized studies have indicated that the BIS monitor is no more reliable in preventing recall of intraoperative events than monitoring of the end-tidal concentrations of inhaled anesthetic agents. The BIS monitor is also not reliable at the extremes of age. In addition, certain anesthetics (nitrous oxide or NMDA antagonists such as ketamine) unquestionably produce anesthesia, but not a decrease in the BIS number because they cause less EEG suppression than other anesthetic drugs (Table 47–3).

Comprehension Questions

47.1. Which of the following statements is accurate regarding the prevention of awareness?

A. A compressed EEG or BIS monitor level of 40 to 60 during general anesthesia guarantees that patients will not have recall of intraoperative events.
B. An end-tidal gas concentration of MAC guarantees that patients will not have recall of intraoperative events.
C. An end-tidal gas concentration of twice MAC guarantees that patients will not have recall of intraoperative events.
D. There are no ways to guarantee that patients will not have recall of intraoperative events.

47.2. Which of the following anesthetics techniques is associated with an increased incidence of intraoperative awareness?

A. Sevoflurane anesthesia
B. Propofol infusion
C. Nitrous oxide
D. Fentanyl infusion
E. Desflurane anesthesia

47.3. A 60-year-old female patient reports that during a previous anesthetic she experienced recall of a conversation occurring during surgery. An appropriate response includes which of the following?

A. Tell the patient that it was all her imagination.
B. Reassure the patient that with new anesthetic agents recall does not really happen.
C. Blame the surgeon for talking too loudly.
D. Reassure the patient and tell her that you will use a BIS monitor so you are sure she will not have recall.
E. Reassure the patient and tell her that you will employ techniques in an attempt to minimize the risks of recall.

ANSWERS

47.1. **D.** Unfortunately there is no way even with monitoring to guarantee that patients will not have recall of intraoperative events. Studies have shown that monitoring the end-tidal concentration of inhalation anesthetic agents is as reliable in preventing recall as using an awareness monitor, and either of these methods is superior to observing for signs of sympathetic stimulation, seeming to indicate pain.

47.2. **D.** Fentanyl infusion. Primarily narcotic-based techniques have been shown to be associated with a higher incidence of intraoperative awareness than inhalation anesthetic techniques. This is because narcotic-based techniques do not provide for amnesia. Anytime a narcotic is used for the primary anesthetic agents, supplemental amnesic agents should be administered as well.

47.3. **E.** Patients who have experienced intraoperative recall are understandably very anxious about subsequent anesthetics. Unfortunately, there is no way to guarantee a patient that they will not experience intraoperative awareness. Using inhalation-based general anesthetic techniques with amnesic agents and careful monitoring of the EEG or end-tidal concentration of inhalation agents are the best way to minimize the chances of intraoperative recall.

Clinical Pearls

- The incidence of intraoperative awareness is estimated to be 0.8%.
- Certain procedures including cesarean section, cardiac surgery with cardiopulmonary bypass, and trauma surgery are associated with an increased incidence of intraoperative awareness.
- Although techniques such as monitoring end-tidal gas concentrations and the compressed EEG reduce the incidence of awareness, there is no monitor which can guarantee against intraopertive awareness.

REFERENCES

Avidan MS, Zhang L, Burnside BA, et al. Anesthesia awareness and the bispectral index. *N Engl J Med*. 2008:358;1097.

Kent CD. Liability associated with awareness during anesthesia. ASA *News*. 2006;70(6):8-10.

Case 48

A 36-year-old G_3P_3 woman, 1 day after vaginal delivery, presents for postpartum tubal ligation. She has no significant past medical or surgical history and states she does not wish to be awake during the procedure. The patient is anesthetized with general anesthesia via a rapid-sequence induction, using propofol and succinylcholine, and is intubated with a 7.0 cuffed endotracheal tube. Anesthesia is maintained with sevoflurane, vecuronium, and fentanyl. The operation proceeds uneventfully, and as the obstetricians close, the sevoflurane is turned off. The patient has two twitches, she is given neostigmine and glycopyrrolate to reverse the effects of her neuromuscular blockade. Twenty minutes later, she is still intubated, has made no ventilatory efforts, and appears unarousable.

➤ What is the differential diagnosis for delayed emergence from anesthesia?

➤ Which monitors may be helpful in discerning the diagnosis?

➤ Which medical condition can mimic delayed emergence, and how is it diagnosed?

ANSWERS TO CASE 48: Delayed Emergence

Summary: A healthy 36-year-old patient, 1 day after vaginal delivery, makes no respiratory effort following general anesthesia for postpartum tubal ligation.

- **Differential diagnosis:** Medication overdose (most commonly opiates), hypoventilation leading to hypercapnia, metabolic abnormalities such as hypoglycemia, and neurologic events.
- **Monitors:** The diagnosis is discerned through physical examination including vital signs, pupillary dilatation, the patient's response to stimulation such as sternal rub, and an observation of respiratory effort. Monitors which may be helpful in this setting include the Train of Four, capnography, and monitors of anesthetic depth. Additional testing such as blood gas analysis, the glucose concentration, and potentially neurologic imaging may also be indicated.
- **Medical condition:** Persistent neuromuscular blockade, reflecting an overdose or inadequate reversal of nondepolarizing muscle relaxants, or atypical pseudocholinesterase, can mimic delayed emergence. In this setting, mechanical ventilation and sedation may be warranted.

ANALYSIS

Objectives

1. Understand the techniques available to evaluate the patient with delayed emergence.
2. Become familiar with the most common causes of delayed emergence.
3. Understand the implications of an atypical pseudocholinesterase enzyme.

Considerations

Before anesthetizing this patient, it is important to realize that a parturient undergoes a number of physiologic changes throughout her pregnancy, and few will have completely returned to normal on the first day post delivery. In addition to the hemodynamic changes associated with pregnancy, the requirements for volatile anesthetics are diminished. Plasma cholinesterase activity decreases throughout pregnancy, and may be impaired up to 6 weeks postpartum. This is usually of little significance.

APPROACH TO Delayed Emergence

Intraoperative Course

This patient received a balanced anesthetic, which means that she received sedation, narcotics, inhaled anesthetic agents, and neuromuscular blocking agents. She has physiologic changes due to pregnancy. There are many reasons why she may have had a delayed emergence.

Overdose. It is possible that a medication has been given in an amount that vastly exceeds a patient's requirements. Therefore, it is important to evaluate what drugs have been given, in what dosage, and ensure there have been no inadvertent drug mix-ups.

Certain groups of patients are prone to drug overdose, so understanding the patient's medical history is of paramount importance. For example, patients suffering from impairments of the kidneys and liver may experience prolonged effects of opiates and some muscle relaxants, since these organs are often the primary sites involved in drug metabolism.

Certain medical conditions and physiologic states also render patients more susceptible to specific drugs. For example, patients with myasthenia gravis have increased sensitivity to nondepolarizing muscle relaxants. Similarly, drug requirements vary with age, with the geriatric patient requirements being much lower doses than an adolescent, and the pregnant or postpartum patient often having a lower drug requirement than the nonpregnant woman.

One of the most common scenarios resulting in a delayed emergence is an overly narcotized patient. While opiates are helpful in managing pain, their side effects include sedation, ventilatory depression, and a blunted ventilatory response to hypercapnia. An opiate overdose is typically associated with pinpoint pupils. However, the presence of pinpoint pupils in and of itself does not necessarily indicate an opiate overdose.

An opiate overdose is treated with naloxone, an antagonist at the opiate receptor. In the absence of an arrest or pending arrest, naloxone should be diluted and administered incrementally in small doses as the sudden reversal of nociceptive inhibition may cause an increased sympathetic response resulting in tachycardia, hypertension, and cardiac dysrhythmias. The duration of action of naloxone is approximately half an hour, so *re-dosing of naloxone is often required until the patient recovers from the opiate*.

Delayed emergence may also be attributed to the effects of benzodiazepines. Midazolam is commonly given preoperatively for anxiolysis and anterograde amnesia. Although the ventilatory depression of benzodiazepines is less than that of opiates or barbiturates, these drugs are long acting, and can be highly sedating in addition to potentiating the effects of other medications leading to airway obstruction and apnea. Benzodiazepines bind to γ-aminobutyric acid type A receptors (GABA), and are antagonized by flumazenil at a dose of 0.2 mg intravenously over 15 seconds in adults. One side effect of flumazenil is seizures.

In addition to the two scenarios mentioned above, a drug overdos is sometimes due to medical errors such as misreading of drug labels, mislabeling of drug syringes, or new or different formulations or strengths of usual medications.

Hypoventilation. Patients with poor ventilation due to airway obstruction, residual muscle paralysis, or excess narcotics can develop hypercarbia leading to sedation and even unconsciousness. This is evaluated by assessing the patient's respiratory rate and tidal volume, and by analyzing the $PaCO_2$ from an arterial blood gas. Hypoventilation also hinders a patient's ability to eliminate (exhale) volatile anesthetics, thus slowing their emergence. Treatment consists of improving the patient's ventilation while administering 100% O_2.

Metabolic abnormality. It is possible the patient is unarousable secondary to some type of metabolic derangement. Hypothermia may reduce the metabolism of, and thereby cause prolongation of, anesthetic agents. This can be assessed with a temperature probe. Blood work can be sent to assess for hypoglycemia, severe hyperglycemia, or electrolyte imbalance. Naturally, the best treatment is to identify and correct the abnormality.

Neurological event. Rare causes of delayed emergence include neurological events such as seizure or an ischemic event from intracerebral hemorrhage, embolism, or thrombosis. Understanding the clinical context, the physical examination, and imaging guide the diagnosis and treatment of these rare but devastating disorders.

Residual neuromuscular blockade. In order to provide optimal surgical conditions, neuromuscular blocking agents are administered to provide muscle relaxation and paralysis. In the case of the patient with delayed emergence, it is possible that the patient has indeed emerged from the anesthetic, but still remains paralyzed.

Nondepolarizing neuromuscular blocking agents require reversal of their action by flooding the synaptic cleft with acetylcholine. If insufficient quantities of neuromuscular reversal had been administered or if the level of blockade had been too great for the agents to overcome, patients may remain paralyzed at the end of surgery. Since the advent of Train-of-Four monitoring, the likelihood of an overdose of neuromuscular relaxant drugs sufficient to cause total paralysis (and thus mimic delayed emergence) is low. More likely, patients will be able to move and communicate that they are awake, albeit weakly. Total paralysis following nondepolarizing muscle relaxants is suggestive of underlying pathology at the neuromuscular junction, such as with myasthenia gravis, multiple sclerosis, etc.

Total paralysis following the administration of succinylcholine, is, on the other hand, a well known complication of following the drug's administration. The effects of succinylcholine are typically short-lived due to hydrolysis by pseudocholinesterase enzymes in plasma. If these enzymes either function abnormally or are present in reduced quantities, then the action of succinylcholine is prolonged and total paralysis may result. The most common form of pseudocholinerase deficiency occurs at a frequency of greater than 1/3,000 cases. Fortunately this type of cholinesterase deficiency only results in a total paralysis of only an hour or so, and since most surgical procedures are longer than 1 hour, it may remain undiagnosed.

First studied by Kalow and Staron in the 1950s, it is now believed that the gene that codes for the pseudocholinesterase enzyme exists on the E1 locus of chromosome 3. It is estimated that 4% of the population carries atypical pseudocholinesterase genes as either heterozygotes or homozygotes. In this population, a much greater dose of succinylcholine arrives at the neuromuscular junction, causing a greatly exaggerated length of time of paralysis. Currently, the only treatment option is continued mechanical ventilation until the paralysis resolves secondary to passive diffusion of succinycholine away from the neuromuscular junction. Administration of fresh frozen plasma or neostigmine is controversial and not recommended.

While preoperative screening for atypical pseudocholinesterase is extremely uncommon, a patient who previously suffered an episode of prolonged paralysis following succinylcholine may be evaluated by a method first described by Kalow and Genest. Dibucaine is a local anesthetic that inhibits normal pseudocholinesterase activity by 70% to 80%, but affects the atypical enzyme by only 20% to 30%. Heterozygotes have about a 50% to 60% inhibition. The amount of enzyme inhibition is termed the "dibucaine number." In contrast, some patients may have lower amounts of pseudocholinesterase due to a decreased synthetic activity such as seen in liver disease, or lower circulating concentrations resulting from the increase in plasma volume such as seen in normal pregnancy.

In addition to their effects at the neuromuscular junction, deficiencies in pseudocholinesterase may also affect the metabolism of ester-based local anesthetics, such as 2-chloroprocaine. There have been case reports of high epidural blockade in parturient with even mildly abnormal dibucaine numbers.

Total muscular paralysis is differentiated from a delayed emergence from anesthesia in several ways. First, patients may show signs of "light" anesthesia from sympathetic stimulation. Tearing, sweating, tachycardia, hypertension, and pupillary dilatation suggest that the patient either has or is beginning to emerge. Second, muscular paralysis can be detected by an absence of the twitch using a Train-of-Four monitor. The level of awareness can also be assessed by a monitor of anesthetic depth, such as the bispectral index (BIS) monitor.

Postoperative Care

The etiology of delayed emergence is ideally discerned in the operating room if at all possible. Otherwise, the patient is left intubated, and transported to an intensive care unit, or if hemodynamically stable, to the PACU. The treatment for delayed emergence is dependent upon the patient's pathology, and is by and large supportive.

Comprehension Questions

48.1. You are called to assess a 58-year-old man, status post left colectomy, who became unresponsive on the floor. As you arrive you are told the patient had accidentally received 10 mg of dilaudid instead of the 1 mg he was prescribed. Which of the following medications can you give to reverse this condition?

A. Naloxone
B. Flumazenil
C. Neostigmine
D. Glycopyrrolate

48.2. A 22-year-old woman undergoes a rapid-sequence induction for her tonsillectomy. Five minutes later she has all four twitches back. Which of the following statements is accurate?

A. Her pseudocholinesterase enzymes are probably low in quantity.
B. Her pseudocholinesterase enzymes may not be functioning properly.
C. Her dibucaine number is probably 30.
D. She is no longer completely paralyzed.

48.3. A 35-year-old type 1 diabetic male undergoes an open carpal tunnel release with an axillary nerve block. The patient received 2 mg of midazolam for sedation prior to the block, but no additional medications in the operating room. He was alert after the midazolam and early in the case, but near the end of the case, he is somnolent and difficult to arouse. Which of the following is the most appropriate treatment?

A. Physostigmine
B. Naloxone
C. Dextrose
D. Midazolam

48.4. Which of the following is the most likely cause for the delayed emergence described at the beginning of the case?

A. Hypoglycemia
B. Pseudocholinesterase deficiency
C. Excessive administration of opiates
D. Residual effects of inhalation anesthetics

ANSWERS

48.1. **A.** This patient has received an overdose of his opiate pain medication. Naloxone will reverse these effects. Most likely, this patient will require a naloxone infusion until dilaudid is metabolized. Flumazenil is a benzodiazepine antagonist. Neostigmine is an acetyl cholinesterase inhibitor. Glycopyrrolate is an anticholinergic.

48.2. **D.** This patient has no signs of prolonged paralysis following succinylcholine administration. For this reason, she should have normal pseudocholinesterase enzymes in both quantity and activity. Since all her twitches have returned to normal, she is no longer completely paralyzed. Since the dibucaine number represents the percent of the enzyme's activity, a normal number would be $\geq$70.

48.3. **C.** This patient is likely hypoglycemic and requires dextrose. Use a glucometer to check the blood glucose level. This patient had a peripheral nerve block and had intraoperative medications. Since no muscle relaxant was given, physostigmine would be an inappropriate choice. For much the same reason, opiate was not administered thus eliminating the need for naloxone. Midazolam is a benzodiazepine and would be of no benefit in this situation.

48.4. **C.** While each of the choices is theoretically a possible etiology for the delayed emergence described at the beginning of the case, the most likely cause is an excessive administration of opiates. Opiates reduce the ventilatory response to CO_2, an effect that is synergistic with the residual effects of any inhalation anesthetics which may not have been eliminated. Hypoglycemia is less likely insofar as the patient is not a diabetic, although it has been observed in young, fasting women undergoing surgery late in the afternoon. Pseudocholinesterase deficiency is also a possibility, especially if this patient never had surgery before. However, the incidence of cholinesterase deficiency is much less frequent than somnolence caused by opiates and retained anesthetic agents.

Clinical Pearls

- Patients may have comorbidities or physical conditions such as normal pregnancy that make them susceptible to prolonged effects from common anesthetic medications.
- Be methodical when evaluating the patient with delayed emergence. Consider their age, medical history, and the intraoperative record including medications given when developing a differential.
- Monitors such as vital signs, the physical examination, a Train-of-Four stimulus, capnograph, monitor of anesthetic depth, imaging, and laboratory tests should be available to you to help guide your diagnosis.
- If an opiate is reversed with naloxone, remember that the opiate's half-life may exceed naloxone's, and that redosing the naloxone may be necessary.

REFERENCES

Miller RD, ed. Anesthesia for obstetrics. *Miller's Anesthesia*. 6th ed. Philadelphia, PA: Churchill Livingston;2005: 2307-2345.

Mondero P, Hess P. High epidural block with chloroprocaine in a parturient with low psuedocholinesterase activity. *Can J Anaesth*. 2001;48(3):318-319.

Nixon JC, Thiel CJ. Apnea due to inheritance of atypical pseudocholinesterase. *Can Med Assoc J*. 1964 9;90:1125-1127.

Savarese JJ, Caldwell JE, Lien CA, Miller RD. Pharmacology of muscle relaxants and their antagonists. In: Miller RD, eds. *Miller's Anesthesia*. 6th ed. Philadelphia, PA: Churchill Livingston;2005: 481-573.

Case 49

An 82-year-old woman presents for cataract surgery. She has a history of hypertension, and an MI some 10 years ago. She reports no change in her health recently, and her functional capacity is excellent for her age. She is an avid gardener. As is custom at your institution, this patient did not visit the preoperative clinic. The ophthalmologist did provided a recent note from the patient's physician stating that her medical conditions were stable, and "clearing her for surgery." Her ECG and laboratory tests from 3 months ago were attached to his note.

- ➤ What is this patient's suitability for cataract surgery?
- ➤ What are the most likely complications which may be observed during the case?
- ➤ What factors influence the need for sedation?

ANSWERS TO CASE 49:
Basic MAC/Anesthesia for Cataract Surgery

Summary: An 82-year-old patient with stable medical conditions presents for cataract surgery.

- **Suitability for surgery:** This patient is stable, followed by her primary physician, and ready to proceed with monitored anesthesia care (MAC) for her cataract surgery.
- **Most common complications:** During a case performed under MAC, there is always the danger that patients will move inappropriately. During eye procedures, this is especially perilous because the procedure is performed using a microscope. The most likely medical events are hypertension, and an arrhythmia, usually bradycardia.
- **Amount of sedation:** The amount of sedation depends on the type of anesthesia for the eye, topical anesthesia versus an eye block, as well as the method of removing the cataract.

ANALYSIS

Objectives

1. Understand how the preparation of patients having cataract surgery differs from other surgical procedures.
2. Become familiar with the anesthetic techniques used for cataract surgery and many eye procedures.

Considerations

Since this patient's medical condition is stable and she is followed by a primary physician, she is ready for cataract surgery. She does not need any additional medical testing prior to surgery, although it is helpful to have access to any tests which have been recently performed. In particular, a recent baseline ECG is helpful since arrhythmias may occur in eye surgery.

Once it is determined that the patient is ready for cataract surgery, a small intravenous is started, and standard monitors are placed. The need for sedation is determined by the type of anesthesia provided to the eye during the case. This patient's cataract is suitable for PHACO extraction, and she is cooperative and able to lie still without the need for sedation. Thus, her surgery can be safely performed using topical anesthesia administered in the form of eye drops.

APPROACH TO
Basic MAC/Anesthesia for Cataract Surgery

DEFINITIONS

MONITORED ANESTHESIA CARE (MAC): The care of a patient by an anesthesiologist, during which time the patient is monitored, and sedative, hypnotic, opioid, or anxiolytic medications may be administered.

TOPICAL ANESTHESIA: Local anesthesia applied as drops or gels to the surface of the eye.

EYE BLOCK: Method of administering local anesthesia to the eye so as to block nerve conduction, both motor and sensory, to the eye.

RETROBULBAR BLOCK: Local anesthesia injected into the muscle cone behind the globe.

PERIBULBAR BLOCK: Local anesthesia injected outside the muscle cone.

SUB-TENONS BLOCK: Local anesthesia injected into the Tenons capsule below the surface of the globe.

CLINICAL APPROACH

Cataract extraction is the most common surgical procedure in the United States today. These procedures are done very quickly, and often, almost in an "assembly line" fashion. Since this type of surgery is so common, the costs of any associated care are multiplied many times over. In a study of over 18,000 patients, Schein et al demonstrated that preoperative testing did not change outcomes in patients undergoing cataract surgery under MAC anesthesia. However, this study cohort was associated with one significant caveat: all of the study subjects were followed by a primary physician for their medical conditions, and had received testing for these conditions when appropriate. So unlike all other surgical procedures, patients followed by a primary physician may undergo cataract extraction without further preoperative evaluation.

During the course of an eye operation, there are several reasons why a patient may benefit from the care of an anesthetist. The patient may be anxious, and require medication to calm or relax them so they can lie still for the procedure; he or she may need medication to treat pain or fright during the surgery; or the patient may experience arrhythmias, hypertension, or tachycardia necessitating a medical intervention.

It is imperative that the patient remain quiet, cooperative, and still during the procedure. In a recent review of closed malpractice insurance claims for MAC cases, 11% of claims involved injury due to movement or inadequate anesthesia during eye surgery. Elderly patients, especially those with medical conditions and ASA III or IV classification, made up a higher percentage of the MAC claims, but were no different from the population as a whole receiving other types of anesthesia. Eye procedures may also pose some additional risk, since the patient is draped around the head and neck making detection of any impairment in respiratory movements difficult, or even a buildup of carbon dioxide may occur under the drapes, which is more difficult to detect. For this reason, when available, measurement of end-tidal CO_2 levels is desirable. Otherwise, standard monitors are all that are necessary for this type of case.

Most cataracts today are removed by PHACO emulsification. The cataract is broken into small pieces by ultrasound waves which are suctioned out through a cannula, requiring only very tiny incisions in the eye. The older technique of extracapsular cataract extraction removes the lens intact through a larger incision. The PHACO procedure is quicker and easier and allows more rapid recovery for the patient.

In many centers, cataract surgeries are now done under topical anesthesia, during which local anesthesia is administered via drops or gels to the surface of the eye. An additional intracameral injection of local anesthesia improves the quality of the anesthesia for the topicalized eye. The patient does not require sedation for the administration of topical anesthesia. However, the emulsification of the lens can cause images that may be frightening. Since the patient's vision is intact, they may see the bright light of the microscope and the surgeon's hands and instruments. They may also feel pain during placement of the speculum on the eyelids, iris manipulation, globe expansion by injection of solution into the eye, and introduction of the new lens. Since the patient's extra-ocular movements are intact, they need to be sufficiently awake to cooperate with the surgeon's instructions during the case.

Many older patients tolerate topical anesthesia for cataract surgery without any sedation. Education for the patient on what to expect during the procedure and careful patient selection results in greater success with topical anesthesia. After cataract surgery under topical anesthesia, patients may have their vision restored immediately, since taping and protective shielding of the eye is not always necessary.

Eye blocks provide anesthesia, analgesia, and motor blockade to the eye. Eye blocks are administered in the operating room as with any regional block, or they may be placed prior to the patient coming into the OR in a holding area or block room where the patient can be sedated and monitored consistent with the same standards applied in the operating room. Although these blocks can be done without sedation, more commonly, the patient is sedated briefly for block placement, often with a small dose of propofol. This practice of doing the block ahead of time ensures that the patient is well recovered from any sedation prior to the start of surgery.

For a retrobulbar block, local anesthesia is injected through the skin of the lower eyelid at the inferior aspect of the orbit, and into the muscle cone behind the globe. Entrance into the muscle cone is confirmed by downward movement of the eye, as the needle travels through the inferior rectus muscle. After a negative aspiration, a small amount of local anesthesia is injected, and travels along the nerves and blood vessels to block nerve transmission at the ciliary ganglion.

The peribulbar technique is similar, but requires a larger volume of local anesthesia and a longer time to work since the drug needs to diffuse further to reach the ganglion. To perform a peribulbar block, the local anesthetic is injected outside the muscle cone, inferior and/or superior to the globe. It is important that the patient does not move during the injection of an eye block due to the proximity of the needle to nerves and blood vessels, as well as to the globe itself.

The sub-Tenons eye block is typically performed by the surgeon after prepping and draping the eye. A small incision is made on the surface of the globe under local anesthesia, then a small blunt cannula is inserted into this space and local anesthesia travels to the retrobulbar space via Tenons capsule.

A patient's extra-ocular movements indicate the quality of all eye injection blocks. All blocks provide superior pain relief during and after cataract surgery as compared to topical anesthesia. Injection blocks prevent the occulo-cardiac reflex, which causes bradycardia during manipulation of the globe. Major complications that may occur after injection blocks include retrobulbar hemorrhage, globe perforation, and brain stem anesthesia if the local anesthesia tracks back along the nerves all the way to their origin.

There are several drugs commonly used for sedation during cataract surgery. Midazolam, a short-acting benzodiazepine, is useful for patients undergoing either topical anesthesia or injection blocks. It provides sedation, anxiolysis, and amnesia. A dose of 0.5 to 2 mg total should be administered slowly in elderly patients to avoid respiratory depression or over dosage. One must avoid oversedation since patient cooperation is necessary to prevent unintentional movement during surgery. Midazolam may cause prolonged psychomotor impairment in the elderly, especially those with pre-existing cognitive dysfunction.

Propofol, an induction agent, is used in smaller doses for sedation during administration of an eye block. The rapid onset and quick recovery profile allow the patient to be awake and cooperative prior to starting the surgery. Propofol can be administered in a dose from 0.3 to 1.0 mg/kg prior to the eye block. The patient will have sedation and amnesia for the eye block but little analgesia is expected. Movement during the block is frequent and sneezing may also occur. This technique is useful for the patient who wants to be "asleep" for the block.

Remifentanil, an opioid agonist, is the newest drug frequently administered to eye surgery patients. This drug displays both fast onset and rapid clearance by the plasma via ester hydrolysis. Given in a dose of 0.3 to 0.5 mcg/kg the patient feels no pain for the injection block. However, respiratory depression and chest wall rigidity can occur when remifentanil is bolused quickly. Also, like any other opiate, remifentanil is not a hypnotic, so patients frequently have recall for the block. Nausea and vomiting may occur, although rarely.

Sedative drugs are often used in combination. However, in the elderly these combinations may result in exaggerated sedation or respiratory depression. The Study of Medical Testing for Cataract Surgery found infrequent adverse medical events during cataract surgery in their study population. However, the administration of a combination of drugs increased the odds ratio for an event significantly. The use of a short-acting hypnotic (such as propofol), combined with an opiate, a sedative, or both elevated the odds ratio for an adverse event from a low of 9.8 with a hypnotic alone to as high as 30.7 for a combination of all three categories. Fortunately, they did not identify any anesthetic regimen that increased the risk of death or unexpected hospitalization.

Patient satisfaction following eye surgery has been associated with specific factors such as surgeon skill and the length of operation. However, there is no evidence that any particular class of sedative or anesthetic improves satisfaction.

The postoperative course for the cataract surgery patient most often is very short and uneventful. The patients usually meet discharge criteria prior to leaving the OR, so it is customary for cataract patients to go directly to a phase 2 or step down unit rather than the main PACU. Since the injection block usually lasts much longer than the procedure, vision is limited and so the patient is instructed to wear an eye shield to protect the eye from injury. Significant postoperative pain is an unusual event. Pain in the cataract surgery patient that is unrelieved with an over-the-counter strength analgesic such as acetaminophen should be considered unusual and that patient should be seen by a physician. If nausea or vomiting occurs, they should be treated aggressively as both retching and vomiting can increase intra-ocular pressure and jeopardize the closure of the incisions.

Comprehension Questions

49.1. A 75-year-old man is being scheduled for an outpatient cataract extraction and lens placement. He is followed by his primary physician for coronary disease with congestive heart failure, which is stable. Which of the following tests are required prior to his anesthesia for cataract surgery?

A. ECG
B. Chest x-ray
C. Hemoglobin
D. Electrolytes
E. No tests are required

49.2. Your patient expresses fear of the injection block for cataract surgery. Which drug or combination is most likely to be associated with recall of the block?
A. Propofol
B. Midazolam
C. Remifentanil
D. Midazolam and propofol

49.3. Which of these statements about topical anesthesia for cataract surgery is most accurate?
A. Extra-ocular movements are a good way to check the quality of the block.
B. Topical anesthesia renders the patient insensate during iris manipulation and lens placement.
C. Patients cannot see instruments or light following topical anesthesia.
D. Patients usually don't require sedation for placement of the topical anesthetic.

ANSWERS

49.1. **E.** Patients who have stable medical conditions that are followed by a primary physician do not need additional testing prior to cataract surgery. An ECG is useful, especially if it is recent (within the last 6 months).

49.2. **C.** Remifentanil, an ultra short-acting opioid agonist, may allow recall of the injection block since it has no amnesic properties. During the block, the patient is analgesic, but not amnestic. He is aware of and remembers the block in many cases. Midazolam usually results in amnesia. Propofol administered prior to the block in small doses allows the patient to sleep through the block, and be unaware of its administration. One caution with propofol: a patient is more likely to move during the block placement.

49.3. **D.** Topical anesthesia is applied to the surface of the eye with drops or gels, providing less analgesia so a patient has more pain during the procedure as well as sensations of light and movement. The administration of the drops is sometimes associated with a burning sensation, but this does not usually require sedation. However, since there is no nerve block with topical anesthesia, movements of the extraocular muscles remain intact.

Clinical Pearls

- Elderly patients undergoing cataract surgery do not need additional preoperative testing as long as they are followed by a primary physician and receive care for any medical conditions.
- Monitored anesthesia care for the eye surgery patient varies greatly with the type of procedure, method of anesthesia for the eye, and the amount of pain or discomfort the patient may encounter.
- There are several methods to deliver anesthesia to the eye for cataract procedures. The patient's sensations during cataract surgery may differ based on the type of block. Often eye blocks are administered by anesthesiologists; sometimes these are performed in the holding area.

REFERENCES

Bhananker SM, Posner KL, Cheney FW, Caplar RA, Lee LA, Domino KB. Injury and liability associated with monitored anesthesia care: a closed claim analysis. *Anesthesiology*. 2006;104:228-234.

Katz J, Feldman MA, Bass EB, Lubomski LH, et al. Adverse intraoperative medical events and their association with anesthesia management strategies in cataract surgery. *Ophthalmology*. 2001;108:1721-1726.

Schein OD, Katz J, Bass EB, et al. The value of routine preoperative medical testing before cataract surgery. *NEJM*. 2000;342:168-175.

Vann MA, Ogunnaike BO, Joshi GP. Sedation and anesthesia care for ophthalmologic surgery during local/regional anesthesia. *Anesthesiology*. 2007;107:502-508.

Case 50

A 58-year-old dialysis-dependent diabetic woman is scheduled to receive a living related kidney transplant from her 40-year-old brother. She has chronic renal failure from diabetes, has been on chronic dialysis for the past 5 years, and was dialyzed yesterday. The patient's medical history includes hypertension, diabetes, and hepatitis B. Her medications include metoprolol, furosemide, insulin, calcium carbonate, ferrous sulphate, epogen, and sevalamer. On physical examination, the patient is 5 ft 7 in, 55 kg, and her physical examination is otherwise normal. Her laboratory results show: Na 135 mEq/L, K 4.9 mEq/L, pH 7.32, and Hct of 29%. Her ECG is normal. The patient's brother is healthy, with the exception of gastric reflux and a hiatus hernia. His laboratory results are normal, and his Hct is 45%.

➤ What are the anesthetic considerations for patients each of the above?

➤ How are the kidney donor and recipient typically managed?

ANSWERS TO CASE 50:
Anesthesia for Renal Transplantation

Summary: A living sibling is donating a kidney to his diabetic sister with kidney failure.

- **Anesthetic concerns:** Renal transplant donors are typically anxious. In addition to the concerns with positioning, such as the potential for nerve compression and pressure sores, their general anesthetic is similar to that for any other healthy patient. Renal transplant recipients typically have comorbid illnesses and may benefit from invasive monitoring. Bleeding may be exacerbated because of platelet dysfunction. Renal recipients require immunosuppressant medications to prevent rejection and possible diuretics to facilitate urine production.
- **Management of donor:** General endotracheal anesthesia with muscle relaxation is usually employed. Since living organ donation is an altruistic act of the highest order, every attempt should be made to provide optimal postoperative analgesia.
- **Management of recipient:** General endotracheal anesthesia with consideration of central and arterial monitoring, and judicious fluid and electrolyte management is vital.

ANALYSIS

Objectives

1. Understand the differences in the surgical approach for renal donor and recipient.
2. Become familiar with the anesthetic considerations and plans for each patient.
3. Become acquainted with the postoperative issues associated with renal transplantation in both donors and recipients.

Considerations

Living donors are often quite anxious. A reassuring approach and anxiolytic therapy are important to the donor. It is important to verify that they are volunteering freely and understand the risks of surgery prior to proceeding.

The recipient's dependence on dialysis lends challenges to fluid management. Most patients undergo dialysis the day before the procedure, resulting in relative and sometimes significant hypovolemia. In addition, electrolytes, and particularly potassium vary markedly depending upon the timing of the most recent dialysis, so the timing of dialysis should be verified and a recent set of postdialysis electrolytes obtained. Failure to dialyze or inadequate dialysis in the preoperative period can predispose to volume overload and electrolyte imbalances such as hyperkalemia.

The recipient's diabetes requires monitoring of blood sugars in the perioperative period. Given her end-stage nephropathy, it is reasonable to assume that diabetes has also affected other organ systems and could lead to gastropathy, neuropathy, and autonomic instability, all of which could complicate the anesthetic.

APPROACH TO Anesthesia for Renal Transplantation

DEFINITIONS

LIVING RELATED RENAL TRANSPLANT: A kidney is removed from the donor who is otherwise healthy and related to the recipient. Living donors may also be unrelated. The other source for donors is cadaveric, where an organ is donated after death.

DONOR: The person giving a kidney to the recipient. Live donors should be healthy and have normal renal function.

DIALYSIS-DEPENDENT RENAL FAILURE: When renal function falls below 10% of normal, patients typically start dialysis to aid in elimination of fluids, urea, potassium, and replace other kidney functions. Hemodialysis is conducted through a large central catheter (Permcath) or AV fistula. Some patients undergo peritoneal dialysis, in which fluid is introduced into the peritoneal cavity and fluids and waste products are filtered through the peritoneal membrane and intermittently drained or exchanged. Hemodialysis is conducted three times a week, whereas peritoneal dialysis is either done continuously or at least nightly.

DONOR SURGICAL APPROACH: Donor receives either a laparotomy or a "hand assisted" laparoscopic nephrectomy under general anesthesia. The donor kidney is dissected carefully and separated from the bladder. It is isolated from the blood supply and removed from the donor.

RECIPIENT SURGICAL APPROACH: Recipient has donor kidney implanted under general anesthesia. The new kidney is placed in the preperitoneal space in the pelvis and generally anastomosed to the iliac vessels. The native kidneys are left in place.

CLINICAL APPROACH

The donor's preoperative evaluation is usually quite straightforward, and in most ways, does not significantly differ from that of a normal, healthy patient.

The evaluation examines their renal function (creatinine, GFR, urinalysis), cardiopulmonary status (history, exercise tolerance, possible ECG, and chest x-ray), compatibility (blood type and antigen match to the recipient), and suitability (emotional and mental status, freedom from coercion to donate).

The recipient requires verification of donor compatibility (blood type and antigen matching), assessment of cardiopulmonary status, and volume and electrolyte status. Patients are often chronically ill. They may be anemic and acidotic, but both these electrolyte disturbances are usually well tolerated. Uremia is also associated with coagulopathy due to platelet dysfunction, which can increase bleeding during surgery. Preoperative tests of particular interest to the anesthesiologist include an ECG, potassium level, complete blood count, and type and screen.

Since donors are healthy patients, standard monitors and a large-bore intravenous are placed prior to the surgery. A general anesthetic is utilized for an open or laparoscopic nephrectomy, and muscle relaxants are administered to facilitate the surgical approach. Fluids are given liberally to maintain urine output. Both laparoscopic and open donor nephrectomies are typically completed in a lateral position, so positioning and padding is important to prevent intraoperative ulcerations and nerve palsies. In addition, if the kidney bar is raised, compression of the inferior vena cava may result in hypotension. Pain control in the postoperative period can be provided with a patient-controlled analgesia (PCA) administration of narcotics, or an epidural. PCA is usually appropriate for laparoscopic approaches, but open procedures may require more aggressive postoperative analgesia.

The recipients are chronically ill, and particularly if the renal failure is the result of diabetes, may have many comorbidities. Decisions can be challenging, and should be based on individual patient characteristics. Most centers utilize general anesthesia for recipient nephrectomies, though some use spinal or combine spinal-epidural techniques as primary anesthetics. The anesthetic considerations in this kidney recipient include likely gastroparesis or reflux which may increase the risk of aspiration, electrolyte abnormalities, particularly with potassium, anemia, and the altered metabolism and excretion of anesthetic drugs in patients with end-stage renal disease.

The choice of induction agents varies with coexisting disease and volume status postdialysis. If volume status or cardiovascular issues are present, etomidate may be preferable since it causes minimal changes in cardiovascular function. Propofol or thiopental may also be used, bearing in mind that these agents decrease SVR, resulting in hypotension in normal patients. These effects would be predicted to be amplified in the hypovolemic patient.

The choice of muscle relaxants is determined by the potassium level and the patient's renal disease. Serum potassium levels vary widely in the freshly dialyzed patient when compared to the patient ready for dialysis. In addition to the risks associated with hyperkalemia in general, hyperkalemia may put the patient at risk of hyperkalemic arrest if succinylcholine is administered. Succinylcholine increases potassium levels by as much as 0.5 mEq/L. So in patients with potassium levels greater than 5.5 mEq/L or evidence of hyperkalemia (peaked T waves on ECG), it is best to avoid succinylcholine. Other neuromuscular blockers with renal clearance such as rocuronium or vecuronium may have prolonged effect in renal failure patients, so dosing with caution and titrating to effect are advisable. Cisatracurium is degraded by Hoffman elimination, so its duration of action is not altered in patients with renal dysfunction. Thus, cisatracurium is the relaxant of choice in patients with end-stage renal disease.

Inhalational agents are often used for maintenance of anesthesia, though their metabolism to compound A and release of fluoride ions limits choices. Enflurane is generally avoided due to risk of nephrotoxicity. Sevoflurane use carries a theoretical risk of compound A–induced nephrotoxicity. Fresh gas flows in excess of 2 L/min should minimize this risk with Sevoflurane. While demonstrated in animal studies, this topic remains controversial in human subjects.

Analgesia is typically provided by narcotics. Morphine and meperidine have active metabolites which require renal excretion, and so should be used with caution. Other narcotics such as fentanyl and sufentanil are reasonable alternatives. Epidural catheters are not typically used in kidney recipients since these patients are immunosuppressed and thus susceptible to infection, and bleeding diatheses are often present.

Both lactated Ringer and normal saline are acceptable choices for fluid administration. Due to concerns over the inability of these patients to clear potassium, some clinicians elect to use normal saline. However, large volumes of normal saline could cause a metabolic acidosis, resulting in potassium migration out of cells.

In addition to standard monitors, arterial access can be beneficial for hemodynamic monitoring and frequent blood sampling. This need must be balanced against the fact that, if the transplant fails, the patient may require subsequent AV fistulas. Thus, preserving arteries from possible injury may be of future benefit. Also, the radial artery should not be cannulated on the side of an existing AV fistula, as the readings may not be an accurate representation of arterial blood pressure, and the blood drawn may be mixed arterial and venous due to the presence of a shunt.

A central venous line may serve a variety of purposes in this patient population. It can provide an estimate of volume status which can be helpful given the frequent volume changes with hemodialysis and superimposed NPO status. It is also helpful to ensure euvolemia or even mild hypervolemia after the transplanted kidney is implanted to provide adequate perfusion and avoid ischemia to the implant. Central venous access may be helpful in chronically ill patients to provide venous access for the administration of immunosuppressant regimens, and frequent blood sampling. However, renal failure patients have often had multiple central lines placed for dialysis, rendering central venous access difficult due to thrombosis or scarring. Ultrasound is helpful in identifying and cannulating vessels in this difficult patient population. In the case of patients who come to surgery with a central dialysis catheter *in situ*, it may also be possible to utilize the indwelling catheter. But since dialysis lines are flushed with concentrated heparin (5000 units/cc), care must be taken to withdraw all the heparin from the catheter to avoid inadvertent anticoagulation. The catheter also should be accessed in sterile fashion to avoid risk of infection. A discussion should be undertaken with the surgical team prior to using this approach.

During the maintenance of anesthesia, close attention must be paid to volume status, electrolyte balance, and hemodynamics. Although volume expansion is preferable once the new kidney is implanted, sometimes pressors such as phenylephine are required for blood pressure support prior to its implantation. In patients with significant cardiac dysfunction, it may be necessary to employ ionotropes such as dopamine or epinephrine to improve cardiac output and deliver an adequate blood flow to the transplanted organ. At the transplant of the new kidney, steroids and other immunosuppressants are given to avoid rejection, while diuretics such as mannitol (osmotic) and furosemide (loop) are often used to facilitate urine production and avoid acute tubular necrosis (ATN). Muscle relaxants should be closely monitored with a goal of reversal and extubation in the operating room.

Postoperative care is typically centered around immunosuppression, analgesia, and plasma volume. CVP and urine output are monitored closely to ensure adequate hydration and urine output. Intravenous fluids are typically aggressive and titrated to maintain supra-normal urine output in the early postoperative period and avoid acute tubular necrosis (ATN). Because the most common site of implantation is the pre-peritoneal space, there is usually less pain in recipients than donors. Narcotics, delivered by patient-controlled analgesia (PCA) are usually adequate for postoperative analgesia.

Comprehension Questions

50.1. Compared with kidney donors, which of the following is most accurate for kidney transplant recipients ?

A. Do not require preoperative dialysis
B. Have more comorbid medical conditions
C. Have normal renal function
D. Require less intraoperative monitoring

50.2. Which of the following is most accurate regarding patients undergoing dialysis?

A. Patients undergoing dialysis typically have stable circulating blood volumes due to the dialysis.
B. Patients undergoing dialysis need to have their serum potassium measured just prior to the procedure.
C. Because of the dialysis, their intravenous access is usually easy.
D. Patients undergoing dialysis must be sufficiently stable to be transported to a dialysis unit.

ANSWERS

50.1. **B.** Kidney transplant recipients typically have more comorbid medical conditions such as diabetes or hypertension. Their renal function is impaired and they require more intraoperative monitoring. Renal failure patients undergo dialysis, whereas donors do not.

50.2. **B.** Dialysis in the patient with renal failure is associated with significant fluxes in serum potassium concentrations. If the patient is near his or her routinely scheduled dialysis time, the serum potassium can exceed 6.0 and even 7.0 g/dL. Similar fluctuations also occur in blood volume, even from relative hypovolemia to hypervolemia. However, in patients immediately postdialysis, hypovolemia should be anticipated. Patients on dialysis often have an arteriovenous fistula(s) in their upper extremity. Because only one arm can be used for blood sampling, their intravenous access is usually difficult. Being sufficiently stable to be transported to a dialysis unit is not a prerequisite for dialysis. Peritoneal dialysis is easily conducted in the ICU setting.

Clinical Pearls

- Donors require no special monitoring. Key points include anxiolysis, adequate hydration, and analgesia.
- Recipients typically have numerous comorbidities and may benefit from invasive monitoring.
- Recipients are immunosuppressed and may require diuretics and/or mannitol to facilitate urine production.
- While both surgeries are typically performed under general endotracheal anesthesia, the level of anesthetic complexity is very different between the two.

REFERENCES

Miller R. Solid organ transplant. *Miller's Anesthesia*. 6th ed. Philadelphia, PA: Churchill Livingstone;2005: 2234-2243.

O'Hara J, Cywinski J, Monk T. The renal system and anesthesia for urologic surgery. In: Barash P, Cullen B, Stoelting R, eds *Clinical Anesthesia*. Philadelphia, PA: Lippincott Williams and Wilkins;2006: 1013-1025.

Sarin Kapoor H, Kauri R, Kaur H. Anesthesia for renal transplant surgery. *Acta Anaesthsiologica Scandinavica*. 2007;51:1354-1367.

Case 51

A 62-year-old woman has just arrived in the post-anesthesia care unit (PACU) following an attempted declotting and subsequent revision of a left forearm arteriovenous (AV) dialysis fistula under general anesthesia. She had presented to the emergency department earlier today for evaluation after difficulty with reduced flow on her dialysis run this morning. Notably, on her first set of vital signs in the PACU, her blood pressure is 70/48 mm Hg, heart rate is 95 bpm, SaO_2 is 98%, and she is afebrile. The patient is somewhat somnolent, but moaning. Intraoperatively, estimated blood loss was 500 mL and she received 1.1 L of normal saline. The patient's medical history is significant for end-stage renal disease (ESRD), chronic anemia secondary to ESRD, hypertension, coronary artery disease with several prior myocardial infarctions, type 2 diabetes mellitus, and lower extremity peripheral vascular disease. Her medications include insulin, atenolol, vitamin B complex (Nephrocaps), iron, vitamin C, and aspirin 81 mg. She has a history of smoking 1 pack/day for 30 years. She does not drink alcohol. Preoperative laboratory values were significant for Hct 24%, K 3.8 mEq/L, Cr 4.4 mg/dL, and an INR of 1.1. Her ECG showed evidence of an old inferior MI, but was otherwise normal. On examination, the patient weighs 64 kg and is 5 ft, 2 in tall. Auscultation of her heart reveals a regular heart rate, normal S1 and S2, no S3 or S4. Auscultation of her lungs reveals a few bibasilar rales, but her respiratory rate is normal.

- ➤ What are the three most common physiologic causes of hypotension in the PACU?
- ➤ How would you evaluate this patient for an acute coronary syndrome?
- ➤ How would you monitor this patient in the PACU?

ANSWERS TO CASE 51:
Hypotension in the Post-Anesthesia Care Unit

Summary: A 62-year-old woman with hypotension (blood pressure 70/48 mm Hg) in the PACU following a left forearm AV fistula revision. Her past medical history is remarkable for ESRD, diabetes mellitus, CAD, and peripheral vascular disease. Her estimated blood loss intraoperatively was 500 mL and she received 1.1 L of normal saline.

- **Three most common physiologic causes of hypotension in the PACU:** Hypovolemia, left ventricular dysfunction, and excessive arterial vasodilation.
- **Evaluation for acute coronary syndrome:** A history, physical examination, vital signs, 12-lead ECG, chest x-ray, troponin, creatine kinase and myoglobin, CBC, and basic chemistry panel.
- **Monitored in PACU:** The patient should receive an ECG, noninvasive blood pressure cuff, pulse oximetry, and an arterial line.

ANALYSIS

Objectives

1. Appreciate the role of the PACU following an anesthetic.
2. Understand the most common physiologic causes of hypotension in the PACU and create a working differential diagnosis.
3. Describe the evaluation and management of acute coronary syndrome.

Considerations

Interventions for the hypotension are shaped by the differential diagnosis. Our patient, described above, has multiple factors which are concerning. Her history of diabetes and CAD with prior infarctions raises the issue of acute coronary syndrome. Her preoperative anemia combined with the intraoperative blood loss, and possible recent dialysis suggest that hypovolemia may be a significant factor. Yet the rales on examination in the PACU suggest that she may have some degree of congestive failure, or alternatively, atelectasis.

The first concern is to increase the patient's (already compromised) myocardial oxygen supply. Oxygen should be administered, if not already in progress. Second, her blood pressure should be increased. Given her previous dialysis, the fact that she was NPO, and judicious fluid administration during the procedure, the most likely diagnosis is hypovolemia. If the rales reflected hypervolemia, then some evidence of hypoxemia would quite possibly have been observed. Moreover, hypotension to this degree, in and of itself, can cause cardiac ischemia. The administration of a small amount of phenylephrine, 50 to 100 g, should increase her blood pressure and augment both myocardial and cerebral perfusion. Once her volume resuscitation has begun, focus should turn toward evaluating the possible presence of an acute coronary syndrome. Almost simultaneously, a 12-lead ECG should be obtained to check for ischemia, and biochemical markers drawn.

Given her persistent hypotension and the need for closely monitoring blood pressure during medication interventions, an arterial line should be considered. If fluid is required, the resuscitation fluid of choice in this patient is cross-matched blood, as she began the case anemic and lost an additional 500 mL intraoperatively.

APPROACH TO
Patients in the Post-Anesthesia Care Unit

CLINICAL APPROACH

The post-anesthesia care unit (PACU) is a relatively recent development in the history of anesthesia and surgical care. Prior to the Second World War, patients were often managed either back on their hospital ward or in the intensive care unit following an anesthetic. As surgical volume and complexity increased, the need for a specialized area for patients to recover from anesthesia became critical. Issues following anesthetic emergence, including airway management and hemodynamic changes, are managed in the PACU by a specialized group of nursing staff working in conjunction with the anesthesiologists (Feeley and Macario, 2005).

Upon admission to the PACU, patients emerging from anesthesia are placed on standard ASA monitors identical to the operating room. These include pulse oximetry, ECG, and blood pressure monitors. Oxygen and suction are available for each patient. Resuscitation equipment is available, including a "crash cart" with medications, a defibrillator, and airway management devices.

Once the initial vital signs have been obtained, the anesthesiologist must provide a full report of the anesthetic to the PACU nurse. Details from the surgery as well as the patient's pre-existing medical conditions, medications, allergies, fluids and blood administered, and any complications that may have been encountered should be included. The anesthesiologist should also provide the nurse with areas of concern specific to the particular patient's recovery.

Patients are monitored in the PACU until they are stable for transfer to a regular medical/surgical ward, the intensive care unit, or the day surgery discharge unit for patients having ambulatory surgical procedures. A number of scales exist for determining a patient's readiness for discharge from the PACU. The most common scale used is the Modified Aldrete Score (Table 51–1), which consists of five items, each with a possible score of 0, 1, or 2. Patients achieving a score of 8 or higher are suitable for discharge to a ward, while those with scores of 7 or less should either be observed longer or transferred to an intensive care unit.

Hypotension

During the recovery period, hypotension is a common urgent issue to be encountered, second only to airway management. It is important to quickly recognize the various factors that may contribute to hypotension, develop a differential diagnosis, and enact appropriate management. The general approach for evaluation of hypotension involves evaluating preload, contractility, and afterload. To expedite the creation of a differential, knowledge of the patient's pre-existing medical conditions along with the intraoperative events and anesthetic management must all be considered.

Table 51–1 THE MODIFIED ALDRETE SCORE

Activity	Able to move four extremities on command	2
	Able to move two extremities voluntarily or on command	1
	Unable to move extremities voluntarily or on command	0
Respiration	Able to breathe deeply and cough freely	2
	Dyspnea or limited breathing	1
	Apneic	0
Circulation	BP ± 20% of pre-anesthetic level	2
	BP ± 20%-49% of pre-anesthetic level	1
	BP ± 50% of pre-anesthetic level	0
Consciousness	Fully awake	2
	Arousable on calling	1
	Not responding	0
O_2 saturation	Able to maintain O_2 saturation >92% on room air	2
	Needs O_2 inhalation to maintain O_2 saturation >90%	1
	O_2 saturation <90% even with O_2 supplementation	0

From Aldrete, 1995.

Hypovolemia is a common finding in patients following anesthesia and frequently contributes to a diminished preload. Patients typically present for elective surgery having fasted for at least the preceding 8 hours. Intraoperative fluid management focuses on repleting the pre-existing deficit, meeting maintenance fluid requirements, and finally replacing losses. These losses take two forms: insensible fluid losses and frank bleeding. Patients lose fluid volume from insensible losses, either through evaporation from large tissue exposures or third spacing of fluid into the extracellular compartment of the body. Bleeding may be easy to appreciate in large incisions such as cardiac operations, but can be quite difficult to assess in other settings such as transurethral prostate resections. Pneumothorax, pulmonary embolus, or cardiac tamponade are less frequent causes of a reduced preload.

Left ventricular dysfunction may have a variety of causes. Hypoxia, hypercarbia, and hypothermia can worsen myocardial function. Arrhythmias may lead to poor filling of the ventricle (with supraventricular arrhythmias) versus intrinsic ventricular dysfunction, such as polymorphic ventricular tachycardia. Acute coronary ischemia can impair myocardial left ventricular contraction. Volume overload may worsen an impaired ventricle, by exceeding the optimal point on the Starling curve. Medications such as beta blockers and calcium channel blockers, can reduce cardiac output by reducing heart rate. Inhalation agents, in particular older agents such as halothane, also had myocardial depressant effects.

Afterload reduction in the form of vasodilation must also be considered. Residual anesthetic, either from a neuraxial block or a general anesthetic, may continue to cause hypotension into the recovery period. Intraoperative medications should be considered, especially antihypertensives or opioids that may have been given in response to surgical stimulus. There is a case report of a patient with persistent postoperative hypotension after this surgeon placed 2% nitroglycerin ointment along wound edges to promote vascular blood flow for wound healing (Siddiqi, 2004). Anaphylaxis should also be considered as it may occur as a result of a reaction to one of the intraoperative medications or as a result of contact with latex or other allergens. Lastly, sepsis can cause severe vasodilatation and result in significant hypotension.

The likelihood of whether each of the above items is going to rise or fall on the differential diagnosis is based on the patient's history combined with the type of surgery and their immediate postoperative state. An otherwise healthy lymphoma patient who underwent a tunneled central venous catheter that complains of new shortness of breath and rapidly worsening hypotension will have a very different differential than a patient with heart failure who just underwent a 4-hour bowel resection.

Acute Coronary Syndrome

Acute coronary syndrome (ACS) describes a wide spectrum of heart diseases ranging from stable coronary disease without angina to unstable angina, acute myocardial infarction, and even sudden death. Awake patients may describe anginal symptoms in the recovery room, but in the diabetic patient, these symptoms may be absent. Other symptoms such as nausea, dyspnea, or alteration in mental status may be present.

After performing a physical examination, one should consider other diagnostic tools. Continuous ECG monitoring is performed in both the operating room and the PACU. ST-segment or T-wave changes may be early signs of ACS. A 12-lead ECG should be obtained for greater diagnostic resolution since the detection of ST-T wave changes is unreliable on a monitor. A chest radiograph should be obtained to exclude other intrathoracic causes of hypotension and ECG changes, and to also evaluate the cardiac size and silhouette. Serum biochemical markers of myocardial injury should be assayed with an order for troponin, myoglobin, and CK-MB.

If the ACS is quite early on, a single negative result from a single marker does not exclude the diagnosis. The markers should be followed over the next 6 to 12 hours. Using these three markers in combination was shown to have 100% sensitivity and 100% negative predictive power for acute myocardial infarction in the emergency department setting (Ng, 2001). Echocardiography provides a very sensitive measure of regional wall motion abnormalities, which may correspond to any underlying ischemia.

The initial management of ACS focuses on increasing oxygen supply to the myocardium and reducing myocardial metabolic requirements. The patient should be given oxygen. Aspirin should be given either orally or rectally depending on the patient's surgery and mental status. Nitrates should be considered, though in the setting of profound hypotension, they may not be well-tolerated. Untreated pain, either from the surgery or from angina, should be treated to reduce catecholamine stress response. Likewise, beta blockade may be considered, though its use may be relatively contraindicated in the setting of severe congestive failure, profound bradycardia, or severe hypotension. Patients with a history of severe asthma may also be poor candidates for beta-blocker therapy. A cardiologist should be contacted as soon as ACS is suspected, as studies have shown that better outcomes are associated with an earlier revascularization intervention, either via thrombolytics or percutaneous coronary intervention (PCI). Patients that are in the immediate postoperative state are generally not candidates for thrombolytic therapy due to the risk of bleeding from the surgical sites. The final focus should be stabilizing the patient for potential transfer to the cardiac catheterization laboratory for PCI.

Comprehension Questions

51.1. A 33-year-old healthy man presented for ACL reconstruction following a skiing injury. He received a femoral nerve block and an uneventful general anesthetic with an LMA. Following his 2-hour operation, he was transferred to the PACU, where he was observed for 45 minutes. His nurse reports that his oxygen saturation is 98% on room air. His blood pressure is 130/79 mm Hg (preoperation 145/80 mm Hg). He is awake and asking questions about his operation. His respiratory rate is normal an unlabored. He is unable to extend his lower leg at the knee. Which of the following is his Aldrete score?

A. 1
B. 4
C. 7
D. 9

51.2. A 44-year-old woman presents for elective total abdominal hysterectomy. She has a history of migraines, GERD, and significant uterine fibroids. She exercises four to five times each week. She received a spinal anesthetic and light sedation during the operation. Operative events were notable for an estimated blood loss of 1 L. She received 1.5 L of crystalloid intraoperatively. On arrival in the PACU, the RN notes a blood pressure of 78/33 mm Hg with a heart rate of 118 bpm. Which of the following is the most likely cause of her hypotension?

A. Hypovolemia from her preoperative fast and intraoperative blood loss
B. Persistent spinal anesthesia-mediated autonomic dysfunction
C. Acute myocardial infarction
D. Persistent postoperative bleeding

51.3. Which of the following is the first therapeutic intervention for a patient with possible acute coronary syndrome in the PACU following a colon resection?

A. Give aspirin.
B. Start nitroglycerin.
C. Administer oxygen.
D. Administer alteplase.

ANSWERS

51.1. **D.** The Aldrete score was developed to help determine which patients may be safely transferred from the recovery room to the ward or the day surgery unit. The score contains five components: activity, respiration, circulation, saturation, and consciousness. Each of the five components receives a score of 0 to 2 with 2 being best. The 33-year-old patient received a femoral nerve block, which will impair movement of his lower extremity and result in an activity score of 1. All of his other components received a 2, thus giving a score of 9. He is ready for discharge.

51.2. **A.** When approaching a patient with hypotension in the recovery room, it is important to quickly form an accurate differential diagnosis to avoid spending time on issues that are unlikely to be responsible for the problem. One must consider the patient's preoperative condition as well as intraoperative events when developing the differential. The 44-year-old woman was on fast since the night before surgery, had a significant intraoperative blood loss, and received a minimal amount of fluids. She also received a spinal anesthetic, which can have persistent autonomic effects into the recovery period. However, by the recovery period, the spinal is beginning to recede, and is not a likely explanation for newly found hypotension. Postoperative bleeding is always a possibility and early contact with the surgeon should be considered. But this is not "first" on the list. The appropriate treatment for this patient is fluid resuscitation and pressors. In this otherwise active patient with few comorbidities, option C, an acute coronary syndrome would be quite unlikely.

51.3. **C.** Acute coronary syndrome can present in the immediate postoperative period and require immediate management by the anesthesiologist and PACU nurse. The initial treatment for suspected acute coronary syndrome emphasizes promotion of myocardial oxygen supply and reduction in myocardial oxygen demand, so oxygen is administered. Next, restoring any abnormal hemodynamics also facilitates maintenance of coronary perfusion. Hypotension can reduce myocardial blood flow; while conversely, hypertension and tachycardia increase the heart's demand for oxygen. Nitroglycerine should be considered, although it may be poorly tolerated in a patient who is hypertensive. Option D, alteplase is a tissue plasminogen activator produced by recombinant DNA technology. It is indicated for acute myocardial infarction, acute ischemic stroke, and pulmonary embolism. Alteplase is contraindicated in the setting of recent major surgery due to the risk of massive hemorrhage.

Clinical Pearls

- The PACU is a specialized unit designed for the recovery of patients following anesthesia and surgery. Patients are observed until they have recovered their mental status, achieved hemodynamic stability, and are achieving adequate oxygenation with minimal supplementation.
- The Modified Aldrete Score is a common scale from 0 to 10 used to determine whether a patient meets criteria for discharge from the PACU to the ward or the day surgery unit. Scores of 8 to 10 suggest the patient will do well outside of the PACU setting.
- Acute coronary syndrome (ACS) describes a wide range of cardiac events ranging from stable coronary artery disease without angina to acute myocardial infarction or even sudden cardiac death. When ACS is encountered in the PACU, the anesthesiologist must focus on therapies to improve myocardial oxygen supply. However, a cardiologist should be contacted as early as possible for the potential need for percutaneuos coronary intervention as postsurgical patients are not candidates for intravenous thrombolytics.

REFERENCES

Aldrete JA. The post-anesthesia recovery score revisited. *J Clin Anesthesiol.* 1995;7:89-91.

Feeley TW, Macario A. The postanesthesia care unit. In: Miller RD, ed. *Miller's Anesthesia.* 6th ed. Philadelphia, PA: Elsevier Churchill Livingstone; 2005.

Ng SM, Krishnaswamy P, Morissey R, et al. Ninety-minute accelerated critical pathway for chest pain evaluation. *Am J Cardiol.* 2001;88:403.

Siddiqi M, Marco AP, Gorp CV. Postoperative hypotension from topical use of 2% nitroglycerin ointment after a total knee replacement procedure. *J Clin Anesthesiol.* 2004;16(1):77-78.

Case 52

You are called to the recovery room because a patient reports difficulty in breathing, and the nurse notes that her O_2 saturation is 89%. She is a 55-year-old woman who has just undergone a bilateral total thyroidectomy for cancer. Her past medical history is significant for hypertension and depression, for which she takes atenolol and fluoxetine (Prozac) respectively. She is a nonsmoker and denies other medical illnesses. She has undergone previous general anesthetics without complications.

The patient's surgery was performed under general endotracheal anesthesia with inhalational sevoflurane, fentanyl 200 g, and cisatracurium for muscle relaxation. Tracheal intubation was uneventful, with a grade I view of the larynx. On examination, the patient is sitting upright with labored breathing and breath sounds are bilateral with inspiratory stridor.

- ➤ What is the first therapeutic step even prior to your evaluation?
- ➤ How do you assess this patient in the recovery room?
- ➤ What is the differential diagnosis of decreased oxygen saturation (hypoxemia) in this patient?

ANSWERS TO CASE 52:

Hypoxemia in Recovery Room after Thyroidectomy

Summary: A 55-year-old woman status post thyroidectomy is reporting difficulty breathing in the recovery room with an O_2 saturation of 89%.

- **First therapeutic step:** Increase the patient's FIO_2. This can be done by replacing nasal cannulae with a "green" mask, replacing a mask with a non-rebreathing mask, or replacing a non-rebreathing mask with a source of 100% oxygen such as an Ambu bag or a Briggs apparatus.
- **Assessment:** The immediate assessment of this patient in the recovery room should include a directed physical examination including auscultation of the lungs and heart, a check for obvious airway obstruction, and assessment of her vital signs. Initial assessment should also include ensuring that the patient is receiving supplemental oxygen via face mask or nasal cannula, and that the oxygen source is turned on and if an oxygen tank is being used, that the tank is not empty.
- **Differential diagnosis of hypoxemia:** This not only includes the usual causes of hypoventilation (Table 52–1) and hypoxemia (Table 52–2) after general anesthesia but also the potential causes unique to thyroidectomy including postoperative bleeding and hematoma causing airway compression, unilateral or bilateral recurrent laryngeal nerve injury, tracheomalacia following tracheal compression by a large mass, and hypocalcemia secondary to parathyroid gland removal.

Table 52–1 CAUSES OF POSTOPERATIVE HYPOVENTILATION IN THE PACU
Central nervous system depression—drug induced (inhalation anesthetics, opioids) or CNS event such as stroke
Residual neuromuscular blocking agents
Impairment of ventilatory muscles or obstructive sleep apnea
Increased production of carbon dioxide
Pre-existing pulmonary pathology such as COPD

Table 52–2 CAUSES OF ARTERIAL HYPOXEMIA IN THE PACU
Right-to-left intrapulmonary shunt (atelectasis)
Ventilation-to-perfusion mismatching (decreased functional residual capacity)
Obesity with obstructive apnea or decreased FRC and vent-perfusion mismatching
Increased oxygen consumption (shivering or sepsis)
Pulmonary embolism
Pulmonary edema (fluid overload, postobstructive or negative pressure pulmonary edema)
Congestive heart failure
Pneumothorax
Congestive heart failure
Adult respiratory distress syndrome
Aspiration of gastric contents
Posthyperventilation hypoxia
Diffusion hypoxia
Transfusion-related lung injury

ANALYSIS

Objectives

1. Develop a framework for evaluating a hypoxic patient in the recovery room.
2. Understand the differential diagnosis of decreased oxygen saturation in the recovery room.
3. Review causes and treatment of hypoxemia after thyroidectomy.

Considerations

In this particular patient, as with any patient presenting with decreased oxygen saturation in the PACU, immediate assessment is required. The first considerations are

- Is the patient receiving oxygen?
- Is she getting better or worse?
- Are there any easily treatable causes of the hypoventilation or hypoxemia?

There are many possible causes of hypoxemia in the recovery room (Tables 52–1 to 52–3). It is essential that the anesthesia provider has an

Table 52–3 CAUSES OF DECREASED OXYGEN SATURATION IN PACU AFTER THRYOIDECTOMY
Unilateral recurrent laryngeal nerve injury
Bilateral recurrently laryngeal nerve injury
Tracheal compression from hematoma or tracheomalacia
Hypocalcemia secondary to removal or parathyroid glands

intimate, working knowledge of this differential, and not just those causes of hypoxia specific to the patients post thyroid surgery.

The first step in evaluating this patient is a directed physical examination and determination of whether the patient's status is improving or deteriorating. If the patient is improving, then she may be observed at the bedside and a differential diagnosis can be established. If the patient's condition is deteriorating, then her airway may need to be secured first and a differential diagnosis established later. Once the need for immediate airway intervention is determined, the provider can look for easily treatable causes of decreased oxygen saturation such as equipment failure, airway obstruction, hypoventilation from inadequately reversed opioids, residual anesthetic agents, or neuromuscular blocking drugs.

This patient appears to be clinically stable in the PACU. However, on physical examination an expanding hematoma is discovered near the site of the surgical dressing. It is determined that this hematoma is most likely causing tracheal compression and airway compromise. While the surgical team is called, the anesthesiologists must decide if the hematoma is expanding rapidly enough that the patient must be reintubated immediately. Ideally, she would be intubated in the operating room using either a fiberoptic (a popular choice for many anesthetics) or direct laryngoscopy with the surgeon in attendance. This situation is ideal because in the event that the trachea cannot be intubated, the surgeon could open the wound under direct vision thus reducing the compression on the tracheal and theoretically improving intubation conditions.

APPROACH TO
The Hypoxemic Patient in the PACU

DEFINITIONS

HYPOXEMIA: Decreased oxygen saturation following anesthesia has two primary causes, hypoventilation (inadequate ventilation) and hypoxemia (decreased delivery of oxygen in the presence of adequate respiratory ventilation). Atelectasis along with hypoventilation is the most common cause of arterial hypoxemia in the recovery room.

RECURRENT LARYNGEAL NERVE PARALYSIS: The most common nerve injury after thyroid surgery is unilateral damage to the recurrent laryngeal nerve, resulting in hoarseness and a vocal cord paralyzed in the intermediate position. If the tecurrent laryngeal nerve paralysis is bilateral, the vocal cords flap together during inspiration, resulting in airway obstruction.

SUPERIOR LARYNGEAL NERVE PARALYSIS: This results in hoarseness and decreased sensation above the vocal cords, making patients vulnerable to aspiration.

TRACHEOMALACIA: It is a softening of the tracheal rings that occurs from prolonged compression and pressure on the trachea from a large mass or goiter. This softening may cause the trachea to collapse, leading to airway obstruction.

NIMS TUBE—A NIMS tube is a specialized endotracheal tube that when positioned properly can monitor the EMG or electromyographic function of the recurrent laryngeal nerves. Studies are in progress to determine if this monitoring will decrease the incidence of recurrent laryngeal nerve injury during thyroid surgery.

CLINICAL APPROACH

When called to assess a patient in the postoperative care unit for decreased oxygen saturation, there is a long differential diagnosis. The most common causes are hypoventilation (Table 52–1), arterial hypoxemia (Table 52–2), or problems specific to the patient's particular surgery (Table 52–3). On initial assessment, it is usually fairly easy to determine if the patient's ventilatory effort is adequate. If the patient is not making good ventilatory effort, then the differential diagnosis includes central nervous system depression from narcotics, volatile agents or central neurologic event, the residual effects of neuromuscular blocking agents, and an increased production of carbon dioxide or pre-existing pulmonary disease—specifically COPD.

If the patient is making adequate ventilatory effort, then the differential diagnosis shifts to causes of arterial hypoxemia. The most common cause of arterial hypoxemia in the recovery period is right-to-left intrapulmonary shunt secondary to atelectasis. Additional causes include ventilation-perfusion mismatching secondary to decreased functional residual capacity or obesity, congestive heart failure, pulmonary edema from fluid overload or negative pressure, pulmonary embolus, aspiration pneumonitis, increased oxygen consumption due to shivering or sepsis, adult respiratory distress syndrome, or transfusion-related lung injury.

Several specific complications from thyroid surgery can lead to postoperative respiratory insufficiency. These include damage (either unilateral or bilateral) to the laryngeal nerves, tracheal compression from hematoma or from tracheomalacia, or accidental removal of the parathyroid glands. The laryngeal innervations are supplied by the two superior and two recurrent laryngeal nerves. The superior laryngeal nerves provide the motor supply to the cricothyroid muscles, and sensation above the vocal cords. The recurrent laryngeal nerves supply motor innervation to all the other muscles of the larynx, and sensation below the vocal cords. The most common nerve injury after thyroid surgery is unilateral damage to the recurrent laryngeal nerve, which can be either temporary or permanent. Unilateral damage to the recurrent laryngeal nerve results in hoarseness and a vocal cord paralyzed in the intermediate position (not completely opened or closed). Bilateral recurrent laryngeal nerve paralysis results in cords that can flap together during inspiration and cause airway obstruction. Superior laryngeal nerve paralysis results in hoarseness and a decreased sensation above the vocal cords, which renders patients vulnerable to aspiration. In addition to complications resulting from nerve damage, compression of the trachea may be caused by hematoma formation or by tracheomalacia.

Finally, an accidental or unrecognized removal of the parathyroid glands is an uncommon but recognized complication which follows thyroid surgery. Patients post removal of the parathyroid glands may develop hyperparathyroidism and hypocalcemia. Signs and symptoms can occur as early as 1 to 3 hours after surgery, but do not typically present until 24 to 72 hours postoperatively. The first symptoms of hypocalcemia may be inspiratory stridor progressing to laryngospasm. Other symptoms include circumoral paraesthesia, carpopedal spasm, tetany, a prolonged QT interval, and/or mental status changes.

Comprehension Questions

52.1. A 47-year-old woman is in the recovery room following general anesthesia for arthroscopic surgery of the knee. You are called because her oxygen saturation is 88% and her respiratory rate is 4 breaths/minute. The most likely cause of her decreased oxygen saturation is which of the following?

A. Residual inhalational anesthetics
B. Inadequate reversal of neuromuscular blocking agents
C. Narcotic overdose
D. Oxygen tank equipment malfunction
E. Equipment malfunction of the pulse oximeter

52.2. A healthy 20-year-old is in the PACU 3 hours after tonsillectomy. Immediately after extubation in the operating room, the patient developed severe laryngospasm with good respiratory effort. Now he has developed hypoxemia, fluffy infiltrates on chest x-ray, and productive cough with watery sputum. Which of the following is the most likely diagnosis?

A. Congestive heart failure
B. Atelectasis
C. Pulmonary embolism
D. Negative pressure pulmonary edema
E. Iatrogenic fluid overload

52.3. A 60-year-old patient appears weak and is struggling to breathe following emergent open cholecystectomy in the PACU. The patient's oxygen saturation is 85%. You suspect inadequate reversal or neuromuscular blocking agents. Your first step should be which of the following?

A. Sit the head of the bed up higher.
B. Assist the patient's ventilation with bag mask.
C. Go to get a neuromuscular stimulator to check for adequate return of neuromuscular function.
D. Administer neostigmine.
E. Administer midazolam for amnesia.

ANSWERS

52.1. **C.** Narcotic overdose. This patient's extremely slow respiratory rate is indicative of narcotic overdose. Her airway can be assisted with an Ambu bag and mask or naloxone can be administered in small titrated doses up to a maximum of 1 to 4 g/kg.

52.2. **D.** The most likely diagnosis in this otherwise healthy patient is negative pressure pulmonary edema. This occurs when a large negative pressure inspiratory breath is attempted against an obstructed or closed airway. Since this patient is symptomatic and hypoxemic, he will require hospital admission and at a minimum overnight observation. Patients are most symptomatic 8 to 12 hours after the negative pressure episode.

52.3. **B.** The most appropriate first step is to assist the patient with ventilation. Once oxygenation is assured, neuromuscular function can be assessed and reversal agents can be given if appropriate.

Clinical Pearls

- Hypoxemia in the post-anesthesia care unit from any cause requires immediate assessment and treatment.
- Extubation of the trachea following thyroid surgery should be performed under ideal conditions.
- Bilateral recurrent laryngeal nerve injury is a potentially devastating complication; though it is extremely rare.
- Laryngeal stridor progressing to spasm may be one of the first indications of hypocalcemic tetany.

REFERENCES

Horn D. *Intraoperative EMG Monitoring of the Recurrent Laryngeal Nerve in Langenbeck's Archives of Surgery*. Berlin: Springer; 1999.

Stoelting RK, Miller RD. *Basics of Anesthesia*. 5th ed. Philadelphia, PA: Churchill Livingstone; 2007.

REFERENCES

Case 53

A 52-year-old woman with end-stage metastatic breast cancer is scheduled for plating of her femur, indicated because of a lytic lesion at risk of fracture. She is anemic and thrombocytopenic, and will likely require transfusion of blood and platelets during the case. The patient has signed papers requesting a DNR/DNI (do not resuscitate/do not intubate) status.

- ➤ What issues need to be considered before an anesthesia plan is made?
- ➤ How is DNR dealt with in the OR?
- ➤ What are some of the other types of ethical issues that anesthesiologists face?

ANSWERS TO CASE 53:
End of Life/Ethics in Anesthesia

Summary: A 52-year-old patient with metastatic breast cancer presents for elective palliative surgery. She has a standing DNR/DNI request. She is anemic and has a low platelet count.

- **Preoperative evaluation:** Includes an assessment of the patient's medical condition(s), their potential impact on the anesthetic plan if any, the type and complexity of the surgery to be performed, and an assessment of the possible need for transfusion of blood or blood products. In addition, prior to entering the OR, this patient warrants a clear and complete discussion of the goals for her treatment. This discussion should include members of the surgical team, family, and primary physician.
- **DNR in operating room:** Given the patient's right to self-determination, it is she who will ultimately determine how the DNR will be dealt with in the OR. One useful technique involves discussing the patient's goals of care, for example, not to be on a ventilator for the rest of their life, which permits the anesthetist to determine the means of best achieving those goals.
- **Other ethical issues:** Anesthesiologists also face other types of ethical dilemmas including issues involving informed consent, patient privacy, a colleague's impaired function, and production pressure.

ANALYSIS

Objectives

1. Become acquainted with the concept of a patient's right of self-determination, and its impact in the operative setting.
2. Understand how the DNR status is managed in the OR.
3. Become acquainted with other types of ethical challenges that may affect an anesthesiologist.
4. Recognize the physician's options when his or her ethical value system differs markedly from the patient's.

Considerations

This patient has a standing request for DNR/DNI status. A discussion with the patient and the rest of her care team should occur well before the scheduled surgery to confirm her wishes, and to determine the need for any accommodation of DNR requests in the operating room. This discussion should optimally include members of the patient's family, the surgery and anesthesia care teams, and the primary physician.

Because of the low platelet count, the patient is not a candidate for regional anesthesia, and will thus require general anesthesia. In the setting of impaired clotting, regional anesthesia, especially neuraxial techniques, could result in bleeding and cause unnecessary harm. Since this patient requires general anesthesia, it is important that she understands and agrees to the possibility of intubation if necessary. A procedure- or goal-directed approach can be taken to suspension of DNR for patients in the operating room.

APPROACH TO End of Life/Ethics in Anesthesia

DEFINITIONS

DNR/DNI: Do not resuscitate/do not intubate. A patient's requests to limit resuscitation from a cardiac arrest, usually verified by a primary physician's order in the patient's medical record. (May also be stated as DNAR: do not attempt resuscitation.)

SELF-DETERMINATION: The right to self-determination allows a patient to make independent, informed decisions about their health care. Also described as the principle of patient autonomy.

ADVANCE DIRECTIVES: Instructions from a patient stating their desires for certain types of care if they are unable to speak for themselves.

INFORMED CONSENT: The autonomous, informed authorization by a patient for a specific procedure.

PRODUCTION PRESSURE: Incentives and pressures on a person to place production and not safety as the priority.

CLINICAL APPROACH

Every patient has a right to self-determination, which refers to the autonomy to decide what kind of care they would or would not like to receive. Indeed, the concept of patient self-determination and principle of patient autonomy guide the ethical practice of medicine. Such dilemmas may involve the ultimate health-care decision: the choice to limit health care at the end of life, including a decision as to whether to be or not be resuscitated from cardiac or respiratory arrest. These decisions may also address whether or not a patient wants to be intubated and placed on a ventilator.

The discussion regarding the patient's DNR status in the OR should occur well before the time of surgery, and should include the surgical and anesthesia team members, the primary physician, and family if the patient desires it. It goes without saying that any such discussions with patients and other physicians must be clearly documented in the patient's record, especially if other anesthesia personnel may be called on to care for the patient in the OR.

Patients may be unaware that routine anesthesia care is often considered resuscitation in other parts of the hospital. In the past, many hospitals automatically suspended DNR requests for patients going to the OR. However, this action does not properly address the patient's right to self-determination in an ethical or legal manner. A measured approach to this issue evolves from a discussion with patient leading to partial or total suspension of DNR. Alternatively, limitations on resuscitation can be made in a goal-directed or procedure-directed fashion. A goal-directed suspension of DNR asks a patient to clarify and state their goals of care, for example, not to be on a ventilator for the rest of their life, and frees the physician to utilize various means to achieve this goal. These goal-directed approaches are often extended into the postoperative period. It is crucial that all medical teams agree upon these goal-directed suspensions of DNR. For example: in a patient who agrees to general anesthesia under the condition that they will not be intubated for a long period after surgery. All specialties need to concur that at a certain time the patient will be extubated, regardless of the medical situation.

A procedure-directed suspension of DNR allows a patient to make a checklist of procedures they would not permit, such as chest compression or defibrillation. A patient who wishes to maintain full DNR/DNI status can go to the OR for a minor procedure requiring minimal sedation. However, even under minor sedation events could occur, for example, a reaction to antibiotics or local anesthesia, which would be reversible with basic resuscitation techniques. General anesthesia, because of the potential need for intubation and paralysis, coupled with the anesthesiologist's responsibility to do no harm, almost always requires at least a partial suspension of the DNR/DNI status. Each hospital has its own policies regarding DNR in the OR, and these policies can vary significantly.

In an urgent situation or when formal discussions are impossible, full resuscitative measures are instituted to meet the tenet of "do no harm." In some cases, where a patient is unable to communicate, either advance directives or a person designated as the health-care proxy decision-maker can convey the patient's desires for resuscitation. The legally accepted method of surrogate decision making varies according to state law. The most complete way to ascertain an incapacitated patient's wishes is from both a written statement such as an advance directive or "living will" and the health-care proxy decision maker, which is often a family member. In most situations, only one of these means of information is available. However, if the patient's wishes are unknown or unclear, full measures are undertaken since the consequences of refraining from resuscitation are usually permanent.

Obtaining consent for routine methods of airway management are sometimes the most difficult part of this process. Patients may not understand that intubation and the use of resuscitative drugs go part and parcel with anesthesia care, and that refraining from their use would be a significant (and possibly even unethical) departure from normal clinical practice. However, an understanding and informative discussion of these points may be sufficiently reassuring for a patient fearing prolongation of life on a ventilator in an ICU.

Even if the use of another type of airway device is planned, consent for possible intubation is required for general anesthesia. This does not mean that the patient's desires cannot be accommodated. However, just because a patient states that they do not want an intervention, such as intubation, a physician is not required to agree to something that they think is unsafe or unethical. For example, even a regional anesthetic may fail requiring conversion to general anesthesia. When disagreements occur, a physician should withdraw and find a replacement, or ask for intervention from a third party, such as the hospital's ethics committee.

For extremity surgery, regional anesthesia may be an option for the patient who does not want to be intubated. However, the medical comorbidities near the end of life often preclude the use of a regional block. Coagulopathy, thrombocytopenia, and lytic lesions at the area of surgery pose a significant risk for bleeding and hematoma formation. If a neuraxial block is utilized, a hematoma could result in paralysis and even require emergent surgery for evacuation.

Informed Consent

Informed consent is another manner in which a patient expresses their right to self-determination. The process of informed consent has several steps. A patient must possess the ability to understand the medical information, must have the capacity to make a decision, and must be acting voluntarily.

The physician needs to provide adequate information for the patient to make an educated decision. The "subjective person standard" requires the physician to be aware of the individual's medical conditions, wants, and needs to provide sufficient information. The ethical standard expects the physician to provide specific information appropriate for that particular patient. For example, the risks and benefits of intubation are different for an opera singer than it is for someone not dependent on vocal nuances for their livelihood. The legal standard for information is the "reasonable person standard," that which any usual person would require to make a decision. The physician is obligated to make a recommendation based on medical knowledge to assist the patient in making an adequately informed decision. This recommendation is often meant to persuade, but coercion or manipulation should be avoided.

Once the patient has an understanding of the information, an autonomous authorization or consent can be obtained. A common limitation on informed consent for anesthesiologists is the rushed or distracted consent process that may occur in the holding area prior to a procedure, when the patient is seen and interviewed only minutes before they go into the OR. The elements of understanding and being voluntary can be limited when a patient is hesitant to ask questions or change their minds moments before a procedure.

Despite a physician's best efforts to inform and recommend, patients occasionally make bad decisions. It is important to remember that they have the right to do so according to the principle of patient autonomy. When physicians disagree morally with a patient's choice or think that it is inappropriate, they may withdraw from caring for that patient, and should attempt to find a replacement. The Ethics Consultation Service or Committee also provides guidance when there are ethical disputes between physicians, or between physicians and patients or families.

Institutions differ with regards to their policies which govern patient care in an emergency. Many hospitals require that a physician provide emergency care in accordance with the patient's wishes until another physician can assume that role. Others allow physicians to withdraw from providing care, or certain types of care. It is important to understand the Medical Staff Bylaws which govern a physician's practice.

Production pressures are overt or covert incentives and pressures on a person to place production, not safety as the priority. There are organizational, economic and social demands on the anesthesiologist, especially in fast paced ambulatory practices. These pressures may lead an anesthesiologist to avoid canceling cases, or to cut corners or work faster to reduce costs or maximize income. Production pressures cause errors, stress and fatigue, which are detrimental to both physicians and patients.

The Right to Privacy

Patient privacy is another common ethical issue encountered by anesthesiologists. Today, many patients receive anesthesia interviews and instructions over the phone. Messages left on answering machines can violate a patient's right to privacy, much as taking a history in front of family members may reveal guarded personal information. Operating room schedules and other documents with patient's medical histories need to be shielded from public view.

Comprehension Questions

53.1. Which of the following statements regarding DNR/DNI is most accurate?

A. It is irrevocable and unchangeable once stated.
B. It is an expression of a patient's choice to limit health care.
C. It can be applied only when expressed by an awake, competent patient.
D. It is invalid in the operating room.

53.2. The concept of self-determination includes which of the following?

A. It requires a physician to do anything a patient requests.
B. It is a replacement for informed consent.
C. It is not valid if the patient is unconscious or incompetent to make decisions.
D. It affirms the principle of patient autonomy.

53.3. Which of the following statements is accurate about the informed consent process?

A. Consent forms should be signed prior to the patient preoperative interview.

B. Consent forms exist solely to meet legal requirements.

C. The process requires both disclosure and a recommendation by the physician.

D. Preferably, this should be done in the holding area immediately before a procedure.

53.4. If a physician disagrees morally or ethically with a patient's decision, or believes that that decision may cause unnecessary harm, the physician should do which of the following?

A. He does not generally have the right to withdraw from providing care.

B. He may assign the hospital administrator to find a replacement for providing care.

C. He may state whatever objections in the chart, but should continue to provide care.

D. He may be aided by the institution's Ethics Service or Committee.

ANSWERS

53.1. **B.** Do not resuscitate/do not intubate is a request by a patient to limit resuscitation, guided by the concept of self-determination. Although it is expressed in the chart as a physician order, all physicians caring for the patient should have their own discussion on how this should be expressed. Sometimes this request needs alteration or suspension when a patient is going to the operating room or undergoing a procedure. When a patient is unconscious or incompetent to make decisions, these desires can be ascertained through advance directives or a health-care proxy decision-maker.

53.2. **D.** Self-determination and the principle of patient autonomy reinforce the same concept: patients have the right to make their own decisions about their health care. Respect for patient autonomy guides the physician to adequately inform the patient, disclose risks and benefits, and make recommendations for their care. A physician is not required to do something unsafe or unethical just because the patient requests it. A patient's advance directives or health-care proxy can assert a patient's right to self-determination when they are unable to do it on their own.

53.3. **C.** Informed consent requires the physician to both gain an understanding of a patient's conditions and needs and to disclose information to provide an individual with adequate understanding of the risks and benefits of a procedure. This discussion is best accomplished when both the patient and physician have the time and voluntariness to do so. When rushed or distracted, the physician may not give the patient adequate information or allow time for the patient to ask questions. Informed consent fulfills not only a legal obligation, but also an ethical one.

53.4. **D.** If a physician disagrees morally or ethically with a patient's decision, or believes that that decision may cause unnecessary harm, the physician has the right to withdraw from providing care. However, if the physician withdraws from providing care, he or she must seek a replacement. The institution's Ethics Service or Committee can be invaluable in providing guidance and support.

Clinical Pearls

- All patients have the right to participate fully in health-care decisions.
- DNR orders are not necessarily suspended automatically when a patient goes into the OR.
- Educating patients as to the typical and usual tools used during an anesthetic and using goal-directed or procedure-directed approach to DNR is helpful for patients anticipating the need for surgery.
- Physicians may withdraw from providing care which they deem likely to cause unnecessary harm, or with which they disagree morally or ethically.
- When in doubt, consult the Ethics Service or Committee.

REFERENCES

ASA Ethical Guidelines for the Anesthesia Care of Patients with Do-Not-Resuscitate Orders. Amended in 2001. asahq.org/publicationsandservices/standards/09.html.

ASA Syllabus on Ethics. asahq.org/publicationsandservices.

Truog RD, Waisel DB, Burns JP. DNR in the OR: a goal-directed approach. *Anesthesiology*. 1999;90:289-295.

SECTION IV

Listing of Cases

Listing by Case Number

Listing by Disorder (Alphabetical)

INDEX

Page numbers followed by *f* or *t* indicate figures or tables, respectively.